T0342505

CMOS Integrated Lab-on-a-Chip System for
Personalized Biomedical Diagnosis

CMOS Integrated Lab-on-a-Chip System for Personalized Biomedical Diagnosis

Hao Yu
Southern University of Science and Technology
China

Mei Yan
Consultant
China

Xiwei Huang
Hangzhou Dianzi University
China

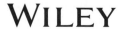

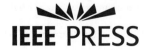

Registered Office(s)
John Wiley & Sons, Inc., 111 River Street, Hoboken, NJ 07030, USA
John Wiley & Sons Singapore Pte. Ltd, 1 Fusionopolis Walk, #07-01 Solaris South Tower, Singapore 138628

Editorial Office
1 Fusionopolis Walk, #07-01 Solaris South Tower, Singapore 138628

For details of our global editorial offices, customer services, and more information about Wiley products visit us at www.wiley.com.

Library of Congress Cataloging-in-Publication Data

Names: Yu, Hao, 1976– author.
Title: CMOS integrated lab-on-a-chip system for personalized biomedical diagnosis / Hao Yu, Southern University of Science and Technology, China, Mei Yan, Consultant, China, Xiwei Huang, Hangzhou Dianzi University, China.
Description: Hoboken, NJ : Wiley, 2018. | Series: Wiley - IEEE | Includes bibliographical references and index. |
Identifiers: LCCN 2017049248 (print) | LCCN 2017050886 (ebook) | ISBN 9781119218357 (pdf) | ISBN 9781119218340 (epub) | ISBN 9781119218326 (hardback)
Subjects: LCSH: Medical instruments and apparatus–Research. | Metal oxide semiconductors, Complementary.
Classification: LCC RA856.4 (ebook) | LCC RA856.4 .J53 2018 (print) | DDC 610.28/4–dc23
LC record available at https://lccn.loc.gov/2017049248

Cover Design: Wiley
Cover Image: © e-crow/Gettyimages

Set in 10/12pt Warnock by SPi Global, Pondicherry, India

Printed in Singapore by C.O.S. Printers Pte Ltd

10 9 8 7 6 5 4 3 2 1

Contents

Preface

Considering the current aging society, the future personalized diagnosis requires portable biomedical devices with miniaturization of bio-instruments. The recent development of lab-on-a-chip (LOC) technology has provided a promising integration platform of microfluidic channels, microelectromechanical systems (MEMS), and multi-modal sensors, which allow non-invasive and near-field sensing functions. The standard complimentary metal-oxide semiconductor (CMOS) process allows a low-cost system-on-chip (SOC) solution to integrate sensors from multimodal domains, which has raised many new design challenges, such as how to develop multimodal sensors for system integration; how to integrate with MEMS and microfluidic channels from the device technology perspective; as well as data fusing and smart processing of multiple domains from system application perspective.

This book will report on the recent progress in CMOS integrated LOC system for personalized diagnosis. The book is organized into 12 chapters. After a background discussion on personalized diagnosis, LOC, and CMOS-compatible multimodal sensors in the first Chapter of introduction, Chapter 2 to Chapter 7 discuss CMOS sensor design and several CMOS sensor technologies, namely CMOS electronic impedance sensor, CMOS Terahertz sensor, CMUT ultrasound sensor, CMOS 3D-integrated MEMS sensor, and CMOS optical sensor for microfluidic contact imaging. Then two dual-mode sensor are illustrated in Chapters 8 and 9, such as dual-mode chemical/optical image sensor and dual-mode energy-harvesting image sensing. Finally, based on the aforementioned sensors, two important applications of DNA sequencing and cell counting are elaborated on. Chapter 10 focuses on DNA sequencing application, Chapter 11 covers cell imaging and counting application, and Chapter 12 briefly summarizes the book.

The authors would like to thank their colleagues Y. Shang, S. Manoj, X. Liu, Hantao Huang, Zichuan Liu, and Hang Xu. The authors also acknowledge with gratitude discussions with Professors Krishnendu Chakrabarty, Tsung-yi Ho, Zhihua Wang, Yong Lian, Guoxing Wang, Mohamad Sawan, Pantelis Georgiou, Dongping Wu, Chenjun Huang, Paul Franzon, Xin Li, and Kenneth Shepard. Their support was invaluable to us during the writing of this book. Finally, the authors acknowledge TSMC's contribution to sensor chips fabrication in the MPW tapeout shuttle.

Hao Yu, Mei Yan, and Xiwei Huang

1

Introduction

1.1 Personalized Biomedical Diagnosis

1.1.1 Personalized Diagnosis

The world's older population continues to grow at an unprecedented rate. The proportion of people aged 60 years and over grows faster than any other age group, as shown in Figure 1.1 [1]. According to the expectation of the World Health Organization [2], between 2000 and 2050, the world's population of over 60 years of age will double from about 11% to 22%, and the absolute number of such people will also increase from 605 million to 2 billion. Among the aging countries, the most dramatic changes are now taking place in low and middle income countries with limited biomedical infrastructure, incomplete healthcare systems, and shortage of funds and resources. The current aging society also comes with special healthcare challenges due to limited hospital resources, doctors and related facilities. A portable and low-cost biomedical diagnosis instrument is thereby in high demand to meet the needs of the growing aging population in the form of personalized biomedical diagnosis.

Over the past several decades, biomedical diagnostic techniques such as the microscope [3], ultrasound [4–6], flow cytometry [7–9], and genetic sequencing [10–12], have improved the accurate monitoring of existing diseases, and also the understanding of the underlying causes of those diseases. However, to obtain highly sensitive measurements, current diagnosis instrument systems are usually bulky and expensive, their complicated operation requiring professional personnel. As such, they are usually only available in established hospitals or clinics, and hence are not flexible for multiple functionality diagnoses for on-site personalized diagnosis. These problems pose significant challenges for the personalized healthcare of aging populations, especially in low-income developing countries. As such, portable and affordable biomedical instruments that can be miniaturized are required to provide a point-of-care (POC) diagnosis [13–15].

A POC biomedical instrument is meant to perform the diagnosis at the site of patient care by a clinician or by the patient without the need for clinical laboratory facilities. The tests are rapid, portable, non-invasive, and easy-to-use, with timely testing results, which allow rapid clinical decision-making and also mitigate treatment delay. The development of these POC diagnostic and monitoring instruments

CMOS Integrated Lab-on-a-Chip System for Personalized Biomedical Diagnosis,
First Edition. Hao Yu, Mei Yan, and Xiwei Huang.

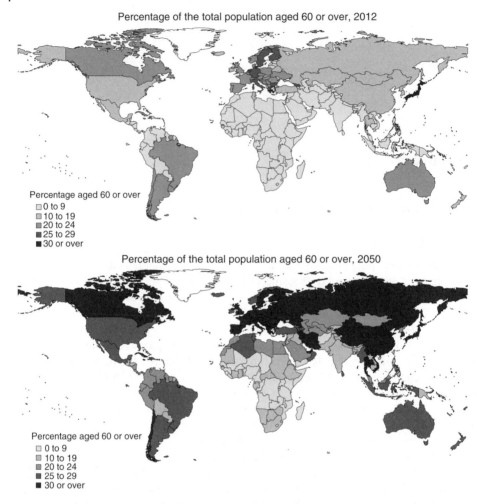

Figure 1.1 Global aging trends for the percentage of the total population at 60 years of age or over in 2012 and 2050 [1].

thereby allow individuals, especially these older people, to monitor their own health. It leads to a paradigm shift from conventional curative medicine, to predictive and personalized diagnostics [16]. Moreover, because factors such as medication adherence, genetics, age, nutrition, health, and environmental exposure can vary, and also the extent of biomedical treatment and drug response of each individual, people are becoming more interested in exploring the biology of the disease and its treatment at his or her own individual level. For example, people can use the information about his or her own genes, proteins, metabolites, etc. at the molecular level, and the leverage with the existing environment to prevent, diagnose, and treat the disease at the individual level. Therefore, such personalized biomedical diagnostics, with the existing supporting instrument platform, has emerged as a significant need for the coming aging world.

1.1.2 Conventional Biomedical Diagnostic Instruments

In the following section, three of the most widely-used traditional biomedical diagnosis instruments, namely the high-resolution optical microscope, flow cytometer, and DNA sequencer, are discussed as the starting point for comparison.

1.1.2.1 Optical Microscope

A microscope is an optical instrument that produces a magnified image of the biomedical object under inspection, compared with what the naked human eye can observe, using visible light with lenses. The optical microscope was invented more than 400 years ago by two Dutch spectacle makers, Hans and Zaccharias Janssen, then improved by Galileo and Antonie van Leeuwenhoek, and is the leading high-resolution visualization tool and the gold standard for biomedical imaging at the cellular level [17].

To achieve micrometer or sub-micrometer resolution, almost all microscopes require precise and expensive optical lenses, as well as a large distance between the object lens and eyepiece lens for the light to travel and reshape, as shown in Figure 1.2. The object to be observed is illuminated by a light source. As light passes through the object, the objective lens (i.e. the lens closest to the object) produces the corresponding magnified object image in the primary image angle. The eyepiece (i.e. the lens that people look into) acts as a magnifier that produces an enlarged image by the objective lens. The overall magnification of the microscope system is the

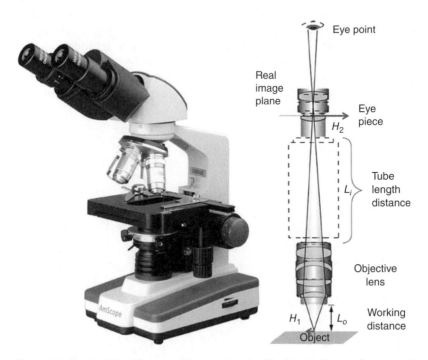

Figure 1.2 A typical microscope and its optical path with objective lens and eye piece. To reach high-resolution imaging capability, bulky, expensive, and sophisticated lenses are required.

multiplication of both the object and the eyepiece. The principle of magnification is based on the thin lens approximation as follows:

$$\frac{1}{L_i} + \frac{1}{L_o} = \frac{1}{F}M = \frac{L_i}{L_o} = \frac{H_2}{H_1} \tag{1.1}$$

where L_i and L_o are the image distance and object distance, F is the focal length of the objective lens, M is the magnification factor of the objective lens, and H_1 and H_2 are the sizes of object and image respectively. Therefore, a significant space L_i is usually required to produce a large microscopic magnification, which is the main difficulty for the minimization of the optical microscope.

Compared with the earliest compound microscope, the current design has evolved to incorporate multiple lenses, filters, polarizers, beam-splitters, sensors, illumination sources, and a host of other components, aimed at improving resolution and sample contrast. However, this basic microscope design has undergone very few fundamental changes over the centuries, so it bulky, expensive, and complicated, hence not suitable for the desired POC diagnosis.

1.1.2.2 Flow Cytometer

Flow cytometer is another widely-used biomedical instrument for applications in, for example, blood cell counting and sorting. Based on basic working principles, there are two types of flow cytometry methods, optical-based and electrochemical-based, as shown in Figure 1.3. With the help of sheath fluid and fluid dynamics effects, the blood cells are injected and passed through the measuring tunnel one at a time. For the optical-based cytometry shown in Figure 1.3(a), each cell along the path interacts with the laser beam respectively and the light intensity of the scattering is measured by the forward and orthogonal optical detectors. The measurement results depend on the size of the cell and its internal complexity, which can be used for cell differentiation and counting. Whereas, for the electrochemical based cytometry shown in Figure 1.3(b), pairs of electrodes are placed on both sides of a narrow orifice and a low-frequency

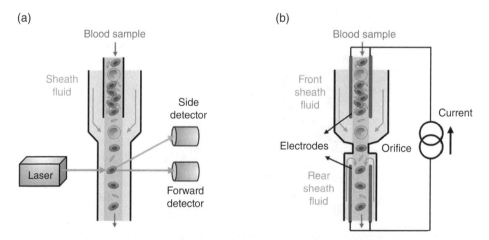

Figure 1.3 Diagrams of: (a) Optical-based; and (b) Electrochemical-based flow cytometry.

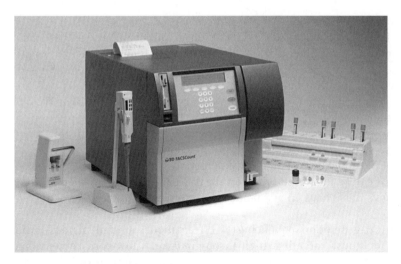

Figure 1.4 BD FACSCount™ cell cytometer system.

current is applied. When blood cells are driven through, the impedance values are measured, which vary with the cell size and composition.

As an example, the FACSCount, as shown in Figure 1.4, is one commercial optical-based flow cytometer system that can provide absolute and percentage counting results of various types of cells, such as red blood cells (RBCs), leukocytes, and CD4 T-lymphocytes. Clinicians rely on this system to diagnose the stage progression of HIV/AIDS, guide the treatment decision for HIV-infected persons, and evaluate the effectiveness of Antiretroviral Therapy (ART) [18]. However, it is only available in laboratory settings due to the limitations of bulky desktop size, prohibitive equipment cost ($27,000), high maintenance and reagent costs ($5–$20), low throughput (30–50 samples/day), and the need for an experienced operator, etc. [19]. Thus, it cannot meet the needs of personalized diagnosis.

1.1.2.3 DNA Sequencer

DNA sequencing, which detects the nucleotide order in DNA strands, enables the study of metagenomics and genetic disorders for diseases in aging people on an individual basis. Therefore, it plays an important role in personalized diagnostics. The first widely-applied DNA sequencing technique was the Sanger sequencing in the 1970s. This technique employs DNA polymerase to synthesize double-stranded DNA (dsDNA) from a primed single-stranded DNA (ssDNA) template. Four standard deoxyribonucleoside triphosphates (dNTPs), adenine (A), cytosine (C), guanine (G), and thymine (T), are used to extend the DNA, whereas four radioactively labeled di-dNTP (ddNTP) elements (ddATP, ddGTP, ddCTP, and ddTTP) are used to cease DNA extension. That is, once a ddNTP is attached to the DNA template, polymerase synthesis of this strand is invalid and no more dNTPs (or ddNTPs) can be added.

During sequencing, four chambers are employed for DNA synthesis. Each chamber is loaded with ssDNA templates, primers, polymerases, all four dNTPs, and one type of ddNTPs respectively. With sufficient dNTPs and a certain volume of labeled ddNTP, DNA extension is randomly stopped, thereby producing a set of dsDNAs of various lengths. Locations of terminating ddNTPs in all four chambers can be visualized with electrophoresis gel. Since ddNTP in each location is complementary to the nucleotide in the template, the DNA sequence can be obtained after combining all the ddNTP types and location information. Sanger's contribution accelerated the process of DNA sequencing from roughly 10 base pairs (bp) per year to about 100 bp/day [20]. Later, the adoption of fluorescent labeling [21] and its associated optical detection hardware further improved Sanger's sequencing efficiency. In this technique, polymerase synthesis can be finished in one chamber by using four types of fluorescent labels. With the help of an optical detection system, each type of labeled ddNTP terminator can be identified based on the different color or wavelength they emit. These improvements have greatly helped the automation of the DNA sequencing process.

Since 2005, the next-generation sequencing (NGS) techniques substantially advanced the sequencing methods, targeting high-throughput and low-cost sequencing. A typical NGS machine is shown in Figure 1.5. Important examples of NGS technologies include the Solexa/Illumina bridge amplification method, which dominates this field currently [22], as well as Roche's pyrosequencing method [23] with bead-emulsified polymerase chain reaction (PCR) [24]. However, most of these methods require bulky and expensive optical instruments, which greatly restrict their use at the patient scale, such that only hospitals and research centers can afford them. In order to reduce the cost and size, new technologies targeted at personalized sequencing should be explored.

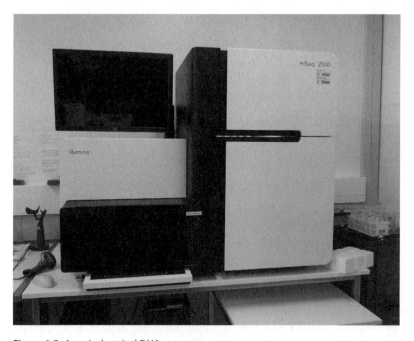

Figure 1.5 A typical optical DNA sequencer.

1.2 CMOS Sensor-based Lab-on-a-Chip for System Miniaturization

1.2.1 CMOS Sensor-based Lab-on-a-Chip

For bio-instrument miniaturization towards personalized diagnosis, effective solutions can only be derived from technologies that can resolve the scaling. One proved technology from the semiconductor industry is based on the complimentary metal-oxide semiconductor (CMOS) process. CMOS technology has been utilized in digital, analog, and mixed-signal integration circuits (ICs), such as microcontrollers, microprocessors, cell-phones, amplifiers, data converters, and transceivers, etc. More recently, the CMOS process has been developed in optical sensing, charge detection, temperature measurement, and electrochemical sensing applications, which can be realized by integrating readout circuits with on-chip sensing devices, such as photodiodes, ion-selected field effect transistors (ISFET), and microelectrodes. The main advantages of CMOS are the scalability in integration but also the variability in sensing. Large numbers or multiple functions of sensing devices (also called multi-modal sensors) can be integrated on one chip, so as to create mass-produced, low-cost, diversified, and miniaturized biomedical sensors for personalized diagnosis.

In most applications, biomedical samples are prepared and detected in an aqueous environment, which means that sensors usually need to be physically interfaced with fluidic samples, so as to realize a portable size. Thus, the emerging Lab-on-a-Chip (LOC) technique can combine a microfluidic system with the CMOS sensor. A microfluidic structure directs fluid samples towards the sensing sites, which are then detected by the underlying CMOS sensing devices. These devices, on the one hand, may act as voltage or current sources for actuating purpose. On the other hand, they may convert interesting biological information into an electric signal for sensing purposes.

As is implied by the name, Lab-on-a-Chip means a minimized chip-scale (a few square centimeters in size) device that has the ability to perform one or several laboratory functions [25–29]. Since LOCs need to deal with chemical or small biological objects, analyses in extremely small fluid volumes (microliters or even picoliters), it greatly relies on microfluidics for sample preparation, delivery, and on-chip processing. The recent advancement of LOC technology has provided a promising solution to integrate microfluidics [14], micro-electro-mechanical systems (MEMS), and CMOS multimodal sensors [30–33] on one platform, which allows a miniaturized biomedical sensing system without bulky mechanical components. For such a CMOS sensor-based LOC method, the reduced sample volume, portability, low cost, and the possibility to integrate multiple analytical devices, are key advantages over the traditional laboratory-scale instruments.

A diagram of the CMOS sensor-based LOC is shown in Figure 1.6. The sensor chip is fabricated through the standard CMOS process for the scaling benefit of low cost and mass production. It usually consists of a large amount (millions) of sensing nodes, or CMOS sensing pixels, to improve the sensing throughput. Thus, it can detect a great number of biological reactions simultaneously. In order to increase sensor density, the pixel design not only needs to consider the performance optimization, but also the scaling capability of continuously shrinking the pixel size. The CMOS sensor array can be further equipped with a fluidic package to carry and separate biomedical samples, so

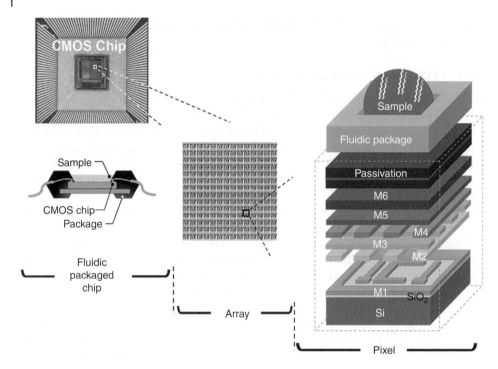

Figure 1.6 CMOS-based LOC integration for biomedical instrument miniaturization.

that a large volume of samples can be detected in parallel by their respective underlying pixels. After the sensor chip is fabricated, post processed, and packaged, it can be integrated with the microfluidic channel with fluidic packages to realize a completed LOC integration. Thus, such CMOS sensor-based LOC microsystems can create tremendous opportunities for future personalized diagnosis applications.

Building such CMOS-based LOC platforms can bring great potential and opportunities. It enables the development of multimodal CMOS sensors. The multimodal sensing types can vary from electrochemical, electric impedance, terahertz, and optical, etc., which will be mainly addressed in this book. Note that CMOS-based LOC platform can further integrate the data analytics part as well.

1.2.2 CMOS Sensor

1.2.2.1 CMOS Process Fundamentals

CMOS circuit design was invented in 1963 by Frank Wanlass at Fairchild Semiconductors. In 1968, a group led by Albert Medwin at RCA invented the first commercial CMOS integrated circuits that consist of 4000 series of CMOS logic gates. During the 1970s, CMOS technology was used in computing processor development, which led to the explosive growth of personal computers. It is estimated that the CMOS transistor is the most manufactured device in the history of mankind. Now, more than 95% of integrated circuits are fabricated in CMOS. One important reason behind this dominance is that CMOS is scalable for system integration.

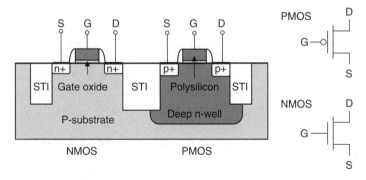

Figure 1.7 Cross-section view (left) and symbol (right) of CMOS technology components: NMOS and PMOS.

A metal oxide semiconductor (MOS) technology can be classified as PMOS (P-type MOS), NMOS (N-type MOS), and CMOS (Complementary MOS). The basic physical structure of MOS devices consists of a semiconductor, oxide, and a metal gate. Nowadays, polysilicon is more widely used as the gate (G). Voltage applied to the gate controls the current between source (S) and drain (D). Since very low power is consumed, MOS allows very high integration.

Figure 1.7 shows the components of a modern CMOS technology. Basically, it includes NMOS and PMOS transistors on the same substrate. For NMOS, the first letter "N" indicates the kind of carrier that carries the current flow between source and drain when the threshold voltage is reached. Thus, NMOS stands for transistors where negatively charged electrons are the current carriers between source and drain. PMOS stands for transistors where positively charged holes are the current carriers. The CMOS circuit uses both NMOS and PMOS transistors for pulling down to ground and up to power supply. The transistors are arranged in a structure formed by two complementary networks, Pull Up Network (PUN) and Pull Down Network (PDN). PUN is a network composed of PMOS transistors between output and power source, whereas PDN is an NMOS-type network between output and ground. Typically, in the CMOS circuit, only one of PUN and PDN is switched on and the other one is switched off with the corresponding gate capacitor to hold the charge information. This physical basic can be utilized in sensing.

CMOS technology requires fabrication of two different transistors – NMOS and PMOS on a single chip substrate. Actually, NMOS and PMOS need substrates with different kinds of doping in one integrated circuit. A silicon wafer always has one doping type and doping level. Hence, to accommodate both NMOS and PMOS transistors, CMOS technology requires creation of special regions, called wells, by impurity implantation in the substrate. The semiconductor type in these regions is opposite to the base substrate type. A p-well is created in an n-type substrate or, alternatively, an n-well is created in a p-type substrate. Thus, if the base substrate is p-type, the NMOS transistor is created in the p-type substrate, while the PMOS transistor is created in the n-well built into the p-type base substrate.

Historically, fabrication started with p-well technology, but now has completely shifted to n-well technology. This is due to the lower sheet resistance of the n-well compared with the p-well, as electrons are more mobile than holes. The simplified n-well process to fabricate CMOS integrated circuits on a p-type silicon substrate works as follows. First, n-well regions are created for PMOS transistors by impurity implantation into the substrate. Next, a thick oxide (Shallow Trench Isolation, STI) surrounding the NMOS and PMOS active regions is grown to isolate each transistor. A thin gate oxide layer is then grown on the surface through thermal oxidation. After this process, n+ and p+ regions (source, drain, and channel-stop implants) are created. Finally, the metallization step creates metal interconnections in this process.

As each processing step requires that certain areas are defined on the chip by appropriate masks, the CMOS integrated circuit can be viewed as a set of patterned layers of doped silicon, polysilicon, metal, and insulating silicon dioxide. A layer is patterned before the next layer of material is applied on the chip. The lithography process is used to transfer a pattern onto a layer, which should be repeated for every layer using a different mask, since each layer has its own distinct requirements.

The main processing steps to fabricate an n-channel MOS transistor on a p-type silicon substrate are as follows. First, the oxidation of the silicon substrate (Figure 1.8(a)) is performed, which creates a relatively thick silicon dioxide layer on the surface, that is, the field oxide (Figure 1.8(b)). The field oxide is then selectively etched to expose the silicon surface on which the transistor will be created (Figure 1.8(c)). Then the surface is covered with a thin, high-quality oxide layer to form the gate oxide of the MOS transistor (Figure 1.8(d)). A polysilicon layer is then deposited onto the thin oxide (Figure 1.8(e)), which is used as both a gate material for MOS transistors as well as an interconnect medium in silicon. The resistivity of polysilicon, which is usually high, is reduced by doping it with impure atoms. Next, the polysilicon layer is patterned and etched to form the MOS transistor gate (Figure 1.8(f)). The thin gate oxide not masked by the polysilicon is also etched away, exposing the bare silicon surface. The drain and source junctions are to be formed, as in Figure 1.8(g).

Diffusion or ion implantation is used to dope the entire silicon surface with a high concentration of impurities (in this case donor atoms to produce n-type doping). Figure 1.8(h) shows two n-type regions (source and drain junctions) in the p-type substrate as doping penetrates the exposed areas of the silicon surface. The penetration of impurity doping into the polysilicon reduces its resistivity. After this stage, the entire surface is again covered with an insulating layer of silicon dioxide after the source and drain regions are completed (Figure 1.8(i)). Then contact windows for the source and drain are patterned into the oxide layer (Figure 1.8(j)). Interconnections are formed by evaporating the metal layer (aluminum/copper) onto the surface (Figure 1.8(k)), which is followed by patterning and etching of the metal layer (Figure 1.8(l)). A second or third layer of metallic interconnections can also be added after adding another oxide layer, by cutting (via) holes, depositing, and patterning the metal.

1.2.2.2 CMOS Sensor Technology

The development of CMOS technology offers the advantage of cost-effective CMOS integrated sensors, and the CMOS process can be applied to realize various CMOS sensors integrated for personalized diagnosis systems. Over the past few decades, many CMOS-based sensors have been developed for analyzing biological or chemical samples. Unlike conventional biomedical diagnostic instruments, new CMOS-compatible

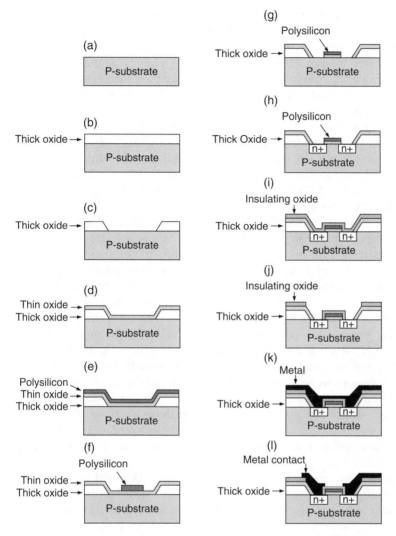

Figure 1.8 Process flow for the fabrication of an n-type MOSFET on p-type silicon.

biochemical sensing methods should be developed, especially for the conversion of biochemical information to circuit understandable languages, such as impedance, voltage, and current. For the CMOS process, the major materials involved are semiconductor materials (e.g. Si, SiO_2, and Si_3N_4) and metalic materials (e.g. Cu and Al); major manufacturing methods are doping, etching, deposition, and photolithography; and major fabricated structures are p-n junction, bipolar, and MOSFET. Thus, new CMOS-sensor-based biomedical sensing methods should evolve from these existing materials, processes, or structures to perform the biochemical-to-electrical conversion. One method is to directly fabricate the biochemical sensing part in standard CMOS processes. Another method is to first fabricate electrical-readout interfaces in standard CMOS processes and then use special surface treatments or post processing to make the biochemical sensing parts.

On the other hand, even though most of existing biomedical diagnostic methods vary, from either the substances used or procedures involved, the basic working principle can be categorized as optical-based and electrochemical-based. For the optical method, one way is to directly capture images to obtain the samples' physical properties such as shape, structure, or density. Another way is to first label or dye the samples and then detect the luminous parts to determine whether the desired reactions have occurred or not. Apart from optical characteristics, each object has its own electrical features that can be represented by impedance, voltage, or current. For the electrochemical method, one way is to directly measure these electrical properties of the target samples. Another way is to monitor the changing environmental conditions due to the samples' reactions or activities. New techniques can also be evolved from these two basic methods.

As examples, three types of CMOS process compatible biochemical sensing structures are illustrated. As shown in Figure 1.9(a), the p-n junction structure is utilized as a photodiode where photons are absorbed and converted into photocurrent. With illumination from the top, light intensity changes caused by the biomedical sample's optical properties are captured by the photodiode. This is a common optical sensing method utilizing a CMOS image sensor. In addition, electrochemical sensing structures are also involved, such as the voltage sensing in Figure 1.9(b) and current/impedance sensing in Figure 1.9(c). The electrode/electrode pair is normally employed to provide a steady biasing environment. Biochemical information will be converted into voltage or current signals that can be observed by CMOS sensors. In Figure 1.9(b), the non-conductive passivation layer (Si_3N_4) works as a sensing membrane. Ion density changes in the sample solution will charge or discharge the membrane. The resulting voltage shifts are detected by CMOS devices, whereas in Figure 1.9(c), an on-chip metal electrode will be fabricated, which forms an electrode pair together with the one in the sample solution. After applying a voltage drop, the current will flow through the electrode. The ion current value depends on the combined effects of sample and background solutions with varying resistance and capacitance. The induced current signals will also be detected by the underlying CMOS devices.

For CMOS sensors, large pixel arrays are preferred to reduce chip cost while improving the throughput, so that the capability to form a large pixel array and detect in parallel are the key issues to be addressed. Apart from the biochemical sensing part, other

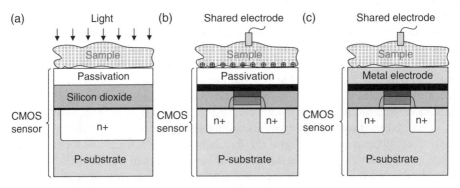

Figure 1.9 Diagrams of biochemical sensing structures; the sensing parts are: (a) p-n junction; (b) Passivation; and (c) Metal electrode pair.

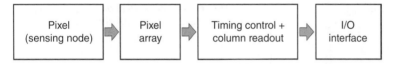

Figure 1.10 A typical architecture diagram of a CMOS sensor.

function blocks should also be involved to read out the converted signals or perform data processing. A typical CMOS sensor architecture is shown in Figure 1.10. The biomedical-to-electrical conversion is conducted in each pixel cell. A large amount of pixels can be arranged in a 2-D and pixel array. The pixel array is operated by timing control blocks and pixel signals are read out or processed by column readout blocks. All communication behaviors between the CMOS sensor and peripheral instruments, such as the voltage source or computer, are through the input/output (I/O) interface on chip.

In the following chapters, we will introduce impedance, terahertz, ultrasonic, MEMS, optical, or electrochemical sensors, etc. The CMOS impedance sensor employs an electrode array on top of the pixel array. It detects the sample's change in impedance magnitude and phase, which can be applied for single-cell detection. The CMOS Terahertz sensor can be applied as a THz spectroscopy for *in-vitro* tissue diagnosis. The CMOS ultrasound sensor can act as the front-end signal conditioner after the ultrasonic transducer for signal transmitting and receiving. The CMOS MEMS sensor can integrate the CMOS readout chip with the MEMS accelerometer to realize data fusion in a low-cost chip size fashion. The CMOS optical image sensor can capture images using a 2-D large pixel array to reach high resolution towards cell counting applications. The CMOS electrochemical sensor, or the CMOS pH sensor, can employ potentiometric ISFET pixels to sense the ion changes for bacteria detection or DNA sequencing application. In addition, the CMOS fabrication technology makes it possible to implement multimodal sensors that integrate multiple biomedical sensing modalities in one sensor chip, such as optical-electrochemical sensor or optical-energy harvesting sensor. In this case, high accuracy and diversified measurement can be realized when further fusing and recovering data from multimodal domains.

1.2.2.3 Multimodal CMOS Sensor

In biomedical testing, some properties of a reaction or biological material can be detected optically but not chemically, and vice versa for other properties. In some cases, it is only when these properties are known together that we can draw conclusions about the state of the reaction or biological material. The field of sensor fusion has received much attention recently as the combining of sensors can improve sensing capability. Thus, multimodal CMOS image sensors are required.

Light and electricity are two important media used in the measurement or control of biological samples such as proteins, neural cells, and DNA. Conventionally, optical imaging is based on microscopy technology, and electrical sensing of neural activity is through micro-electrode technology. In [34] or [35], a dual-mode CMOS image sensor is demonstrated. It can simultaneously capture optical and potential/electrochemical images of targeted biomedical samples, such as DNA or neural cells. As shown in Figure 1.11, the pixel array is composed of optical sensing pixels and potential sensing pixels that are interleaved. These two different types of pixels share the same timing and

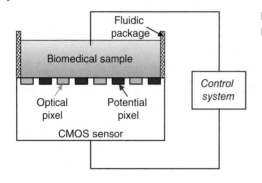

Figure 1.11 The concept of the optical and potential dual-mode CMOS image sensor.

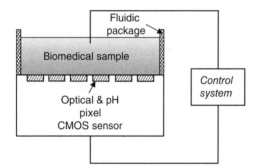

Figure 1.12 Schematic of the multimodal optical and pH CMOS image sensor.

column readout circuits, communication interface, package, and peripheral control system. In this way, system cost and size are minimized compared to the situation when these two sensor chips are separately fabricated.

For a CMOS sensor with a large pixel array, a small change in pixel size will make a large difference to the whole sensor chip. Thus, another attractive structure is to integrate multiple biochemical sensing devices into one pixel. Compared with the separately placed pixels in Figure 1.11, the pixel-level readout circuit can be shared by different types of sensing modes. In this way, chip size and cost can be further reduced. For example, in [36], a multimodal CMOS image sensor for pH and light sensing in real time is proposed. A photo sensor and a pH sensor are fused in the same pixel, as shown in Figure 1.12, enabling the optical and pH signals to be detected simultaneously in the same sensing area. As the pH sensing and optical sensing are built into the same area, more accurate chemical information can be extracted without loss of spatial resolution.

The fusion of various types of sensors has been receiving more attention recently, aiming to achieve high performance in the detection of signals from multiple domains. Next, more details about the LOC system components are introduced.

1.2.3 Microfluidics

1.2.3.1 Microfluidic Fundamentals
Microfluidics is a multidisciplinary engineering field where chemistry, physics, engineering, and biotechnology intersect to develop microscale chips, where the fluid analysis can

Figure 1.13 A typical microfluidic channel.

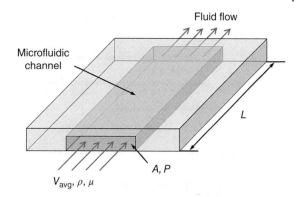

take place. The control and manipulation of the micro fluids are usually precisely and geometrically constrained to a microscale or nanoscale volume. For the typical microfluidic channel shown in Figure 1.13, the flow of the fluid can be characterized using the Reynolds number as follows:

$$Re = \frac{LV_{avg}\rho}{\mu} \tag{1.2}$$

where L is the most relevant channel length scale, V_{avg} is the average flow velocity, ρ is the fluid density, and μ is the fluid viscosity. For many microchannels, $L = 4A/P$, where A is the channel cross-sectional area, and P is the wetted channel perimeter. Re is usually much less than 100 (often < 1.0), due to the small dimensions of microchannels. In this Re regime, microfluidic flow is completely laminar without turbulence. Thus the micro sample can be transported in a relatively predictable manner through microchannels. When the Re increases to the range of 2000, the micro flow starts to change to a turbulent flow.

There are usually two methods of fluid actuation, namely electrokinetic flow and pressure driven flow. In electrokinetic flow, the fluids are driven by electroosmotic pumping. In pressure driven flow, the fluid is driven through the channel by positive displacement pumps such as syringe pumps. The advantage of electrokinetic flow over pressure driven flow is that it can couple other on-chip electronic applications. However, electrokinetic flow often requires very high voltages. Without off-chip power supplies, it is difficult to miniaturize. One other significant disadvantage of electrokinetic flow is the variability in surface properties. For example, the proteins absorbed into the channel walls can substantially change the surface charge characteristics, and hence lead to a change in fluid velocity. This problem will result in unpredictable and irregular long-term time dependency on the fluid flow

There is also another kind of microfluidics, droplet-based digital microfluidics. This employs electrowetting-on-dielectric to precisely manipulate discrete droplets of biochemical samples and reagents at microliter or picoliter volumes under digital clock control. It can combine electronics with biology, and integrate together a number of bioassay operations, such as sample preparation, separation, mixture, analysis, and detection to form a miniaturized digital microfluidic biochip (DMFB) and automate laboratory procedures in immunoassays, biochemistry, and molecular biology.

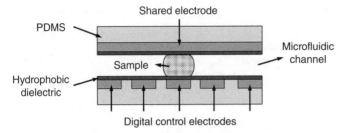

Figure 1.14 Cross-sectional schematic of a unit cell on digital microfluidic arrays.

An example of DMFB is shown in Figure 1.14. Compared to conventional expensive and cumbersome laboratory procedures, DMFBs show the advantages of lower cost, higher sensitivity, easier system integration, and less likelihood of human error.

There are several advantages of using microfluidic devices in clinically useful technologies to perform biomedical diagnosis:

1) Microfluidic technologies make it possible to fabricate highly integrated devices so that several different functions, such as blood or saliva filtering, desalting, denaturation, concentration, and derivatization, can be performed on the same chip.
2) Small volumes lead to fast analyses; moreover, the small amount of reagents and analytes used is especially important for expensive reagents.
3) Material cost is negligible in micro-systems. The techniques used to fabricate microfluidic devices are relatively inexpensive and suitable for highly multiplexed devices and mass production.

After the fundamentals of fluid flow and sample transportation becoming well developed, microfluidics has recently developed towards integrated devices that incorporate multiple fluidic, mechanical, and electronic components as well as various chemical processes onto a single chip. There has been a major push towards bio-imaging instrument miniaturization.

1.2.3.2 Microfluidics Fabrication

To fabricate microfluidic channels, polymers, instead of silicon and glass, are commonly used. Specifically, the poly-dimethylsiloxane (PDMS) is widely used as it is inexpensive, flexible, optically transparent, and biological compatible. The fabrication of microfluidic channels using the conventional soft-lithography process is presented here:

1) **Photolithography Mask**

   Some examples of the designed microfluidic channel masks are shown in Figure 1.15. First, the channel microstructures or features are designed in a computer-aided design (CAD) program, such as the AutoCAD (Autodesk, San Rafael, CA). Using commercial services, the CAD-generated patterns are printed onto a transparent photolithography mask. The photolithography mask is an opaque film or plate template with transparent areas that allow light to shine through in the designed pattern. The feature size (or the lateral resolution) of the mask is determined by its material; three types of base materials are commonly used to make photolithography masks, namely Quartz, Soda Lime (SL), and polyester film. Quartz and SL masks are high resolution, easy to clean, stable, but expensive. Polyester film masks have less resolution, but are low cost and much easier to handle.

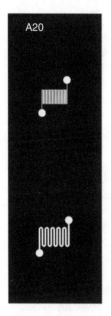 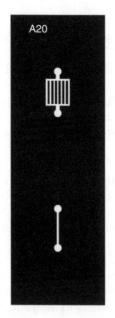 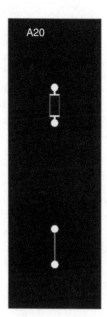

Figure 1.15 Microfluidic channel masks designed by AutoCAD.

2) **SU-8 Mold**

After the turnaround time, the designed masks are sent back for microfluidic channel mold fabrication. Here, the negative photoresist SU-8 (SU-8 25, Microchem, MA) is used, which is a high contrast and epoxy-based photoresist for micro-machining. The SU-8 has superb chemical and temperature resistance and can build a thickness from 1 to 200 μm with the single spin coat process. A normal process is shown in Figure 1.16:

1) *Substrate Pretreat*

Both a silicon wafer and glass slide can be used as the SU-8 substrate. Here we take the glass slide as an example due to its low cost. To obtain the maximum process reliability, substrates need to be clean and dry before applying the SU-8 resist. The glass slide is pretreated in the following way:

1) Soak and wash the glass slide with acetone for at least 1 h for solvent cleaning.
2) Use distilled water to rinse the glass slide, and then use a stream of air or nitrogen to blow to dry.
3) To dehydrate the surface, bake the cleaned glass slide at 200 °C for 5 min on a hotplate.
4) Plasma treat for 10 min to further clean and dehydrate the glass slide surface.

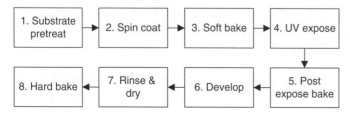

Figure 1.16 PDMS mold fabrication process.

2) *Spin Coat*

Next, the SU-8 is spin-coated using a spin machine (SCS G3P-8, Indianapolis, IN) onto the clean glass slide. The spin speed directly determines the height of the mold, which is also the height of the final PDMS microfluidic channel. The detailed steps are:

5) Pour SU-8 onto the glass slide (~10–15 ml per glass slide for static dispense), then degas in a vacuum oven for 1 h to remove air bubbles.

6) Spin coat for thin film deposition; the spin speed needs to be set to correspond to different film heights.

3) *Soft Bake*

After the photoresist is spin-coated onto the glass slide substrate, it should be soft-baked on a hot plate to evaporate the solvent as well as to densify the film. As the solvent evaporation rate is affected by the heat transfer and ventilation rate, baking times should be optimized for proximity and the convection oven bake process. The process is:

7) Bake on a 65 °C hot plate for 5 min, then at 95 °C for 15 min.

4) *UV Exposure*

The soft-baked glass slide with SU-8 film is exposed to UV. SU-8 is practically transparent and insensitive above 400 nm, but has high actinic absorption below 350 nm. The exposure dose also affects the film thickness. The process is:

8) UV exposure of 200 mJ/cm^2 energy for 30 s.

5) *Post Expose Bake*

Following exposure, post expose bake (PEB) needs to be performed to selectively cross-link the exposed portions of the film. This is realized through a two-step contact hot plate baking process, as indicated below:

9) Post UV exposure bake on a 65 °C hot plate for 1 min, then at 95 °C for 4 min.

6) *Develop*

After PEB, the SU-8 is developed using an SU-8 developer. The approximate developing time is 6 min, but it can vary widely as a function of temperature or agitation rate, i.e.:

10) Develop the PEB glass slide using the SU-8 developer for 6 min.

7) *Rinse and Dry*

Following the development, the substrate should be rinsed using isopropyl alcohol (IPA), and then dried under a gentle stream of air or nitrogen. It then undergoes a final hard bake. The detailed steps are:

11) Rinse the substrate using IPA and dry.

12) Bake the substrate on a 200 °C hot plate for 10 min.

13) Cool the slides and place them into the culture dish.

3) **PDMS Replica**

After the SU-8 mold is ready, we can cast the PDMS replica, that is, the microfluidic channel. The whole mask, mold, and PDMS channel fabrication process flow is shown in Figure 1.17.

The steps are:

a) Prepare the PDMS mixture for casting, a volumetric ratio of 10:1 mixture of PDMS (Sylgard 184, Dow Corning, MI) and curing agent, and pour into the SU-8 mold.

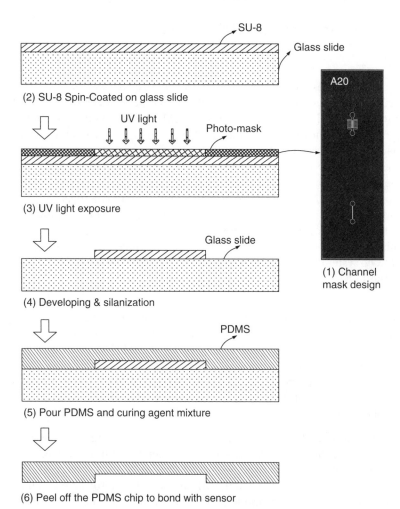

Figure 1.17 Microfluidic channel fabrication process using the soft lithography technique.

b) Degas for 1 h in a vacuum oven to remove any bubbles from the PDMS mixture.

c) Take out the glass slide and bake in the oven for 2 h.

d) After the PDMS replica becomes dry and hard, take out and prepare to cut the channel out and peel off from the glass substrate.

e) Use a puncher to punch holes in the top of the PDMS replica for inlet and outlet channels, which are to be connected with silastic laboratory tubes to a syringe pump and waste bin.

f) Use IPA and de-ionized (DI) water to rinse the PDMS channel. Dry the channel for the final bonding with the CMOS sensors.

Now, the PDMS microfluidic channel fabrication process is complete.

1.3 Objectives and Organization of this Book

1.3.1 Objectives

Towards the personalized diagnosis for the aging society, miniaturized bio-instrumentation is demanded. As such, the conventional bulky optical lens and other mechanical components can no longer be applied. We need to develop CMOS-based LOC integrated systems that integrate microfluidics, MEMS, and CMOS sensors, as well as smart data analysis for biomedical diagnosis. The standard CMOS process provides an low-cost system-on-chip (SOC) solution to integrate sensors from multimodal domains, which has raised many new design challenges, such as how to develop multimodal sensors for system integration; how to integrate with MEMS and microfluidic channels from a device technology perspective; as well as data fusing and smart processing of multiple domains from the system application perspective.

Therefore, in this book, we have particularly reported on the recent progress in the CMOS integrated LOC system for personalized diagnosis [38–61]. The CMOS sensors we developed for the LOC integrated biomedical diagnostic system include multiple modes, which are:

1) CMOS electronic impedance sensor for rare cell detection and counting;
2) CMOS Terahertz sensor for non-invasive imaging;
3) CMOS capacitive-micromachined-ultrasonic-transducer (CMUT) sensor for non-invasive 3-D ultrasound imaging;
4) CMOS ISFET sensor for ion imaging towards DNA sequencing application; and
5) CMOS optical sensor for microfluidic imaging towards cell detection, recognition, and counting applications.

We will illustrate the need and application of the five corresponding bio-imaging diagnosis methods, as well as design problems addressed when being miniaturized. In addition, for MEMS integration, we further present a 3-D CMOS MEMS integration method for high-throughput sensing data readout with smaller form factor, latency, and power consumption. Moreover, two dual-mode sensors are presented. One is from the sensing capability point of view, where the CMOS optical sensing and CMOS ion sensing are integrated together in the same sensing pixel for higher accuracy and lower noise diagnosis. The other is to tackle the problem of energy, where a CMOS image sensor with both energy harvesting mode and optical sensing mode is illustrated. Finally, the smart data analytics are integrated into the discussion of optical image sensor-based lensless cell counting applications.

Our thorough study to explore multimodal CMOS sensors in LOC for the portable personalized diagnosis system could pave the way towards a variety of personalized diagnosis applications. As a conclusion, the CMOS multimodal sensor-based LOC system has shown great potential in providing future personalized e-healthcare solution for the coming aging society.

1.3.2 Organization

The rest of the book is organized into three major parts. Chapters 2 to 7 discuss CMOS sensor design and several CMOS sensor technologies, namely CMOS electronic impedance sensor, CMOS Terahertz sensor, CMUT ultrasound sensor, CMOS 3D-integrated MEMS sensor, and CMOS optical sensor for microfluidic contact imaging. The two dual-mode sensors are illustrated in Chapters 8 and 9, that is, dual-mode chemical/optical image sensor and dual-mode energy-harvesting image sensing. Finally, based on the aforementioned sensors, two important applications, DNA sequencing and cell counting, are elaborated upon. Chapter 10 focuses on DNA sequencing applications. Chapter 11 covers cell imaging and counting applications. Finally, Chapter 12 concludes the whole book.

References

1 WHO Global Brief for World Health Day (2012) Available at: http://www.who.int/ageing/publications/whd2012_global_brief/en/

2 WHO Ageing and Life Course. Available at: http://www.who.int/ageing/en/

3 T. Wilson (1990) *Confocal Microscopy*, vol. 426 Academic Press: London, pp. 1–64.

4 X. Huang, J.H. Cheong, H.-K. Cha, H. Yu, M. Je, and H. Yu (2013) A high-frequency transimpedance amplifier for CMOS integrated 2D CMUT array towards 3D ultrasound imaging. In: *International Conference of the IEEE Engineering in Medicine and Biology Society (EMBC)*, pp. 101–104.

5 I. Kim, H. Kim, F. Griggio, R.L. Tutwiler, T.N. Jackson, *et al.* (2009) CMOS ultrasound transceiver chip for high-resolution ultrasonic imaging systems. *IEEE Transactions on Biomedical Circuits and Systems (TBCAS)*, 3(5), 293–303.

6 G. Gurun, P. Hasler and F.L. Degertekin (2011) Front-end receiver electronics for high-frequency monolithic CMUT-on-CMOS imaging arrays. *IEEE Transactions on Ultrasonics, Ferroelectrics and Frequency Control (TUFFC)*, 58(8), 1658–1668.

7 H.M. Shapiro (2003) *Practical Flow Cytometry*, 4th edition. John Wiley & Sons.

8 A.L. Givan (2001) *Flow Cytometry: First Principles*, 2nd edition. John Wiley & Sons.

9 M. Brown and C. Wittwer, (2000) Flow cytometry: Principles and clinical applications in hematology. *Clinical Chemistry*, 46(8), 1221–1229.

10 J. Shendure and H. Ji (2008) Next-generation DNA sequencing. *Nature Biotechnology*, 26, 1135–1145.

11 M. Margulies, M. Egholm, W.E. Altman, S. Attiya, J.S. Bader, *et al.* (2005) Genome sequencing in microfabricated high-density picolitre reactors. *Nature*, 437, 376–380.

12 D.R. Bentley, S. Balasubramanian, H.P. Swerdlow, G.P. Smith, J. Milton, C.G. *et al.* (2008) Accurate whole human genome sequencing using reversible terminator chemistry. *Nature*, 456, 53–59.

13 G.J. Kost (2002) *Principles and Practice of Point-of-care Testing*. Lippincott Williams & Wilkins: Philadelphia.

14 S.K. Sia and L.J. Kricka (2008) Microfluidics and point-of-care testing. *Lab on a Chip*, 8(12), 1982–1983.

15 P. Yager, G.J. Domingo and J. Gerdes (2008) Point-of-care diagnostics for global health. *Annual Review of Biomedical Engineering*, 10, 107–144.

16 B. Korte (2010) *NIH Fact Sheet: Point-of-Care Diagnostic Testing*. https://report.nih.gov/NIHfactsheets/ViewFactSheet.aspx?csid=112.

17 C. Yang and D. Psaltis (2007) Building a Microscopic Microscope. *ENGenious*, 6, 44–47.

18 C.F. Gilks, S. Crowley, R. Ekpini, S. Gove, J. Perriens, *et al.* (2006) The WHO public-health approach to antiretroviral treatment against HIV in resource-limited settings. *The Lancet*, 368(9534), 505–510.

19 S.J. Moon, H.O. Keles, A. Ozcan, A. Khademhosseini, E. Hæggstrom, *et al.* (2009) Integrating microfluidics and lensless imaging for point-of-care testing. *Biosensors and Bioelectronics*, 24(11), 3208–3214.

20 L. Hartwell, L. Hood, M.L. Goldberg, A. Reynolds, L. Silver and R. Veres (2008) *Genetics: from Genes to Genomes*. McGraw-Hill: New York.

21 L.M. Smith, J.Z. Sanders, R.J. Kaiser, P. Hughes, C. Dodd, *et al.* (1986) Fluorescence detection in automated DNA sequence analysis. *Nature*, 321(6071), 674–679.

22 S. Balasubramanian (2003) Polynucleotide sequencing, Google Patents.

23 P. Nyren (2001) Method of sequencing DNA based on the detection of the release of pyrophosphate and enzymatic nucleotide degradation, Google Patents.

24 M. Margulies, M. Egholm, W.E. Altman, S. Attiya, J.S. Bader, *et al.* (2005) Genome sequencing in microfabricated high-density picolitre reactors. *Nature*, 437(7057), 376–380.

25 R. Daw and J. Finkelstein (2006) Lab on a chip. *Nature*, 442(7101), 367–367.

26 G.M. Whitesides (2006) The origins and the future of microfluidics. *Nature*, 442(7101), 368–373.

27 D. Mark, S. Haeberle, G. Roth, F. von Stetten and R. Zengerle (2010) Microfluidic lab-on-a-chip platforms: requirements, characteristics and applications. *Chemical Society Reviews*, 39(3), 1153–1182.

28 Y. Zhao, D. Chen, H. Yue, J.B. French, J. Rufo, *et al.* (2013) Lab-on-a-chip technologies for single-molecule studies. *Lab on a Chip*, 13(12), 2183–2198.

29 M. Medina-Sanchez, S. Miserere and A. Merkoci (2012) Nanomaterials and lab-on-a-chip technologies, *Lab on a Chip*, 12(11), 1932–1943.

30 Y.-S. Lin, D. Sylvester and D. Blaauw (2008) An ultra low power 1 V, 220 nW temperature sensor for passive wireless applications. In: *IEEE Custom Integrated Circuits Conference (CICC)*, pp. 507–510.

31 S. Hanson and D. Sylvester (2009) A 0.45–0.7 V sub-microwatt CMOS image sensor for ultra-low power applications. In: *IEEE Symposium on VLSI Circuits (VLSIC)*, pp. 176–177.

32 Y.-S. Lin, D.M. Sylvester and D.T. Blaauw (2009) A 150 pW program-and-hold timer for ultra-low-power sensor platforms. In: *IEEE International Solid-State Circuits Conference (ISSCC)*, pp. 326–327.

33 S. Hanson, Z. Foo, D. Blaauw and D. Sylvester (2010) A 0.5 V sub-microwatt CMOS image sensor with pulse-width modulation read-out. *IEEE Journal of Solid-State Circuits (JSSC)*, 45(4), 759–767.

34 T. Tokuda, A. Yamamoto, K. Kagawa, M. Nunoshita and J. Ohta (2006) A CMOS image sensor with optical and potential dual imaging function for on-chip bioscientific applications. *Sensors and Actuators A: Physical*, 125(2), 273–280.

35 T. Tokuda, K. Tanaka, M. Matsuo, K. Kagawa, M. Nunoshita and J. Ohta, (2007) Optical and electrochemical dual-image CMOS sensor for on-chip biomolecular sensing applications. *Sensors and Actuators A: Physical*, 135(2), 315–322.

36 J. Matsuo, K. Sawada, H. Takao and M. Ishida (2008) Multimodal pH and light imaging devices for dynamic chemical reaction observation. In: Proceedings of the μTAS, pp. 326–328.

37 M.P. McRae, G. Simmons, J. Wong and J.T. McDevitt (2016) Programmable bio-nanochip platform: A point-of-care biosensor system with the capacity to learn. *Accounts of Chemical Research*, 49(7), 1359–1368.

38 Y. Jiang, X. Liu, T.C. Dang, M. Yan, H. Yu, *et al.* (2016) A 512 × 576 65-nm CMOS ISFET sensor for food safety screening with 123.8 mV/pH sensitivity and 0.01 pH resolution. pp. 1–2.

39 Y. Jiang, X. Liu, X. Huang, Y. Shang, M. Yan and H. Yu (2016) Lab-on-CMOS: A multi-modal CMOS sensor platform towards personalized DNA sequencing. In: IEEE International Symposium on Circuits and Systems (ISCAS), pp. 2266–2269.

40 X. Huang, Y. Jiang, Y. Shang, H. Yu and L. Sun (2015) A CMOS THz-sensing system towards label-free DNA sequencing. In: IEEE 11th International Conference on ASIC (ASICON), I pp. 1–4.

41 Y. Jiang, X. Liu, X. Huang, J. Guo, M. Yan, *et al.* (2015) A 201 mV/pH, 375 fps and 512 × 576 CMOS ISFET sensor in 65 nm CMOS technology. In: IEEE Conference on Custom Integrated Circuits (CICC), pp. 1–4.

42 D. Jeon, Q. Dong, Y. Kim, X. Wang, S. Chen, *et al.* (2015) A 23 mW face recognition accelerator in 40 nm CMOS with mostly-read 5 T memory. In: VLSI Symposium on VLSI Circuits (VLSI Circuits), pp. C48–C49.

43 X. Liu, L. Yao, P. Li, M. Yan, S.-C. Yen, *et al.* (2015) A 16-channel 24-V 1.8-mA power efficiency enhanced neural/muscular stimulator with exponentially decaying stimulation current. In: IEEE International Symposium on Circuits and Systems (ISCAS), pp. 2992–2995.

44 Y. Shang, H. Yu, C. Yang, Y. Liang and W.M. Lim (2014) 239–281 GHz sub-THz imager with 100 MHz resolution by CMOS direct-conversion receiver with on-chip circular-polarized SIW antenna. In: IEEE Proceedings of the Custom Integrated Circuits Conference (CICC), pp. 1–4.

45 Y. Shang, H. Yu, C. Yang, S. Hu and M. Je (2014) A high-sensitivity 135 GHz millimeter-wave imager by differential transmission-line loaded split-ring resonator in 65 nm CMOS. In: 44th European Conferences on Solid State Device Research (ESSDERC), pp. 166–169.

46 S. Chua, A. Razzaq, K. Wee, K. Li, H. Yu and C. Tan (2014) 3D CMOS-MEMS stacking with TSV-less and face-to-face direct metal bonding. In: Symposium on VLSI Technology (VLSI-Technology): Digest of Technical Papers, pp. 1–2.

47 X. Huang, F. Wang, J. Guo, M. Yan, Y. Hao and K.S. Yeo (2014) A 64 × 64 1200 fps CMOS ion-image sensor with suppressed fixed-pattern noise for accurate high-throughput DNA sequencing. In: Symposium on VLSI Circuits Digest of Technical Papers, pp. 1–2.

48 S. Chua, A. Razzaq, K. Wee, K. Li, H. Yu and C.S. Tan (2014) TSV-less 3-D stacking of MEMS and CMOS via low temperature Al–Au direct bonding with simultaneous formation of hermetic seal. In: IEEE 64th Conference on Electronic Components and Technology Conference (ECTC), pp. 324–331.

49 R. Nadipalli, J. Fan, K. Li, K. Wee, H. Yu and C. Tan (2011) 3D integration of MEMS and CMOS via Cu–Cu bonding with simultaneous formation of electrical, mechanical and hermetic bonds. In: 2011 IEEE International Conference on 3D Systems Integration Conference (3DIC), pp. 1–5.

50 M. Yan, X. Huang, Q. Jia, R. Nadipalli, Y. Shang, *et al.* (2012) High-speed CMOS image sensor for high-throughput lensless microfluidic imaging system with point-of-care application. In; SPIE 8298, Sensors, Cameras, and Systems for Industrial and Scientific Applications XIII, 829804.

51 N. Li, H. Yu, C. Yang, Y. Shang, X. Li and X. Liu (2015) A high-sensitivity 135 GHz millimeter-wave imager by compact split-ring resonator in 65-nm CMOS. *Solid-State Electronics*, 113, 54–60.

52 X. Huang, H. Yu, X. Liu, Y. Jiang and M. Yan (2015) A single-frame superresolution algorithm for lab-on-a-chip lensless microfluidic imaging. *IEEE Design & Test*, 32(6), 32–40.

53 X. Huang, H. Yu, X. Liu, Y. Jiang, M. Yan and D. Wu (2015) A dual-mode large-arrayed CMOS ISFET sensor for accurate and high-throughput pH sensing in biomedical diagnosis. *IEEE Transactions on Biomedical Engineering*, 62(9), 2224–2233.

54 I. Cevik, X. Huang, H. Yu, M. Yan and S.U. Ay (2015) An ultra-low power CMOS image sensor with on-chip energy harvesting and power management capability. *Sensors*, 15(3), 5531–5554.

55 J. Guo, X. Huang, D. Shi, H. Yu, Y. Ai, *et al.* (2014) Portable resistive pulse-activated lens-free cell imaging system. *RSC Advances*, 4(99), 56342–56345.

56 Y. Shang, H. Yu, S. Hu, Y. Liang, X. Bi and M.A. Arasu (2014) High-sensitivity CMOS Super-regenerative receiver with quench-controlled high-Q metamaterial resonator for Millimeter-Wave Imaging at 96 and 135 GHz. *IEEE Transactions on Microwave Theory and Techniques*, 62(12), 3095–3106.

57 Y. Shang, H. Yu, H. Fu and W.M. Lim (2014) A 239–281 GHz CMOS receiver with on-chip circular-polarized substrate integrated waveguide antenna for sub-terahertz imaging. *IEEE Transactions on Terahertz Science and Technology*, 4(6), 686–695.

58 X. Huang, X. Wang, M. Yan and H. Yu (2015) A robust recognition error recovery for micro-flow cytometer by machine-learning enhanced single-frame super-resolution processing. *Integration, the VLSI Journal*, 51, 208–218.

59 X. Huang, J. Guo, X. Wang, M. Yan, Y. Kang and H. Yu (2014) A contact-imaging based microfluidic cytometer with machine-learning for single-frame super-resolution processing. *PloS one*, 9(8), e104539.

60 T.S. Pui, Y. Chen, C.C. Wong, R. Nadipalli, R. Weerasekera, *et al.* (2013) High density CMOS electrode array for high-throughput and automated cell counting. *Sensors and Actuators B: Chemical*, 181, 842–849.

61 Y. Chen, C.C. Wong, T.S. Pui, R. Nadipalli, R. Weerasekera, *et al.* (2012) CMOS high density electrical impedance biosensor array for tumor cell detection. *Sensors and Actuators B: Chemical*, 173, 903–907.

2

CMOS Sensor Design

2.1 Top Architecture

Before using a CMOS sensor in the personalized diagnosis field, the first step is to understand its components and working principles. Figure 2.1 gives an overview of CMOS sensor architecture, involving a large pixel array, column readout blocks, and row/column timing control blocks. Other blocks are also needed, such as current digital-to-analog converter (IDAC) for system bias, status register (SREG) for working mode setting, and input/output (I/O) and PADs as a communication interface with FPGA. This chapter focuses on the main readout path from pixel to system output.

The pixel array part is composed of 2-D sensing nodes. Each sensing node includes a biochemical-to-electrical conversion device and a pixel-level readout circuit. Each column of sensing nodes shares the same column-level readout path. Unlike the pixel-level readout, where transistor amount should be minimized to realize a large array, the column-shared readout can realize more complex functions. Basic column circuit blocks, such as the column amplifier and single-slope analog-to-digital converter (ADC), are introduced. In addition, readout strategies, correlated double sampling, and correlated multiple sampling, are introduced for high-performance sensing. Also, row or column timing control blocks are introduced that determine operations and readout of the pixel array, such as row decoder, row driver, and column decoder. The widely used low-power and high-speed interface, low-voltage differential signaling (LVDS), is also introduced that meets the requirements of modern high-throughput applications.

2.2 Noise Overview

Noise determines the performance and detection limit of a sensor. It is essential to have a basic knowledge of noise sources and analysis before designing a sensor. This section briefly illustrates the definition and origin of thermal noise, flicker noise, and shot noise in circuit design. In addition, the MOSFET noise model in the saturation region and sub-threshold region are introduced.

CMOS Integrated Lab-on-a-Chip System for Personalized Biomedical Diagnosis,
First Edition. Hao Yu, Mei Yan, and Xiwei Huang.
© 2018 John Wiley & Sons Singapore Pte. Ltd. Published 2018 by John Wiley & Sons Singapore Pte. Ltd.

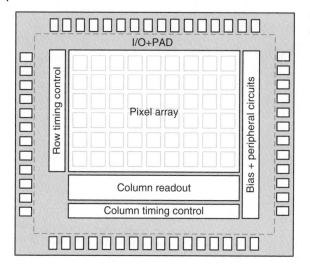

Figure 2.1 A typical CMOS sensor architecture.

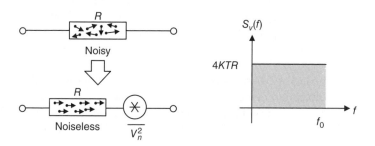

Figure 2.2 Resistor thermal noise model.

2.2.1 Thermal Noise

Thermal noise is also known as white noise, and is caused by the thermal agitation of charge carriers in a conductor. The noise spectral density is constant over a given frequency and proportional to absolute temperature.

Thermal noise is the major noise source in a resistor. As shown in Figure 2.2, a noisy resistor can be modeled as a series of noiseless resistor R and a noise voltage $\overline{V_n^2}$. The spectral density $S_V(f)$ is described as:

$$S_V(f) = \overline{V_n^2} = 4KTR, \quad f \geq 0 \tag{2.1}$$

where K is the Boltzmann constant, and T is the absolute temperature. The unit of $S_V(f)$ is V^2/Hz. The root-mean-square (RMS) value $V_{n(rms)}$ over the frequency range $0 \sim f_0$ is given by:

$$V_{n(rms)} = \sqrt{\int_0^{f_0} \overline{V_n^2}\, df} = \sqrt{4KTRf_0} \tag{2.2}$$

Figure 2.3 MOSFET thermal noise model in strong inversion region.

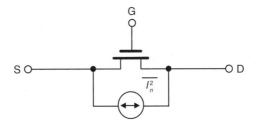

A noise current in parallel with the noiseless resistor can also be employed, and the spectral density is given by:

$$\overline{I_n^2} = \overline{V_n^2}/R^2 = 4KT/R \tag{2.3}$$

For a MOSFET, a conductive channel is formed in the strong inversion region, where the gate-source voltage V_{GS} is larger than the threshold voltage V_{th}. As already described, the channel is the main thermal noise source. It can be modeled as a noise current $\overline{I_n^2}$ between the device source and drain, as shown in Figure 2.3. Figure 2.4(a) shows that when MOSFET works in the triode region, the conductive channel is homogeneous and can be regarded as a resistor r_{ds}. The thermal noise can be simplified as $\overline{I_n^2} = 4KT/r_{ds}$. However, when a MOSFET works in the saturation region, the conductive channel is not homogeneous, as shown in Figure 2.4(b). The spectral density $S_I(f)$ is given by:

$$S_I(f) = \overline{I_n^2} = 4KT\gamma g_m, \quad f \geq 0 \tag{2.4}$$

where g_m is the transconductance of MOSFET. The thermal noise coefficient is $\gamma = 2/3$ for the long-channel transistor and $\gamma \approx 1$ for the short-channel transistor. From Equation 2.4, a long channel length and a minimum g_m is preferred to decrease the thermal noise.

2.2.2 Flicker Noise

Flicker noise is also known as the $1/f$ noise. As the name indicates, this noise is inversely proportional to frequency. The spectral density of noise voltage can be given by:

$$\overline{V_n^2} = K_V^2/f, \quad f \geq 0 \tag{2.5}$$

where K_V is the flicker noise coefficient and of a constant value.

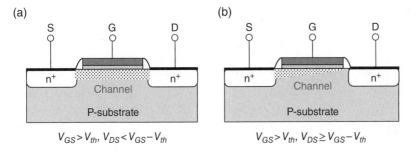

(a) $V_{GS} > V_{th}, V_{DS} < V_{GS} - V_{th}$

(b) $V_{GS} > V_{th}, V_{DS} \geq V_{GS} - V_{th}$

Figure 2.4 MOSFET conductive channel cross-section view in (a) triode and (b) saturation region.

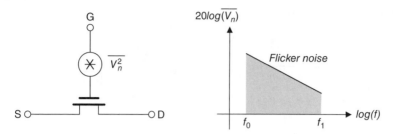

Figure 2.5 MOSFET flicker noise model.

For a MOSFET structure, the gate-oxide and silicon substrate interface has many "dangling" bonds. They will randomly trap and release charge carriers, which introduce flicker noise to the drain current. As shown in Figure 2.5, it can be modeled as a noise voltage connected to the MOSFET gate. The noise voltage is given by:

$$\overline{V_n^2} = K / (C_{OX} WLf), \quad f \geq 0 \tag{2.6}$$

where K is a process-dependent factor and varies between transistors in the same process. C_{OX} is the gate-oxide capacitance per unit area, and W and L are the transistor width and length respectively. The RMS value $V_{n(rms)}$ over the frequency range $f_0 \sim f_1$ is given by:

$$V_{n(rms)} = \sqrt{\int_{f_0}^{f_1} \overline{V_n^2} \, df} = \sqrt{\left[\frac{K}{C_{OX} WL} \right] (lnf_1 - lnf_0)} \tag{2.7}$$

Since flicker noise is inversely proportional to W*L, a larger transistor area can decrease the flicker noise level with an increase of chip cost. Therefore, a tradeoff between noise and cost should be considered during sensor design.

2.2.3 Shot Noise

Shot noise is caused by the non-continuous DC current flow. Due to a lack of energy, charge carriers randomly cross a potential barrier, such as a reversely biased p-n junction. As shown in Figure 2.6, it can be modeled by a noise current in parallel with a noiseless small-signal diode resistance r_d, where $r_d = KT/qI_D$. The spectral density of noise current can be given by:

$$\overline{I_n^2} = 2qI_D, \quad f \geq 0 \tag{2.8}$$

where q is one electron charge and I_D is the diode current. The RMS value $I_{n(rms)}$ over the frequency range $0 \sim f_0$ is given by:

$$I_{n(rms)} = \sqrt{\int_0^{f_0} \overline{I_n^2} \, df} = \sqrt{2qI_D f_0} \tag{2.9}$$

It can be observed that a larger current has a larger noise.

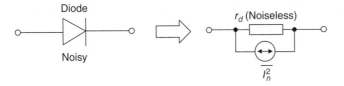

Figure 2.6 Diode shot noise model.

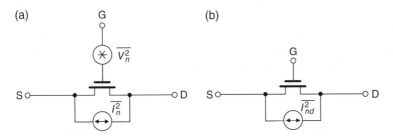

Figure 2.7 MOSFET noise model with: (a) separate; and (b) equivalent noise.

For MOSFET in the sub-threshold region, the conductive channel is weakly inversed. Unlike strong-inversion region with large drift current, it is the diffusion current that is dominant in sub-threshold MOSFET. It exhibits shot noise instead of thermal noise.

2.2.4 MOSFET Noise Model

According to the previous discussion, thermal noise and flicker noise are the main noise sources of MOSFET. The noise model with thermal noise current and flicker noise voltage is shown in Figure 2.7(a). To simplify the analysis in low and moderate frequencies, an equivalent output noise current model is shown in Figure 2.7(b).

For linear and saturation region MOSFET, the drain noise current is given by:

$$\overline{I_{nd}^2} = \overline{I_n^2} + g_m^2 \overline{V_n^2} = 4KT\gamma g_m + g_m^2 K / (C_{OX} WLf), \quad f \geq 0 \tag{2.10}$$

For sub-threshold region MOSFET, the drain noise current is given by:

$$\overline{I_n^2} = \overline{I_n^2} + g_m^2 \overline{V_n^2} = 2qI_D + g_m^2 K / (C_{OX} WLf), \quad f \geq 0 \tag{2.11}$$

2.3 Pixel Readout Circuit

For a cost-efficient CMOS sensor, a large multi-row and multi-column pixel array is preferred. It means that multiple pixels will share the same column readout path. In order to simultaneously read converted biochemical signals, in-pixel transfer circuit is needed. It is typically composed of several transistors that transfer or amplify the sensed biochemical signals, so as to drive the heavily loaded column bus. Several readout structures are described here, such as source follower (SF), sub-threshold G_m integrator, and capacitive transimpedance amplifier.

2.3.1 Source Follower

MOSFET can work in cut-off, sub-threshold, linear, and saturation regions. Most of the pixel readout circuits employ a saturation-region transistor due to its high gain factor and excellent driving capability. There are three types of configurations for a saturated MOSFET: source follower, common source amplifier, and common gate amplifier.

For a saturated MOSFET, the gate-source voltage bias V_{GS} is larger than the transistor threshold voltage V_{th}, and the drain-source voltage V_{DS} is larger than the "overdrive voltage" $V_{sat} = V_{GS} - V_{th}$. The drain current I_D is described as:

$$I_D = \frac{1}{2}\mu C_{ox}\frac{W}{L}\left(V_{GS} - V_{th}\right)^2 \tag{2.12}$$

where μ is the electron (for n-type metal oxide semiconductor, NMOS) or hole (for p-type metal oxide semiconductor, PMOS) mobility, C_{ox} is the gate oxide capacitance per unit area, W is the gate width, and L is the gate length. The current-to-voltage transconductance g_m is calculated as:

$$g_m = \frac{\Delta I_D}{\Delta V_{GS}} = \mu C_{ox}\frac{W}{L}\left(V_{GS} - V_{th}\right) = 2I_D/\left(V_{GS} - V_{th}\right) \tag{2.13}$$

A larger transconductance g_m always results in a high performance amplifier. There are several ways to increase g_m. First, electron mobility is almost twice that of the hole, so that NMOS is easier to realize a higher sensitivity than PMOS. Second, a more commonly used method is to enlarge the W/L value. This is the reason why most of the analog circuits use a large transistor size.

The SF is widely used in pixel design as a voltage buffer. A typical NMOS type structure is shown in Figure 2.8(a). MN_0 is the SF that converts the gate voltage variation to drain current. MN_B also works in the saturation region as a current source and active load. The sensed drain current pass through the overall output resistance and cause an output voltage variation ΔV_{col}.

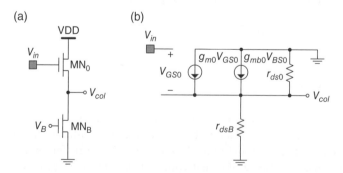

Figure 2.8 (a) Source follower with active load; and (b) The corresponding small signal circuit.

To better understand the working principles of the SF, a small signal circuit is shown in Figure 2.8(b). Apart from the drain current represented by $g_m V_{GS}$ in Equations (2.12) and (2.13), second-order effects, such as body effect and channel length modulation, also play important roles in the small signal model.

NMOS transistors are fabricated on the grounded P-type substrate. When there is a potential difference between source and body, the transistor threshold voltage V_{th} is affected, which is described as:

$$V_{th} = V_{th0} + \gamma \left(\sqrt{|2\phi_F + V_{SB}|} - \sqrt{|2\phi_F|} \right) \qquad (2.14)$$

where V_{th0} is the transistor threshold voltage when the body-source bias is zero, γ is the body effect coefficient, $2\phi_F$ is the silicon surface potential in strong inversion, and V_{BS} is the body-source bias. An additional current source is used to describe this effect, which is represented by $g_{mb} V_{SB}$. The body transconductance g_{mb} is given by:

$$g_{mb} = \partial I_D / \partial V_{BS} = g_m \gamma / \left(2\sqrt{2\phi_F + V_{SB}} \right) \qquad (2.15)$$

Considering channel length modulation, the saturation drain current can be rewritten as:

$$I_D = \frac{1}{2} \mu C_{ox} \frac{W}{L} \left(V_{GS} - V_{th} \right)^2 \left(1 + \lambda V_{DS} \right) \qquad (2.16)$$

where $\lambda V_{DS} = \Delta L / L$, L is the channel length and ΔL is the channel variation due to the pinch-off in the high drain-source electrical field. This effect is represented by the output resistance r_{ds}, which is calculated as:

$$r_{ds} = \partial V_{DS} / \partial I_D = 1 / \lambda I_D \qquad (2.17)$$

In Figure 2.8(b), MN_0 and MN_B are modeled with a small signal circuit, in which g_{m0} and g_{mb0} are the drain and body transconductance, V_{GS0} and V_{BS0} are the gate-source and body-source bias, and r_{ds0} and r_{dsB} are the output resistance of MN_0 and MN_B, respectively. We can obtain the gain A_v from Equations 2.18 and 2.19:

$$V_{col} / r_{dsB} = g_{m0} \left(V_{in} - V_{col} \right) - g_{mb0} V_{col} - V_{col} / r_{ds0} \qquad (2.18)$$

$$A_v = V_{col} / V_{in} = g_{m0} / \left(g_{m0} + g_{mb0} + 1 / r_{ds0} + 1 / r_{dsB} \right) \qquad (2.19)$$

In sensor design, the pixel-level SF readout structure is shown in Figure 2.9(a). To realize a large pixel array, each pixel contains only two transistors (2 T). MN_0 works in the saturation region as a SF. The sensed biochemical signal is connected to the gate of MN_0. MN_1 is a row-select transistor that can be regarded as a switch with linear resistance. Each SF MN_0 can be separately connected to the column bus by turning on the transistor MN_1 and disconnected by turning off MN_1. The current source I_0 in the figure works as a bias block that modifies the drain current of MN_0. The voltage transfer curve is shown in Figure 2.9(b). To make sure that both MN_0 and current source I_0 (normally a biased NMOS transistor) work in the saturation region, the minimal input voltage V_{in} is near to $V_{th} + V_{sat}$. In biomedical applications, the weak input voltage change ΔV_{in} is linearly transferred to the output ΔV_{col}, which is given by:

$$\Delta V_{col} = A_{SF} \cdot \Delta V_{in} \qquad (2.20)$$

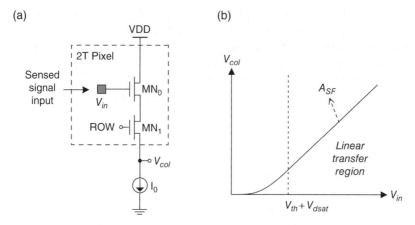

Figure 2.9 (a) Pixel readout structure of a 2T source-follower pixel; and (b) The corresponding transfer curve.

where A_{SF} is the NMOS SF gain that is typically $0.7 \sim 0.8$. According to Equation 2.20, there is no amplification effect presented. The main function of this pixel structure is to linearly transfer input voltage while providing enough driving ability.

In some applications, additional in-pixel transistors may be needed for signal conversion purposes. Take optical sensing as an example, where the photodiode is employed to absorb light and produce photocurrent, where photons are converted to electrons in a reversely biased p-n junction. A typical photocurrent value is at the fA $\sim$ nA level. This current value is too small to be sensed. A common solution is to integrate this small current into a detectable voltage. To operate the photodiode and transfer the collected electron charges, apart from the SF and row-select transistors, additional reset and transfer transistors are also required, as in the 4 T pixel structure shown in Figure 2.10(a). However, more transistors mean a larger pixel area. When forming a pixel array, a little pixel area increment will lead to a considerable increase in the array area.

An effective method to reduce the pixel transistor number is to share part of readout transistors, such as the 4-shared pixel shown in Figure 2.10(b). A total of four sensing nodes are implemented in one pixel. Each sensing node can be separately operated through their dedicated transfer transistors ($TX_0 \sim TX_3$). After biochemical-to-electrical conversion, the sensed signals ($V_{in0} \sim V_{in3}$) are connected to the drain of transfer transistors. They share the same SF MN_0, row-select transistor MN_1, and reset transistor controlled by RSTG. In this way, each pixel is composed of seven transistors with four sensing nodes. It can be regarded that each sensing node occupies only 1.75 transistors (1.75 T). Therefore, a compact and large pixel array can be realized. This methodology can also be utilized in other sensing applications, where more transistors may be involved.

Each sensing node of the 4-shared pixel structure is connected to the gate of SF sequentially, and the sensed voltage is transferred to the column bus respectively. The timing diagram of a sensing node is shown in Figure 2.10(c). A reset phase is first conducted by enabling signals RSTG and ROW, and the reset voltage RSTV is measured as V_{col_r} at the column bus. Then the sensed input signal V_{in0} is transferred to the SF gate by enabling signal TX_0, which is measured as V_{col_s0}. The corresponding transfer curve

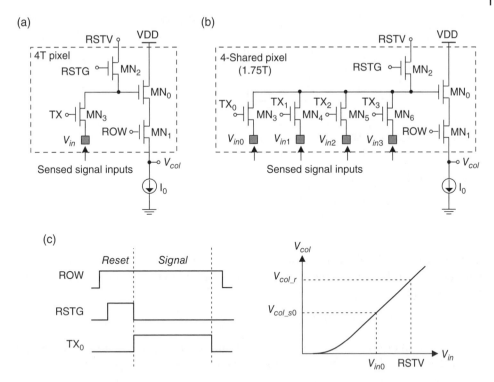

Figure 2.10 Pixel readout structures of (a) a 4T SF pixel; and (b) a 1.75T 4-shared source-follower pixel. (c) Timing diagram and transfer curve of (b).

is also shown in Figure 2.10(c). Normally, both the output reset level V_{col_r} and signal level V_{col_s0} are useful information for high-performance correlated sampling, which will be introduced in the following correlated sampling section.

2.3.2 Sub-threshold Gm Integrator

Apart from the saturation region, MOSFET can also operate in the sub-threshold region. From the previous discussion, the SF cannot provide signal amplification. It is not suitable for applications where the optical or biochemical signal is very weak and the sensed voltage is small (e.g. <1 mV), unless an additional amplifier is employed.

A simplified sub-threshold in-pixel readout scheme can be used to amplify the sensed voltage in the earliest sensing stage; the schematic is shown in Figure 2.11. Similar to the SF structure, each pixel contains only two transistors: MN_0 is the sub-threshold transistor, and MN_1 is the row-selected transistor. The remaining transistors can be implemented at either the pixel level or at the column level, including a reset transistor MP_0, a transfer switch S_0 composed of a complementary NMOS and PMOS transistor pair, an integration capacitor C_0, a SF MN_2 for driving and isolation purposes, and a current source bias I_0.

Sub-threshold region is a transition stage between the cutoff and linear region, where the conductive channel is not completely formed. MOSFET in sub-threshold region can

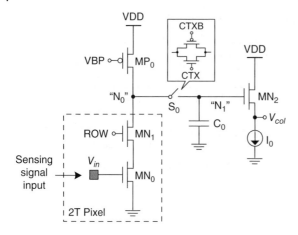

Figure 2.11 Schematic of a sub-threshold Gm integrator pixel readout structure.

be regarded as a simple transconductor. The drain current I_D is exponential to gate voltage V_{in}. A little gate voltage shift can induce an exponential drain current change, which is given by:

$$I_D = I_{D0} \cdot \exp\left[V_{in}/(n \cdot U_r)\right] \tag{2.21}$$

where I_{D0} is a constant characteristic current, and $n = 1 + C_d/C_{ox}$ is a non-ideal slope factor. Therefore, the current-to-voltage transconductance G_m is calculated as:

$$G_m = \Delta I_D/\Delta V_{in} = I_D/(n \cdot U_r) \tag{2.22}$$

For the condition where V_{in} changes within a relatively small range, G_m can be approximately considered as a constant.

Here we briefly explained the operation timing, as shown in Figure 2.12. Before each readout phase, capacitor C_0 is pre-charged to the power supply when turning on the device MP_0 and the transfer switch S_0, which are controlled by the signal VBP and CTX respectively. At the second stage, C_0 is discharged through MN_0 to ground by turning on the row-select device MN_1 while turning off MP_0. The drain current of the weak-inversion MN_0 is integrated on the capacitor C_0, whose value is a function of the gate voltage V_{in}. At the third stage, by turning off S_0, the voltage of node "N_1" can be read out, which is determined by the remaining charge on the capacitor C_0.

A shift in optical- or biochemical-dependent voltage ΔV_{in} will lead to the output voltage ΔV_{col} change, which is given by:

$$\Delta V_{col} = \left(\Delta t/C_0\right) \cdot G_m \cdot \Delta V_{in} \tag{2.23}$$

From the equations above, we can see that a programmable amplification factor $(\Delta t / C_0) \cdot G_m$ is introduced. The factor can be improved by employing a larger transconductance G_m, prolonging the discharging time Δt, or decreasing the capacitance C_0.

The corresponding transfer curve is shown in Figure 2.12. For a sub-threshold transistor, the working region is small and the voltage range is typically $0.1 \sim 0.3$ V. When the input gate voltage V_{in} is small, the conductive channel is not formed. Since there is no discharging path, the output voltage V_{col} retains its pre-charge level, whereas when V_{in} traverses threshold voltage V_{th}, the conductive channel is completely formed.

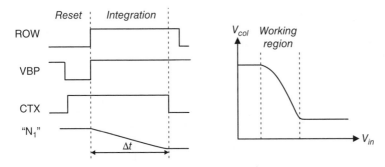

Figure 2.12 The corresponding timing diagram and transfer curve.

The output voltage V_{col} will quickly reach its low level due to the large discharging current. Therefore, this sub-threshold amplification method is suitable for weak signal detection without large dynamic voltage change.

In the previous structure, the current integration takes place at the column level, which means that pixels in the same column should perform this integration one by one. It may slow down the array sampling rate when pixel queuing for the usage of column bus. A solution is to implement the sub-threshold amplification at pixel level, as shown in Figure 2.13(a). In this way, each pixel can perform the integration without occupying the column bus. To make a compact pixel size, an NMOS transfer switch MN_3 is employed instead of the complementary switch S_0. In addition, an NMOS reset transistor is used MN_2.

Consequently, the pixel is composed of pure five NMOS transistors that can save a lot of pixel area compared to the one with both NMOS and PMOS. Another effective method is to adopt the sharing methodology. Similar to SF, a 4-shared pixel readout structure is employed to fully use the pixel area, as shown in Figure 2.13(b). There are a total of 11 transistors with 4 sensing nodes (2.75 T). Each sensed signal within one pixel will be sequentially integrated on the capacitor C_0, while this integration between different pixels is in parallel. In this way, a high throughput sensing method can be realized.

2.3.3 CTIA

For some applications, the sensed signal is the current instead of voltage. For example, in optical sensing, photons are first converted to the photocurrent. It is then converted to voltage by the integration on intrinsic or external capacitor. However, there are situations where the intrinsic capacitance is very large (e.g. 1 pF ~ 100 pF), whereas the current signal is extremely small (e.g. 50 fA ~ 10 pA). Examples are fluorescence imaging [1,2] and nanopore sequencing [3–5]. Therefore, it is not applicable to integrate the current signal in the intrinsic capacitor. The only solution is to employ a small external capacitor and isolate the effects of intrinsic capacitor.

A possible solution is to use Capacitive Transimpedance Amplifier (CTIA), as shown in Figure 2.14(a). It is composed of an Operational Transconductance Amplifier (OTA), a small feedback capacitor C_{fb}, a reset switch controlled by the signal RST, and a row-select switch controlled by the signal ROW. The sensed current signal is connected to

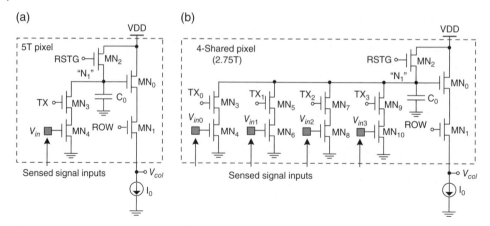

Figure 2.13 Schematic of a 4-shared sub-threshold Gm integrator pixel readout structure.

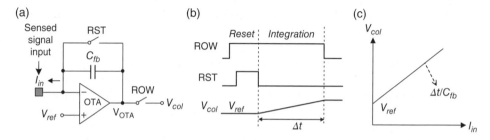

Figure 2.14 (a) Schematic of capacitive transimpedance amplifier (CTIA); The corresponding; (b) Timing diagram; and (c) Current-to-voltage transfer curve.

the negative terminal of OTA, whereas a bias voltage V_{ref} is connected to the positive terminal. The operation shown in Figure 2.14(b) is described as follows:

First, the reset phase is performed. The OTA negative terminal is connected to the output terminal, and both are equal to the positive terminal voltage V_{ref}. Second, the reset transistor is turned off, and the input sensed current I_{in} is input to CTIA. Since the OTA input draws no current, according to Kirchhoff Current Laws (KCL), an opposite current $-I_{in}$ will flow from the OTA output terminal to the negative terminal. In this way, the sensed current is integrated on the feedback capacitor regardless of possible large intrinsic optical- or biochemical-capacitance. The output voltage is given by:

$$\Delta V_{col} = \left(\Delta t / C_{fb} \right) \cdot \Delta I_{in} \tag{2.24}$$

The corresponding current-to-voltage transfer curve is also shown in Figure 2.14(c). A larger amplification can be realized when longer integration time Δt or smaller feedback capacitance C_{fb} is employed.

A typical OTA schematic is shown in Figure 2.15(a). It consists of five transistors, where MP_0 and MP_1 are the active loads that consist of a current mirror; MN_0 and MN_1 are the positive and negative input transistors; and MN_2 is a bias transistor that works as a current source for both MN_0-MP_0 and MN_1-MP_1 paths. This OTA structure is simple but does not give too much gain. There are several ways to increase the gain

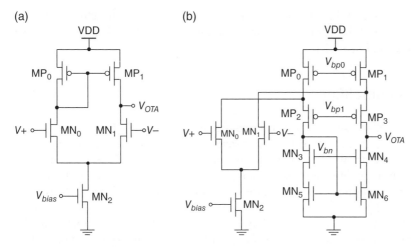

Figure 2.15 Schematic of: (a) A simple 5-T operational transconductance amplifier (OPA); and (b) Folded-cascode OTA.

factor, such as 2-stage OTA, telescopic OTA, folded-cascode OTA, etc. As an example, a folded cascode OTA structure is shown in Figure 2.15(b). At the output terminal, four stacked transistors (MP_1, MP_3, MN_4, and MN_5) are employed, which result in a high gain due to the increased output resistance. However, for the differential input pair MN_0 and MN_1, a large width/length ratio is preferred. Also, it is not cost-efficient to include this OTA structure at the pixel level, since it will occupy a large area.

A possible solution is to move some part of the CTIA to the column bus, as shown in Figure 2.16(a) [1]. Each pixel consists of five transistors that largely reduce the area. Combined with the loading part in the column bus, a single-end common-source cascode amplifier is achieved. In order to maintain a high open-loop gain, the input transistor that accepts the sensed signal works in the sub-threshold region, due to the high gain-to-current ratio in this region. Similar to the 4-shared SF pixel structure, a shared architecture can also be applied here to further reduce the pixel area.

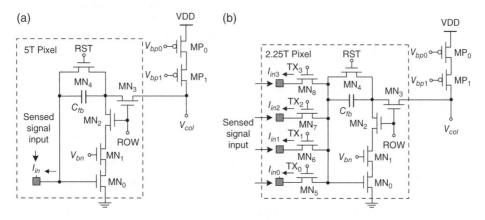

Figure 2.16 Schematic of an in-pixel CTIA readout structure.

As shown in Figure 2.16(b), each pixel contains a total of nine transistors with four sensing nodes (2.25 T). Each sensing node is accessed one by one via their respective transfer transistors ($TX_0 \sim TX_3$).

2.4 Column Amplifier

From the above discussions, the sensed biochemical signal is first converted or integrated to voltage by pixel-level readout circuits, and then transferred to the column bus for further operation. Most biomedical signals are very weak. Even though an early-stage in-pixel amplification may be adopted, the output voltage can still be very small. Therefore, a column-level amplifier is normally employed to improve the Signal-to-Noise Ratio (SNR).

Since the column amplifier can be shared by all rows of pixels connected to the column bus, there is no strict limitations on transistor amount and size. A high-performance amplifier can be used. A multi-gain switched capacitor amplifier is introduced, as shown in Figure 2.17(a). It can satisfy most applications where multiple gains are preferred.

The amplifier is composed of an OTA, an input capacitor (C_{in}), two feedback capacitors (C_{fL} and C_{fH}) that are selected by switches S_L and S_H respectively, an auto-zero (AZ_{amp}) switch, and a sampling switch (S_{sample}). C_L is the parasitic capacitance. The timing diagram is shown in Figure 2.17(b). Before each testing, the amplifier is reset by the AZ_{amp} switch. This operation clears the charges on feedback capacitors. Besides, the offset between two OTA input terminals is canceled out, since the offset voltage is stored in the input capacitor C_{in} before sampling. After selecting the total feedback capacitance, the sampling switch is turned on. Then the column bus voltage change ΔV_{col} is amplified to output voltage ΔV_{amp}. The amplification is determined by the input and feedback capacitance ratio, which is given by:

$$\Delta V_{amp} = -\left(C_{in}/C_f\right) \cdot \Delta V_{col} \tag{2.25}$$

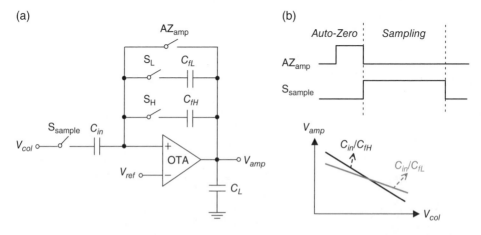

Figure 2.17 (a) Schematic of a multi-gain switched capacitor amplifier. (b) The corresponding timing diagram and voltage transfer curve.

where C_f is selected from one of $\{C_{fL}, C_{fH}, C_{fL} + C_{fH}\}$ $(C_{fL} > C_{fH})$. The voltage transfer curves of high-gain (C_{fH} is selected) and low-gain (C_{fL} is selected) modes are shown in Figure 2.17(b). Normally, the amplified output voltage is large enough to be detected by the following circuit blocks. The sign "−" represents that the direction of voltage change ΔV_{amp} is opposite to ΔV_{col}. More feedback capacitance combinations can be realized by introducing more capacitor-switch groups to the feedback chain, thus able to meet various requirements.

2.5   Column ADC

To facilitate data storage, transfer and analysis, on-chip ADC is required. The function of an ADC is to first sample the continuous-time analog signal to discrete-time voltage points at a certain sampling rate, and then match the voltage points to quantized discrete voltage levels. Many column-parallel ADC structures have been implemented, which can be categorized as Nyquist-rate ADC and oversampling ADC based on the sampling rate. For a signal with a bandwidth of f_B, the sampling rate f_S should be at least twice that of f_B, denoted as $f_S \geq 2f_B$. When f_S is equal or slightly higher than $2f_B$, the converter is called Nyquist-rate ADC, like integrating converters, successive approximation (SAR) converter, cyclic converter, pipelined converter, etc. When f_S is much higher than $2f_B$, the converter is called oversampling ADC, such as a sigma-delta ($\Sigma\Delta$) converter. In this section, two types of the most popular structures are introduced, including the Nyquist-rate single-slope ADC for area-efficient sensing and oversampling sigma-delta ADC for low-noise and high-resolution detection.

2.5.1   Single-Slope ADC

For a large pixel array, column readout paths are independent of each other and each one has its own ADC block. It means that complex ADC structures cannot be used due to the column pitch and chip area limitation. Single-slope ADC meets the requirements that can be implemented in a long and narrow shape.

A basic single-slope ADC schematic is shown in Figure 2.18(a). It is basically composed of a comparator and a 10-bit counter. The input voltage V_{amp} is connected to the comparator's negative terminal. Meanwhile, the RAMP signal is connected to the positive terminal. Normally, the ADC can detect an input voltage between 1 V and 2 V. An on-chip ramp generator is employed to provide the reference ramp signal. The main timing diagram is shown in Figure 2.18(b). Before sampling, auto-zero is performed by turning on AZ_{comp}, thus cancelling out the offset between the comparator negative and positive terminals. After sampling, switches (P_{comp}) are turned on and the ramp generator starts to work. The amplifier output voltage V_{amp} is compared with the ramp signal. The comparison result is output to the 10-bit counter, whose value can be initiated to "0" when reset signal C_RST is high. It works as an enable signal of the counter. The count direction is controlled by the up/down (U/D) signal. In this way, V_{amp} is converted to 10-bit digital data D_{ADC}.

As shown in Figure 2.19(a), the comparator is implemented in a 3-stage structure. Considering that undesired noise may appear in the input signals, with induced error altering the comparison result, two differential pre-amplifier and one Schmitt Trigger

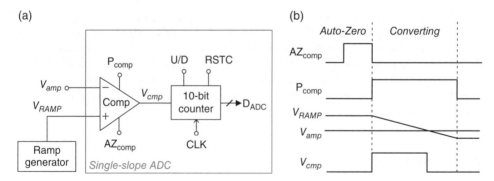

Figure 2.18 (a) Schematic of a single-slope ADC; and (b) The corresponding timing diagram.

circuit are applied. The pre-amplifier in Figure 2.19(b) is composed of differential input pair MN_0 and MN_1, current bias MN_2, active loads $MP_0 \sim MP_3$, and internal positive feedback loops are realized through the drain-gate connections of MP_1 and MP_2. The Schmitt Trigger comparator is shown in Figure 2.19(c). It includes a 5-T pre-amplifier to form a differential input and single-end output structure, where MN_3 and MN_4 are the differential input transistors, MN_5 is a bias transistor, and MP_4 and MP_5 are the active loads. The single-end output is connected to a Schmitt Trigger circuit for better defined switching points. MP_6 and $MN_6 \sim MN_8$ act like an inverter, and a positive feedback is introduced by MN_9. The Auto-zero (AZ) switch and C_{AZ} capacitor pairs are

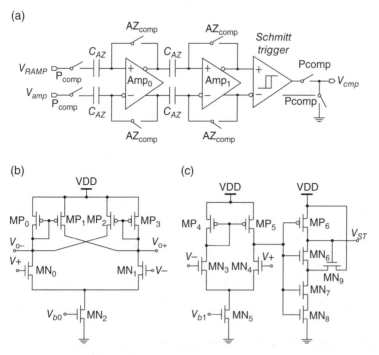

Figure 2.19 (a) Diagram of the 3-stage comparator, including two (b) differential pre-amplifiers; and one (c) Schmitt Trigger comparator.

applied to eliminate comparator offsets between input terminals. The P_{COMP} signal is used to activate the comparator.

A typical ramp generator makes use of current integration on a capacitor, whose slope is determined by the correlated current and capacitor value. As shown in Figure 2.20, a bias voltage V_{adj} is added to the resistor R_0 through OPA_0 and MN_0. Then a current value $I_0 = V_{adj}/R_0$ is generated that is mirrored to the negative terminal of OPA_1 through MP_0 and MP_1. During the auto-zero period, the P_{comp} signal is low, and ramp output and node N_2 is reset to V_{start} through OPA_1. The current I_0 is disconnected from OPA_1 and node N_1 is connected to V_{start}. Ramp generator is disabled. When P_{comp} is high during the conversion period, the current I_0 is connected to node N_2 and integrated on the feedback capacitor of OPA_1. Since nodes N_1 and N_2 are initialized to the same voltage level as before, there is no sudden voltage drop at node N_2. The output voltage V_{RAMP} keeps decreasing from the initial voltage V_{start}, which results in a ramp-down curve. The time-to-voltage slope K_{RAMP} is given by:

$$K_{RAMP} = \Delta V_{RAMP}/\Delta t = -V_{adj}/(R_0 \cdot C_r) \qquad (2.26)$$

where the feedback capacitance C_r is selected from one of $\{C_{rL}, C_{rH}, C_{rL} + C_{rH}\}$ $(C_{rL} > C_{rH})$, controlled by switches S_{rL} and S_{rH}. Therefore, the ramp slope can be adjusted by the bias voltage V_{adj} and integration capacitance C_r.

A general OTA can be employed as a comparator due to its high open loop gain. When there is a slight difference between the two OTA input terminals, it will be greatly amplified at the output terminal until reaching its upper (VDD, V_{OH}) or lower (GND, V_{OL}) voltage level. Considering that undesired noise may appear in the input signals and incorrectly alter the comparison result, a hysteresis comparator is widely used; an example is shown in Figure 2.21(a). It is composed of MN_0 and MN_1 as input transistor pair of V_+ and V_-, MN_2 to provide current bias, and $MP_0 \sim MP_3$ as active loads. Hysteresis is realized by introducing internal positive feedback loops through drain-gate connections of MP_1 and MP_2. As shown in the voltage transfer curves in Figure 2.21(b), there are two separate transition points. When V_+ continues to increase and becomes larger than V_-, $V_+ - V_- > 0$. The MN_0 drain current is larger than MN_1 and V_{o1} is smaller than V_{o2}. MP_0 and MP_1 drain current values are larger than MP_2 and MP_3. But the output voltage V_{o2}

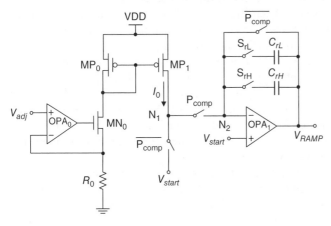

Figure 2.20 Schematic of a ramp generator.

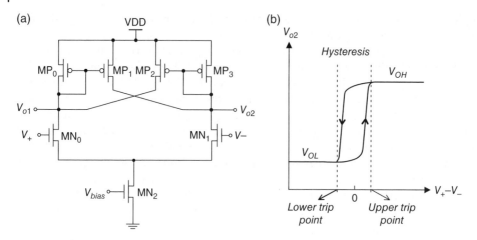

Figure 2.21 (a) Schematic of a simple hysteresis comparator; and (b) The corresponding hysteresis voltage transfer curves.

does not go from low to high immediately. It only transits when the difference between V_+ and V_- exceeds the upper trip point.

On the other hand, when V_+ continues to decrease and becomes smaller than V_-, $V_+ - V_- < 0$. Similarly, V_{o2} only goes from high to low when $V_+ - V_-$ is smaller than the lower trip point. As a result, when $V_+ - V_-$ is within the transition points, V_{o2} tends to retain its value. This bistable characteristic makes the hysteresis comparator noise-tolerant. To obtain better defined transition points, V_{o1} and V_{o2} can also be further modified by circuits like the Schmitt Trigger, inverter, etc.

The comparison result V_{cmp} is converted to digital data through a counter. As an example, a 3-bit bidirectional counter is introduced here, as shown in Figure 2.22(a). It is composed of AND, flip-flops (FF0 ~ FF2), and multiplexers (MUX0 ~ MUX1) logic blocks. Each flip-flop is triggered at the rising edge of signals at the "CK" terminals. This structure can count in two directions, up and down, that is controlled by the signal U/D. The timing diagram is shown in Figure 2.22(b). First, the counter is reset to an initial condition by asserting the signal RSTC. Then the counter is ready for further operations. When V_{cmp} is high, clock signal CLK is enabled and the flip-flops begin to read the input "D" terminal data and reversely output at the "Q" terminals controlled by the clock CLK.

When the U/D signal is low, the "QN" terminals are selected and connected to the "CK" terminals. As a result, a count-up effect can be observed. Similarly, when the U/D is high, the Q terminals are selected and connected to the CK terminals. The counter changes its count direction so that the output data $D_{ADC} < 0{:}2 >$ is decreasing at each rising edge of the clock signal CLK. This 3-bit bidirectional counter can be expanded to a 10-bit counter. This counter can do an on-chip subtraction that is useful in the correlated sampling described in next section.

For a 10-bit counter, there are totally $2^{10} = 1024$ steps. Each step represents a voltage level, which is called the least significant bit (LSB). It denotes the minimal voltage level required to change one bit of output code D_{ADC}, which is determined by:

$$1\,LSB = K_{RAMP} \cdot t_{clk} \tag{2.27}$$

(a)

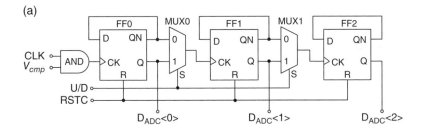

(b)

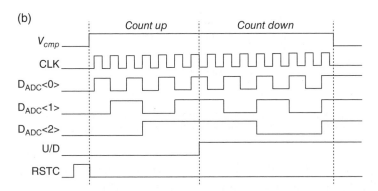

Figure 2.22 (a) Schematic of a 3-bit bidirectional counter; and (b) The corresponding timing diagram.

where t_{clk} is the time period of clock. A high resolution (mV/bit) can be realized by adopting a small ramp slope K_{RAMP} or a fast clock with small t_{clk}. The input voltage V_{amp} can be solely converted to a digital code D_{ADC}:

$$D_{ADC} = t_{tran}/t_{clk} = \left(V_{start} - V_{amp}\right)/\left(K_{RAMP} \cdot t_{clk}\right) \tag{2.28}$$

where t_{tran} is the transition time that the comparator takes to change its output state from high to low.

Single-slope ADC has a simple structure that is suitable for large array applications. When performance and speed are key parameters of the design, other structures can also be implemented, such as sigma-delta ADC, SAR ADC, pipelined ADC, etc. Trade-offs should always be made between area, resolution, and speed.

2.5.2 Sigma-Delta ADC

Sigma-delta ADC is a well-known oversampling converter. It can achieve much higher resolution than Nyquist-rate converters, due to its excellent noise shaping property. To understand this, the first thing is to be aware of quantization noise.

As an important part of ADC, a quantizer translates continuous signal voltages to discrete digital codes. As shown in Figure 2.23(a), an input ramp signal V_{amp} is quantized to four discrete levels D_{ADC}. Quantization error E_Q is inevitable, since one digital value is used to represent a number of input voltage values. To simplify analysis, a quantizer can be represented by a linear model where the quantization error is regarded as a noise

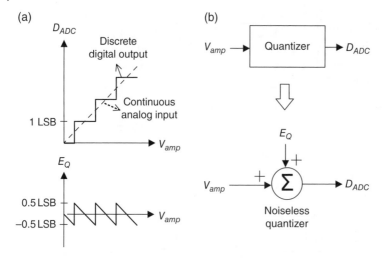

Figure 2.23 (a) Quantization transfer curve with a continuous ramp as input signal and the corresponding quantization error during conversion; and (b) Block diagram of a linear model of quantizer.

source, as shown in Figure 2.23(b). In this way, the output D_{ADC} is equal to $V_{amp} + E_Q$. Quantization error E_Q can be approximated as white noise with a uniform probability density function (PDF) between ±0.5 LSB. The noise power can be calculated as:

$$\sigma_{EQ}^2 = \frac{1}{LSB} \int_{-0.5LSB}^{+0.5LSB} E_Q^2 dE_Q = LSB^2 / 12 \tag{2.29}$$

The corresponding quantization noise power spectrum density (PSD) within the sampling frequency $\pm f_s/2$ is given by:

$$S_{EQ}(f) = \sigma_{EQ}^2 / f_S = LSB^2 / (12 f_S) \tag{2.30}$$

For a Nyquist-rate converter with a sampling frequency of f_S, where $f_S = 2f_B$, the quantization noise power is equally distributed within the frequency range $[-f_S/2, + f_S/2]$, as shown in Figure 2.24. For an oversampled converter with a higher sampling frequency of Nf_S, the noise power is re-distributed to a larger range

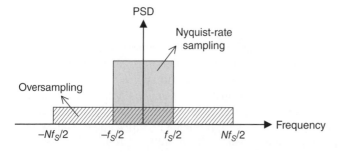

Figure 2.24 Quantization noise power spectrum density distribution of Nyquist-rate sampling and oversampling.

$[-Nf_S/2, + Nf_S/2]$. Since the signal bandwidth of interest is $[-f_B, + f_B]$, the noise power of oversampling within this region is calculated as:

$$N_{\sigma_{EQ}^2} = \int_{-f_s/2}^{+f_s/2} S_{EQ\_OS}(f)df = \text{LSB}^2/(12N) \qquad (2.31)$$

$$S_{EQ\_OS}(f) = \sigma_{EQ}^2/(Nf_S) = \text{LSB}^2/(12Nf_S) \qquad (2.32)$$

From the equations above, when applying a low-pass filter, the quantization noise power can be effectively attenuated and a higher resolution can be achieved due to the improved signal-to-noise ratio (SNR).

The key point of oversampling is to reduce the noise power within the interested signal bandwidth. It is easy to understand that a higher SNR can be obtained if the low-frequency noise can be further pushed to higher frequencies. This can be realized by a sigma-delta modulator. It combines oversampling (sigma) and noise-shaping (delta) techniques. A first-order $\Sigma\Delta$ modulator is shown in Figure 2.25(a). It contains an integrator and a low-resolution ADC (quantizer) in the forward path and a digital-to-analog converter (DAC) in the feedback path. This structure can "memory" previous sampling voltage levels V_{DAC} recovered from SD_{out}, which is subtracted from the current input analog signal V_{amp}. This feedback loop forces the mean value of V_{DAC} to be equal to the input signal V_{amp}.

To explain the noise shaping effect, a simple frequency domain example is shown in Figure 2.25(b). Assuming that the integrator has a transfer function of $1/s$, the quantization error of ADC is $E_Q(s)$, and the DAC is ideal. The output signal $SD_{out}(s)$ can be calculated as:

$$SD_{out}(s) = \frac{1}{1+s} \cdot V_{amp}(s) + \frac{s}{1+s} \cdot E_Q(s) \qquad (2.33)$$

(a)

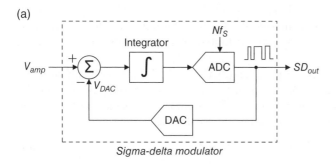

Sigma-delta modulator

(b)

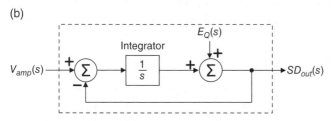

Figure 2.25 (a) A first-order sigma-delta modulator; and (b) The corresponding frequency domain model.

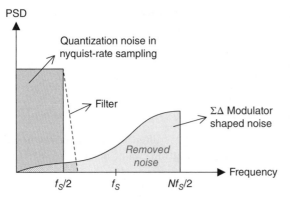

Figure 2.26 Noise shaping property of sigma-delta modulator.

The signal transfer function *STF(s)* and noise transfer function *NTF(s)* can be extracted as:

$$STF(s) = SD_{out}(s) / V_{amp}(s) = 1/(1+s) \tag{2.34}$$

$$NTF(s) = SD_{out}(s) / E_Q(s) = s/(1+s) \tag{2.35}$$

STF(s) follows the function of a low pass filter, whereas *NTF(s)* follows a function of a high pass filter. Therefore, within the interested bandwidth, signal V_{amp} is fully transferred while noise is suppressed. At high frequencies, even though the noise power increases, the conversion performance is not affected, since it is normally out of the signal bandwidth. The oversampling and noise shaping effect of sigma-delta modulator is shown in Figure 2.26. The original quantization noise in Nyquist-rate sampling is re-distributed and re-shaped to a more wide frequency range. When applying a low-pass filter, the large dominant noise power outside the signal bandwidth is removed.

The integrator works as a loop filter. It can be realized by the continuous time (CT) Gm-C or the active-RC filter, as well as the discrete time (DT) switched capacitor. Both integrators have their merits and demerits. The CT integrator is normally used in high-speed applications, and the DT integrator is adopted when precision and accuracy are the required.

For the CT Gm-C filter shown in Figure 2.27(a), the key cell transconductor works as a current source whose output current I_{int} depends on the transconductance G_m and the input voltage V_{amp}. In the frequency domain, the integration capacitance C_{int} can be represented by $1/sC_{int}$. The transfer function can be calculated as:

$$H(s) = V_{int}/V_{amp} = (G_m/C_{int}) \cdot 1/s \tag{2.36}$$

For the CT active-RC filter shown in Figure 2.27(b), the generated current value depends on the resistance R_{int}, which is integrated on the operational amplifier (OPA) feedback capacitance C_{int}. The transfer function can be calculated as:

$$H(s) = V_{int}/V_{amp} = [1/(R_{int}C_{int})] \cdot 1/s \tag{2.37}$$

A DT switched capacitor filter is shown in Figure 2.28(a). It substitutes the resistor R_{int} in Figure 2.27(b) with a switched capacitor, which is composed of a capacitor C_{int1} and four switches controlled by a non-overlapped clock pair ϕ_1 and ϕ_2 with a period of T.

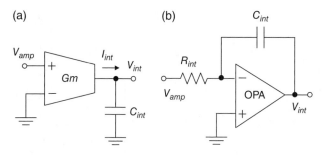

Figure 2.27 Schematic of continuous-time: (a) Gm-C filter; and (b) Active-RC filter.

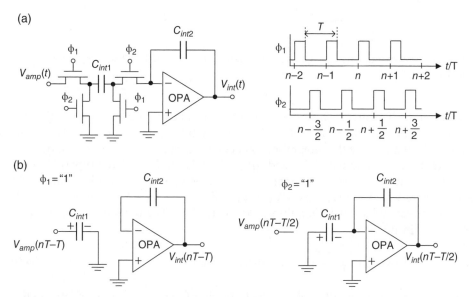

Figure 2.28 (a) Schematic of a discrete-time switched-capacitor filter; and (b) Its operations in different clock phases.

The corresponding operations are shown in Figure 2.28(b). When $\phi_1 = $"1", C_{int1} is charged to $C_{int1} \cdot V_{amp}(nT - T)$. When $\phi_2 = $"1", the capacitor C_{int1} is reversely connected to the virtual ground terminal of OPA. The charge stored in C_{int1} is fluxed into the ground, which results in the same amount of charge added to the feedback capacitor C_{int2}. We have:

$$C_{int2}V_{int}\left(nT - T/2\right) = C_{int2}V_{int}\left(nT - T\right) + C_{int1}V_{amp}\left(nT - T\right) \tag{2.38}$$

$$C_{int2}V_{int}\left(nT\right) = C_{int2}V_{int}\left(nT - T/2\right) \tag{2.39}$$

The transfer function in the z-domain is given by:

$$C_{int2}V_{int}\left(z\right) = C_{int2}V_{int}\left(z\right)z^{-1} + C_{int1}V_{amp}\left(z\right)z^{-1} \tag{2.40}$$

$$H\left(z\right) = V_{int}\left(z\right)/V_{amp}\left(z\right) = \left(C_{int1}/C_{int2}\right) \cdot \left[z^{-1}/\left(1 - z^{-1}\right)\right] \tag{2.41}$$

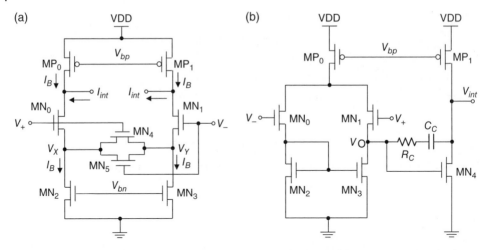

Figure 2.29 Implementation of: (a) A triode-based transconductor; and (b) A 2-stage operational amplifier.

Unlike the OTA already introduced, the transconductor used in the G_m-C filter requires a linear and controllable G_m. One implementation circuit is shown in Figure 2.29(a), where the integration capacitor C_{int} can be placed between the two I_{int} current output terminals. MP_0 and MP_1, and MN_0 and MN_1 are properly biased, so that their drain current values are equal to I_B. MN_4 and MN_5 work in the triode region, where $V_+ - V_X - V_{thn} > V_X - V_Y$ or $V_- - V_Y - V_{thn} > V_Y - V_X$, supposing that all NMOS transistors have the same threshold voltage V_{thn}. The transconductance G_m is determined by [6]:

$$G_m = 4k_{MN0}k_{MN4}\sqrt{I_B}/\left[\left(k_{MN0} + 4k_{MN4}\right)\sqrt{k_{MN0}}\right] \tag{2.42}$$

The OPA used in active-RC and switched capacitor filters can be implemented in the classical 2-stage amplifier, as shown in Figure 2.29(b). The first stage is a 5-T differential amplifier with a gain of $A_{v1} = g_{m(MN0)}(r_{ds(MN1)} || r_{ds(MN3)})$. The second stage is a common-source amplifier with a gain of $A_{v2} = g_{m(MN4)}(r_{ds(MN4)} || r_{ds(MP1)})$. A high output gain A_v can be realized and is described as:

$$A_v = g_{m(MN0)}g_{m(MN4)}\left[r_{ds(MN1)} || r_{ds(MN3)}\right]\left[r_{ds(MN4)} || r_{ds(MP1)}\right] \tag{2.43}$$

The capacitor C_c and resistor R_c are employed for phase compensation, which improves the stability of OPA.

As an example, a simple first-order sigma-delta ADC is implemented with a switched capacitor integrator, a comparator (1-bit ADC), a 1-bit DAC, a low-pass filter, and a decimator, as shown in Figure 2.30. The difference between analog signal V_{amp} and the feedback voltage V_{DAC} is read by the switched-capacitor integrator with an oversampling rate Nf_s. The integrated output V_{int} is compared with zero voltage by the 1-bit ADC. The comparison result is translated to corresponding voltage V_{DAC} by the 1-bit DAC. When V_{amp} is larger than zero, then $V_{int} > 0 \rightarrow SD_{out} = 0 \rightarrow V_{DAC} = V_{REF}$. Therefore,

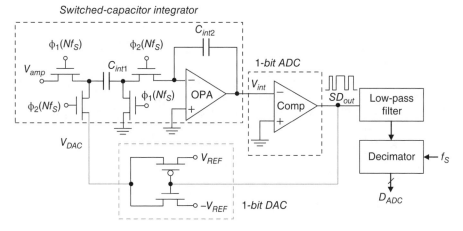

Figure 2.30 Implementation of a first-order sigma-delta ADC.

V_{amp} is subtracted by V_{REF} in the next sampling phase. Similarly, when V_{amp} is smaller than zero, $V_{int} < 0 \rightarrow SD_{out} = VDD \rightarrow V_{DAC} = -V_{REF}$. Therefore, V_{amp} is added by V_{REF} in the next sampling phase. The average value of V_{ADC} translated from SD_{out} is equal to V_{amp}. The sigma-delta modulator output is first modified by a low-pass filter and then numbered by a decimator, such as a counter, with a lower sampling rate of f_s. In this way, a high-resolution sigma-delta ADC is realized.

Apart from the introduced first-order sigma-delta ADC, a higher-order modulator can also be employed to further reduce noise power in the bandwidth of interest, but it will occupy a larger area. In addition, a high resolution also means a slow conversion rate, since it requires a lot of oversampling time. Consequently, there should be a trade-off between resolution, area, and speed. Sigma-delta ADC is suitable for applications where the input signal is very weak.

2.6 Correlated Sampling

2.6.1 Correlated Double Sampling

Correlated double sampling (CDS) is a useful technique to reduce process variation, non-idea offsets, or flicker noise. It detects two voltages and outputs their difference. The previously-mentioned auto-zero operation also serves this purpose. Typically, a reset voltage is measured or stored as a reference voltage. It is later subtracted from the sensed signal voltage. CDS is performed at the system level. Blocks from pixel to ADC are involved. A complete readout path is required to explain the CDS technique. As shown in Figure 2.31, a simple 4 T pixel structure with a reset transistor and a transfer transistor is used, for example, a SF pixel structure is employed. Pixel voltage is transfer to the column bus. It is then amplified by the column amplifier. The resultant voltage V_{amp} is converted to 10-bit digital data by the column single-slope ADC.

The timing diagram of CDS is shown in Figure 2.32. First, the gate of the SF MN0 is reset to RSTV. The corresponding column amplifier output voltage V_{amp} is initialized.

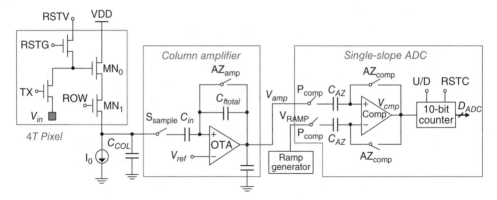

Figure 2.31 A schematic example that CDS and CMS are performed.

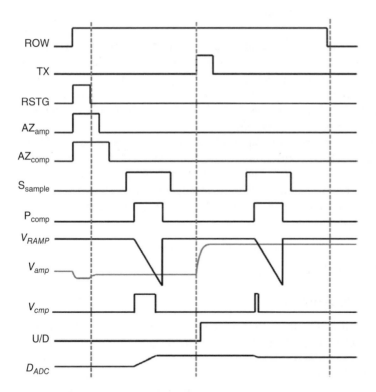

Figure 2.32 Timing diagram of correlated double sampling (CDS).

When RSTG is open, a slight voltage drop at MN_0 gate is observed due to charge injection of switching. It leads to a slight voltage rise in V_{amp}. After auto-zeroing of column amplifier and ADC, the reset level of V_{amp} is measured by ADC. The converted result is stored in the counter. Second, the pixel sensed signal is read by turning on the transfer transistor (TX). The signal level may be smaller than the reset level, so there should be an obvious voltage drop at the MN_0 gate, and V_{amp} is increased. Then the count direction is changed from up to down. The converted sensed signal level is subtracted from the reset level. Therefore, the final data in the counter is actually the difference between the reset and sensed signal level.

The CDS procedure described here can be regarded as digital CDS, since subtraction is performed in the counter. There are also analog CDS where the subtraction occurs on capacitors, as with the auto-zero technique. CDS can be implemented in many forms. For example, the adoption of sequential auto-zero, as shown in Figure 2.32, is also a kind of CDS.

2.6.2 Correlated Multiple Sampling

Another effective way to reduce noise and offset is correlated multiple sampling (CMS). As the name indicates, the sampling times are not limited to two, as shown in Figure 2.33. The basic idea is averaging, which means that the reset level V_{reset} is measured for M times before reading the signal level. Then in the signal reading phase, the sensed signal level V_{sensed_signal} is also measured for M times. The CMS output voltage V_{CMS} can be calculated by [7]:

$$V_{CMS} = \frac{1}{M}\sum_{i=1}^{M}V_{reset,i} - \frac{1}{M}\sum_{i=1}^{M}V_{sensed\,signal,i} \qquad (2.44)$$

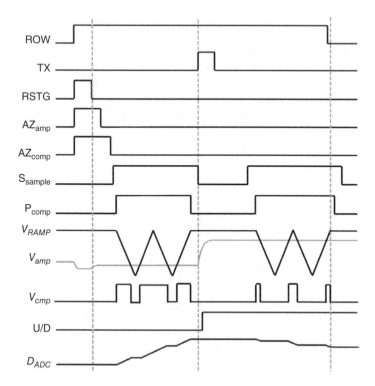

Figure 2.33 Timing diagram of correlated multiple sampling (CMS).

CMS can also be realized in the circuit, as shown in Figure 2.25. The timing diagram is shown in Figure 2.16. The operation is almost the same as with CDS. The difference is that in the reset phase, the column amplifier voltage V_{amp} is detected four times by multiple ramping while maintaining the count direction. This means that the count results keep increasing. In the sensed signal read phase, multiple ramping is also perform in an opposite count direction. Therefore, the remaining data in the counter is the sum of voltage difference in each detection. When dividing the data by four, the noise level is also divided.

Similar to CDS, there are also analog CMS techniques. The multiple voltage levels are stored and accumulated in two capacitors with the help of a sample-hold module. A comparator can be used to output their difference. An obvious issue of CMS is the decrease in dynamic range, so the sampling times cannot be very large.

2.7 Timing Control

For a pixel array, one row of pixels are selected and operated simultaneously. The sensed signals are first transferred to the column bus, and then amplified and converted to digital data. Each column data of the row is read out one by one. Then a new row is selected until the whole pixel array is measured. This row-by-row and column-by-column operations are realized by row or column timing control blocks.

2.7.1 Row Timing Control

Row-level timing control is typically composed of row decoder and row driver. The row decoder is employed so that each row can be solely accessed according to its row address. It is realized by logic blocks such as NAND, AND, OR, NOR, XOR, INV, etc. Taking the 5-input NAND as an example, there are two ways to realize it. As shown in Figure 2.34, one method is to directly configure from pull-up PMOS and pull-down

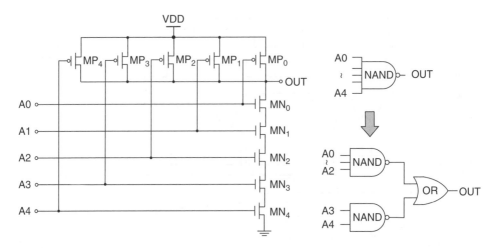

Figure 2.34 Two ways to realize a 5-input NAND logic block.

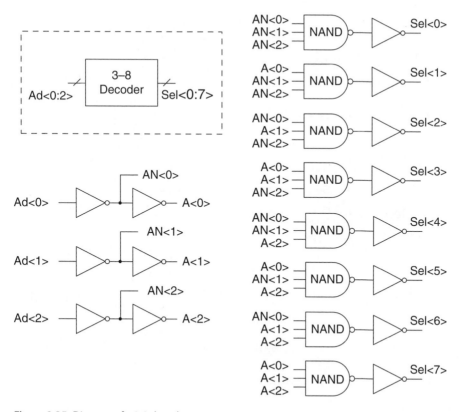

Figure 2.35 Diagram of a 3-8 decoder.

NMOS networks based on the logic equation $\text{OUT} = \overline{A0 \cdot A1 \cdot A2 \cdot A3 \cdot A4}$. In this structure, the output signal may experience a large latency due to the long serial NMOS discharging path. It is not suitable when there are large input numbers. Another method is to adopt a 3-input NAND, a 3-input NAND, and a 2-input OR derived from the equation $\text{OUT} = \overline{A0 \cdot A1 \cdot A2} + \overline{A3 \cdot A4}$. This structure ensures a more balanced signal latency performance compared to the former one.

For a decoder with an address number of N, we can obtain 2^N outputs. A 3-8 decoder is introduced in Figure 2.35 for a better understanding of how to design a decoder. The input address $\text{Ad} < 0{:}2 >$ can be expanded to three pairs of signals, $A < 0{:}2 >$ and $\text{AN} < 0{:}2 >$. There are a total of eight combinations, and each one is correlated to an output terminal $\text{Sel} < i >$, $i = \{0,.., 7\}$. By employing eight 3-input NAND blocks and inverters, a 3-8 decoder is realized. Based on this method, a 5-32 decoder can also be realized, where the 5-input NAND blocks described above are needed.

When N is large enough, a hierarchy decoder structure is required. As an example, a 7-128 decider is introduced here, as shown in Figure 2.36. It employs a 3-8 decoder and 8 5-32 decoders. First, three high address $\text{Ad} < 4{:}6 >$ is translated to eight enable signals (Sel0 ~ Sel7) through the 3-8 decoder. Each enabled signal controls a 5-32 decoder with a four low address $\text{Ad} < 0{:}3 >$. In this way, we can obtain a total of 128 output signals $\text{Sel} < 0{:}127 >$. This hierarchy structure is widely used in large pixel array design.

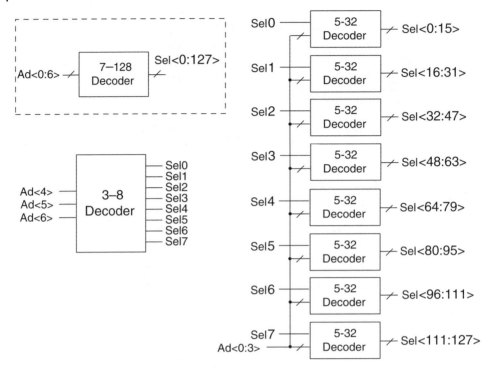

Figure 2.36 Diagram of a hierarchy 7-128 decoder.

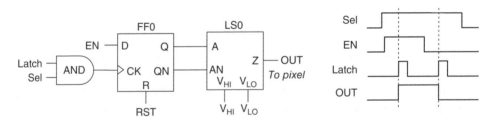

Figure 2.37 Block diagram and timing diagram of a row driver.

Each row can be accessed by row address, but each row may have multiple control signals, such as reset signal RST, transfer signal TX, row-select signal ROW, etc. Therefore, a row driver block is needed to implement various row-level control signals. A typical row driver is shown in Figure 2.37. It is composed of an AND block, a flip-flop FF0, and a level shifter LS0. This row driver is implemented per row per signal. The timing diagram is shown in Figure 2.37. The Sel signal comes from the row decoder that is shared with each row signals. When Sel is high, signal Latch is used to sample the EN signal. On the rising edge of Latch signal, the state of EN is sampled and maintained until the next rising edge of Latch. This structure can effectively reframe the glitch or noise issue. Each row-control signal (e.g. RST, TX, ROW) has its own dedicated EN and Latch signals.

Figure 2.38 Schematic of a typical level shifter.

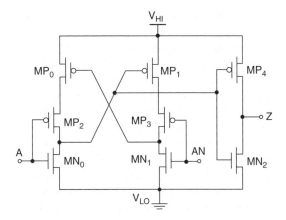

The employment of level shifter allows a more flexible control. Each signal output voltages can be separately adjusted through terminals V_{HI} and V_{LO}. The complementary output of FF0 is used as the input of level shifter. The schematic is shown in Figure 2.38. Normally V_{LO} is connected to ground (GND). When input signal (A) is high and (AN) is low, the MN_0 and MP_3 are turned on, MN_1 and MP_2 are turned off, and the output node (Z) will be charged to V_{HI}. Similarly, when (A) is low and (AN) is high, the output node (Z) will be discharged to V_{LO}.

2.7.2 Column Timing Control

Column-level timing control is composed of column decoder and SRAM, and SA. Similar to the row decoder, a large column decoder can be realized by hierarchy decoder structure. Following ADC conversion, several blocks are involved for column-by-column data readout, as shown in Figure 2.39. First, a flip-flop is used to trigger ADC data on the rising edge of WR signal. Meanwhile, the data is written to the SRAM block. Then the data stored in SRAM is read out by the column SA.

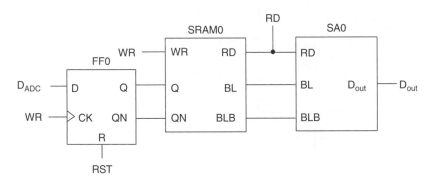

Figure 2.39 Schematic of data readout blocks following ADC.

The schematic of SRAM is shown in Figure 2.40. It is composed of eight transistors, where write and read paths are separated. It simplifies the operations compared to convention 6-T SRAM. During the write phase, the WR signal is high, and the complementary data from "Q" and "QN" terminals of flip-flop FF0 are stored in SRAM inner nodes. During the read phase, BL and BLB are first pre-charged to VDD, then MN_4 and MN_5 are turned on. The inner node with low voltage will discharge the bit line, which results in a voltage difference between BL and BLB. This difference is detected by an SA.

The schematic of SA is shown in Figure 2.41. When the read phase is not activated, the RD signal is low. $MP_2 \sim MP_6$ are pre-charging transistors of bit lines or inner sensing nodes. MP_4 is introduced to balance the inner voltage levels. When RD is high, $MP_2 \sim MP_6$ are turned off and MN_2 is turned on. SA begins to amplify and compare the difference between BL and BLB. The signal RD comes from the output column decoder, so that column-by-column readout can be realized by sweeping the column address.

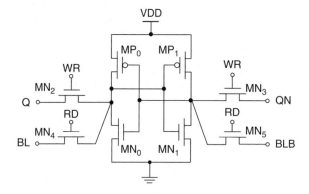

Figure 2.40 Schematic of a SRAM cell.

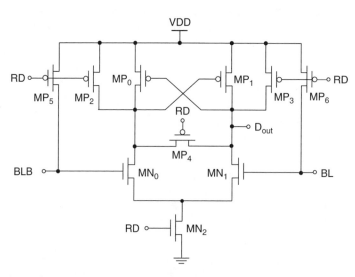

Figure 2.41 Schematic of Sense Amplifier (SA).

2.8   LVDS Interface

Many interface standards have been proposed, such as voltage-mode logic (VML), current-mode logic (CML), and LVDS). In this section, the widely-used LVDS readout strategy found in most large array CMOS sensors is introduced.

The LVDS readout strategy is a high-speed and low-power communication interface between sensor and data receiver. As shown in Figure 2.42, basic components include an on-chip CMOS driver, two differential transmission lines, and a receiver. The driver translates "0" and "1" digital levels to constant current or potential drop in two directions, which is then applied to the differential transmission lines. Compared to a single transmission line, differential typed have a high rejection to common-node noise. Even though signals in both lines fluctuate with common noise, the relative difference between them remains the same. In addition, these two tightly coupled lines can reduce electromagnetic noise, due to the equal and opposite electromagnetic fields created between them. Consequently, signals can be propagated over a long distance.

A termination resistor (R_T) is employed for impedance matching with the transmission line (R_L), where $R_T = 2R_L$ guarantees signal integrity. The transmission line can be realized by a printed circuit board (PCB) interconnection or cable. Assuming that the receiver has a large input impedance, the current will flow through the termination resistor. The voltage drop produced is sensed by the receiver. The receiver can be realized by a hysteresis comparator that is sensitive to a small voltage swing. Therefore, a low dynamic range at the output terminals of the driver is enough for detection. It can greatly reduce the power consumption and enhance the data transition time. The voltage direction is translated to D_{LVDS}, so that the sensor data D_{ADC} is recovered.

The on-chip driver design is now discussed. First, the input single-end data D_{ADC} is split into two opposite signals, D_{ADC+} and D_{ADC-}. The realization circuit is shown in Figure 2.43. The basic component is the inverter, where the input signal is first buffered or reversed through INV0 ~ INV4. INV5 and INV6 are cross-coupled for transition synchronization. INV8 and INV9 are used as buffer blocks before adding to the main driver part.

A schematic of an LVDS driver is shown in Figure 2.44(a). MP$_2$ and MN$_2$ are a pair of current sources that control the output current I_0 to the receiver termination resistor. They determine the voltage swing of LVDS. For example, a 3.5 mA current source is used to generate a normal 350 mV voltage swing with $R_T = 100\ \Omega$. For a higher voltage

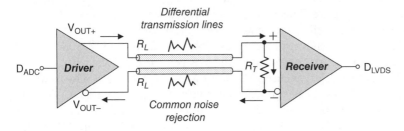

Figure 2.42 Diagram of a typical LVDS.

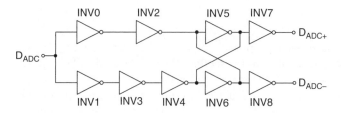

Figure 2.43 Differential input signals generation circuit.

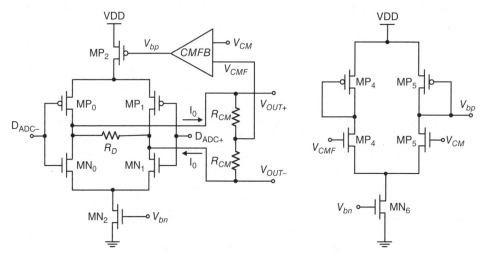

Figure 2.44 (a) Diagram of a LVDS driver circuit; and (b) Simple common-mode feedback circuit.

swing, a larger current source is used. MP_0, MP_1, MN_0, and MN_1 form a bridged switching network. When the input signal V_{ADC} is high, MP_0 and MN_1 are turned on. Current will flow through the V_{out+} terminal and return back through V_{out-} terminal. When V_{ADC} is low, MP_1 and MN_0 are turned on and current flows in the opposite direction. A double termination technique is adopted by employing an additional termination resistor (R_D) at the driver end. It can be used to reduce round-trip reflection and improve signal integrity resulting from crosstalk or imperfect termination. A common-mode feedback circuit (CMFB) is adopted to stabilize the output common mode voltage at a desired value V_{CM}. Two identical resistors with a high resistance R_{CM} form a resistive divider. It senses the output common mode voltage V_{CMF}, where $V_{CMF} = (V_{OUT+} - V_{OUT-})/2$ and the bypass current is negligible. This voltage is compared with the desired value V_{CM} and the comparison result regulated the bias voltage of transistor MP_2.

A simple CMFB circuit is shown in Figure 2.44(b). Similar to the LVDS circuit, its MN_6 NMOS tail current is also controlled by the bias voltage V_{bn}. When $V_{CMF} > V_{CM}$, the MP_4 and MN_4 path has a larger current than the MP_5 and MN_5 path. The feedback output voltage V_{bp}, the bias voltage of the current source MP_2, is increased. LVDS output current I_0 is reduced and V_{CMF} is decreased until $V_{CMF} = V_{CM}$. Similarly, when $V_{CMF} < V_{CM}$, the MP_5 and MN_5 path has a larger current than the MP_4 and MN_4 path. V_{bp} is reduced and eventually increases I_0 and raises V_{CMF} until $V_{CMF} = V_{CM}$.

Serial and parallel LVDS output can be employed. For example, there are 10 output terminals for a 10-bit ADC. For a parallel readout, 10 LVDS drivers can be realized on-chip with each one occupying an output PAD. A high-speed column readout clock can be employed. In the serial readout, one LVDS driver is adopted that can serially output the 10 ADC bits since a 10 times higher sampling clock is possible. It can be used in applications where the PAD amount is limited.

In conclusion, a high throughput sensor can be achieved by increasing the pixel array size, but the resulting problem is the massively produced data size and power consumption. Therefore, a low-power and high-speed readout strategy is essential. The LVDS readout strategy is a high-speed communication interface between sensor and data receiver. It greatly improves the CMOS sensor performance in bio-medical applications, such as DNA sequencing and bio-imaging.

References

1 K. Murari, R. Etienne-Cummings, N.V. Thakor and G. Cauwenberghs (2011) A CMOS in-pixel CTIA high-sensitivity fluorescence imager. *IEEE Transactions on Biomedical Circuits and Systems*, 5(5), 449–458.

2 L. Hong, S. McManus, H. Yang and K. Sengupta. A fully integrated CMOS fluorescence biosensor with on-chip nanophotonic filter. pp. C206–C207.

3 S. Kumar, C. Tao, M. Chien, B. Hellner, A. Balijepalli, J.W. Robertson, *et al.* (2012) PEG-labeled nucleotides and nanopore detection for single molecule DNA sequencing by synthesis. *Scientific Reports*, 2, 684.

4 D. Kim, B. Goldstein, W. Tang, F.J. Sigworth and E. Culurciello (2013) Noise analysis and performance comparison of low current measurement systems for biomedical applications. *IEEE Transactions on Biomedical Circuits and Systems*, 7(1), 52–62.

5 A. Balan, B. Machielse, D. Niedzwiecki, J. Lin, P. Ong, *et al.* (2014) Improving signal-to-noise performance for DNA translocation in solid-state nanopores at MHz bandwidths. *Nano Letters*, 14(12), 215–7220.

6 D.A. Johns and K. Martin (2008) *Analo_g Integrated Circuit Design*. John Wiley & Sons.

7 A. Boukhayma (2016) *Ultra Low Noise CMOS Image Sensors*. École Polytechnique Fédérale De Lausanne.

3

CMOS Impedance Sensor

3.1 Introduction

Electrical impedance sensing, which detects the change in impedance magnitude and phase, is one widely-used biomedical sensing technique for cell detection and counting applications. Existing cell detection usually relies on bulky and expensive optical instruments that are also subject to operator variance. Non-optical methods such as the capacitance-based sensor, electric-cell-substrate impedance sensing, field-effect transistor-based sensor, and voltammetric transduction sensor have been used for detection and enumeration of living cells [1–4].

Among these methods, the electrical-impedance spectroscopy (EIS) method has gained much attention, able to estimate cells even at an accuracy of the single-cell level. The EIS used to quantify the heterogeneity in breast cancer cell lines, as well as to differentiate abnormal cells from normal cell types, has been reported [5,6]. Several research groups have deployed macro-electrode-based impedance sensing to capture cell signals [7–9]. In [9], Manickam *et al.* describe a 10×10 array with integrated measurement circuitry. As such, the size of the electrode is much larger than the size of an individual cell, hence the measurement reflects the total influence of all cells on one electrode. The resulting estimations are thereby only reliable for a large numbers of cells, but with a significant error for rare cell detection. As a result, cell counting with consistent accuracy still remains the primary challenge to be resolved. For the sensor to be useful in early cancer diagnosis or prognosis, the limit of the single cell is required, because five Circulating Tumor Cells (CTCs) can make a difference in a prognosis [10].

Efforts have been made to achieve the single-cell precision counting by designing the electrode size, which can be comparable to the single-cell diameter [11,12]. Recently, for the detection of MCF-7 cells specific to breast cancer, the effect of electrode size on single-cell detection has been reported, which suggests that the sensor can respond with the best results when the size of electrode is comparable to the size of one single cell [11]. Note that it has been hypothesized that the use of a microelectrode array with electrode size comparable to the single cell size will be useful for precise counting of tumor cells over a wide dynamic range. For example, Jiang *et al.* demonstrated a single cell detection resolution with an electrode pixel size of 7 µm by 7 µm in CD4+ cell counting [12]. However, their approach, while improving on the existing detection resolution, has a significant limitation, as the passive electrodes built on the chip are not

CMOS Integrated Lab-on-a-Chip System for Personalized Biomedical Diagnosis, First Edition.
Hao Yu, Mei Yan, and Xiwei Huang.
© 2018 John Wiley & Sons Singapore Pte. Ltd. Published 2018 by John Wiley & Sons Singapore Pte. Ltd.

scalable to accommodate enumeration of a wide dynamic range of cells, owing to the complexity in the channel floor plan and electrode routing. As such, the chip can handle a very limited amount of cells with 200 passive electrodes. For a patient with metastatic cancer, the number of CTCs in the peripheral blood can vary by three orders of magnitude. Therefore, an active electrode array that can count CTCs with single-cell resolution over a large number of cells has become an emerging need.

Extensive research has been carried out and reported in the literature for the active CMOS-based biosensor microelectrodes array [13–15]. For example, Berdondini *et al.* reported CMOS arrays featuring 64 by 64 electrodes for recordings of the spontaneous activity of rat cardiomocyte cultures [15]. On-chip electrode arrays with a 128-electrode array for recording neural activity have also been demonstrated [16]. These devices take advantage of CMOS electronics, which offers on-chip rapid electrical detection, and a capability for handling a large number of closely spaced electrodes.

In this chapter, a high-density CMOS EIS biosensor array for precise counting of breast cancer MCF-7 cells has been developed. The device consists of a 96×96 array of densely packed active microelectrodes in an area of $3\,mm \times 3\,mm$ to enable counting over a wide range of MCF-7 cells. Small electrode size comparable to a typical single tumor cell at $11-17\,\mu m$ enables high counting accuracy down to the scale of single-cell detection. Investigations were made to record the impedance spectrum of electrodes over the wide frequency range with the presence of a cell. A binary "on" and "off" type response of the electrode has been achieved based on impedance change for detection at single-cell resolution. Moreover, the cell counting is accomplished by the sum of the electrode in the "on" type response. The mapping accuracy of EIS compared to optical measurement was also studied.

3.2 CMOS Impedance Pixel

For cell impedance sensing, the CMOS impedance pixel, or CMOS microelectrode, was realized on an 8-inch wafer with standard $0.18\,\mu m$ CMOS technology [17]. The CMOS impedance pixel array diagram and the sensing scheme are illustrated in Figures 3.1(a) and (b). The CMOS impedance pixel array includes 96×96 exposed squares of Al electrodes $17\,\mu m$ in diameter and a centre-to-centre pitch size of $30\,\mu m$, as shown in Figure 3.1(c). A $2\,\mu m$-thick film stack of SiN/SiO_2 dielectrics passivates the underlying metal lines and isolates these Al electrodes. An electronic demultiplexing scheme was implemented with row/column decoder to address the individual electrode. A common electrode, also known as a Counter Electrode, is used for excitation of the cells. When a sinusoid voltage is applied, the amplitude and phase of the current response are sensed by the EIS measurement unit.

The cell impedance measurement is based on the recording of changes in impedance of Au electrodes to AC current flow when the electrodes are covered by cells. Figure 3.2 shows a schematic view of an electrode covered by an MCF-7 cell. The cell adherence to the electrode is mediated by protein molecules that protrude from the membrane. These proteins keep the membrane a certain distance from the electrode, creating a cleft between them. This cleft is conductive as the electrolyte fills in the opening space. The conductance of the cleft depends on the cell-to-electrode distance, because of the shielding effect of cells to electrode [18,19].

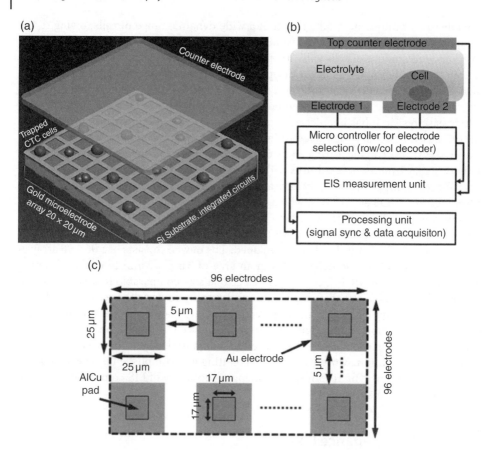

Figure 3.1 (a) CMOS impedance sensor pixel array; (b) Cross-sectional illustration of the sensing and addressing scheme of the CMOS impedance pixel; and (c) 96 × 96 impedance sensing electrode array.

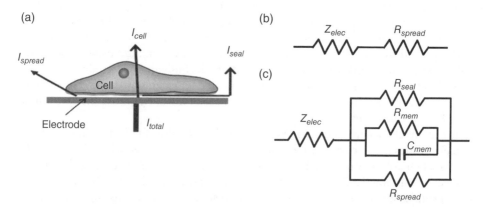

Figure 3.2 (a) Sectional view of an electrode covered with an MCF-7 cell. The total current is split into three pathways: I_{spread}, I_{cell}, and I_{seal}. The equivalent circuit of (b) Electrode without cells; and (c) Electrode with cells.

When an AC current is applied through the electrode, the total current I_{total} is split into three pathways: current through the cell (I_{cell}); current flow through the cleft region (I_{seal}); and the rest of the current, I_{spread}, which easily flows outwards from the electrode to the electrolyte [20]. Figure 3.2(c) shows an equivalent circuit that models the relevant phenomena. In this equivalent circuit, cell impedance consists of membrane capacitance (C_{mem}) and membrane resistance (R_{mem}). R_{seal} is the sealing resistance between cells and the electrode and is inversely proportional to the averaged cell-to-substrate separation distance [18]. R_{spread} represents the resistance to the current spreading from working electrode to the counter electrode.

The total impedance of the system when the electrode is immersed in the electrolyte can be modeled as a series combination of impedance electrode Z_{elec} and spreading resistance R_{spread} (Figure 3.2(b)) [20]:

$$Z = Z_{elec} + R_{spread} = \frac{K}{(i\omega)^m} + R_{spread} \tag{3.1}$$

where K is a size-dependent constant, and m denotes the power constant of Z_{elec}, which is usually around 0.5–1.0. The first term in Equation (3.1) represents the equivalent impedance of the electrode-electrolyte interface that is frequency dependent. For a square electrode (in our case), the spreading resistance is given by [20]:

$$R_{spread} = \frac{\rho ln(4)}{\pi \ell} = \frac{\rho ln(4)}{\pi A^{1/2}} \tag{3.2}$$

where ℓ is the edge length of the electrode and A is its area.

It is also well-known that the spreading resistance is increased when the cell is present [18]. A modified equation of R_{spread}^{*} with the electrode covered with cells is given by [14]:

$$R_{spread}^{*} = R_{spread} \sqrt{\frac{A}{A - A_{cell}}} \tag{3.3}$$

where A is total electrode area, and $A - A_{cell}$ is the electrode area not covered by the cell. Such is the equivalent circuit model for CMOS impedance sensing.

3.3 Readout Circuit

With the above-described CMOS impedance pixel array, equivalent circuit model, and the working principle, we employ a readout scheme, as shown in Figure 3.3. The EIS at the core receives its input signals on its top electrode from an external ac-signal source. After passing through an electrolyte, possibly containing cells, the signal reaches selected electrodes. As the changes of current are to be read out, a transimpedance amplifier (TIA) is employed at the pixel level to amplify the received signal at the pixel level. Then the TIA output signal is buffered through a column amplifier and finally passed to an external measurement system for evaluation of cell impedance. Control of the system is done through a microcontroller connected to a host PC for post-data processing.

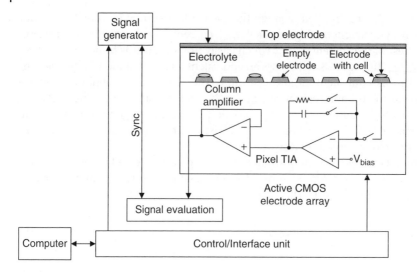

Figure 3.3 Block diagram of the CMOS impedance sensor readout circuit.

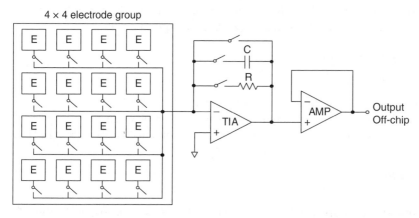

Figure 3.4 Block diagram of a transimpedance amplifier as readout circuit for the shared pixel array.

Considering the layout size as well as to retain the distance between the electrodes and TIA short without requiring a larger electrode size, a group of 4×4 electrodes share one common TIA, as shown in Figure 3.4. The tiling also improves the scalability of the design, because fewer elements need to be combined in each output channel. Within each electrode array, combinational logic is used to select various transimpedance levels and to activate the electrodes based on row and column signals and also global settings. When not selected, the electrodes are kept floating to avoid unnecessary current leakage. If none of the electrodes in the pixel are selected, the output of the amplifier is also decoupled from the column line. The TIA has a selectable transimpedance gain to suit the measurement range of the target biological assay.

The design of the TIA is shown in Figure 3.5, which consists of a PMOS input stage with a folded-cascode design and a class-A output stage. Cascode Miller compensation is used to improve the frequency behavior. Feedback is an implemented variable through

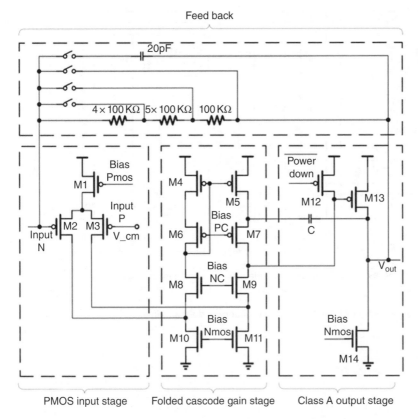

Figure 3.5 Circuit schematic of pixel-level transimpedance amplifier.

a chain of ten 100 kΩ resistors that can be partially bypassed by activating transmission gates. This method is needed to adapt the amplifier to different input impedances. Similarly, a capacitor of 0.86 pF can be added in parallel to adapt the frequency behavior.

For the column level readout amplifier, it is conceptually similar to the pixel amplifiers. However, as shown in Figure 3.6, the input stage includes both an NMOS and PMOS path that are combined in the folded cascode stage. This modification is needed to achieve rail-to-rail input. The column-level column readout amplifier is used in a unity gain configuration and serves as a buffer to drive off-chip loads of up to 20 pF.

3.4 A 96×96 Electronic Impedance Sensing System

3.4.1 Top Architecture

The overall architecture of the 96 × 96 impedance sensing system is shown in Figure 3.7. Due to the nature of slow scanning speeds inherent in processing one electrode at a time, the whole array is split into two independent halves, designated as top and bottom, to double the readout speed. The circuitry in both halves is identical and built up from basic 4 × 4 blocks of electrodes sharing one common TIA. They are arranged in

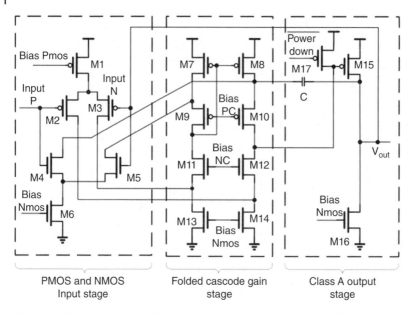

Figure 3.6 Circuit schematic of the column-level column-readout amplifier.

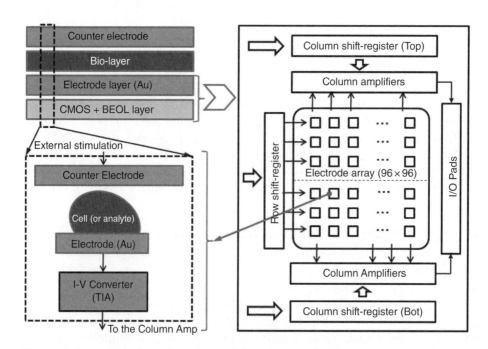

Figure 3.7 Architecture of the 96 × 96 Electronic Impedance Sensing System.

columns of 12 blocks that share a common column amplifier. There are 24 pixel columns in each half to create an array of 96 × 48 electrodes. The individual electrodes are addressable by the use of row shift registers. After each column of electrodes is read out through the column amplifier, the final output is read out off-chip through I/O pads for further processing. Bias currents required by the amplifiers are generated externally and distributed internally through a tree of current mirrors. Bias voltages are also generated externally and distributed without buffers.

3.4.2 System Implementation

3.4.2.1 System Setup

The impedance sensor chip is fabricated in a 0.18 μm standard CMOS process by Global Foundries, featuring six metal layers and a supply voltage of 3.3 V (Figure 3.8(a)). The 96 × 96 electrodes are arranged within a total sensor area of 3.0 mm by 3.0 mm. After fabrication, the electrodes consist of Al as the uppermost metal layer. As this is subject to oxidization and incompatible with bio-testing, post processing is needed. The post-processing steps of the electrode array include a metal deposition step and a single mask lithography step followed by wet etching of the deposited metal. The first step involves the use of an *in-situ* Ar-sputtering process to remove native aluminum oxide from the surface of Al before depositing 100 nm of titanium (Ti) and 1 μm of gold (Au). A 2 μm-thick photoresist (Sumiresist PFI26A, Sumitomo, Japan) is exposed by UV i-line Hg light using an EVG 6200 mask aligner (EV Group, Schärding, Austria). The exposed Au areas are subsequently etched in Au-etchant (Au-600, CLC, ROC) for 90 s, while the 100 nm-thick Ti adhesion film is etched with Ti-etchant (Ti-890, CLC, ROC) for a duration of 60 s. The wet etching process incurs an undercut of approximately 1.5 μm on the Au electrodes, producing arrays of patterned Au electrodes of 22 μm × 22 μm in size.

The counter electrode area is kept much larger than the working electrode, to ensure that impedance is dominated by the surface properties of the working electrode. As depicted in the zoom-in optical image in Figure 3.8(b), Au electrodes are uniformly separated at 8-μm intervals and the size of the Au electrode is 22 μm × 22 μm, which is comparable to single MCF-7 cell (~20 μm diameter). A scanning electron microscopy (SEM) of a slice of cross-sectioned electrode (Figure 3.8(c)), taken using focus ion beam (FIB), indicates 1-μm thick Au deposited on top of a 2.5-μm thick Al layer.

The chip was attached to a ceramic 68 pin grid array (PGA) carrier using silver epoxy (H20E, Epoxy Technology, Inc.) and wire bonded, as shown in Figure 3.8(d). The glob top silicone encapsulant (Silicone 3140, Dow Corning), which is biocompatible, was used to make a chamber (200 μm high) and insulate the bonded wire. Indium-tin-oxide (ITO) coated glass was positioned on top of the chamber to act as a counter electrode. Owing to transparency and good electrical properties, ITO coated glass provides ease of optical imaging and produces an uniform electric field between the Au working electrodes and the counter electrode. Before EIS measurement, the packaged chip was treated in oxygen-plasma for 5 min for final cleaning and to make the chip hydrophilic, so that the solution can easily flow into the chamber by capillary forces.

The CMOS chip mounted on a disposable ceramic PGA carrier was plugged into the socket of a printed circuit board (PCB)-based control unit. The control unit is intended to address working electrodes organized in an array with 96 rows and 96 columns.

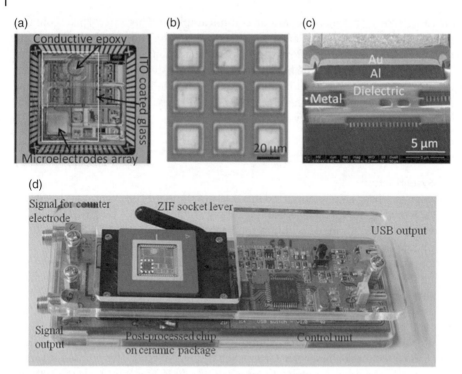

Figure 3.8 Electrical-impedance spectroscopy (EIS) platform for the detection and enumeration of CTCs: (a) Optical image of high-density CMOS electrodes surrounded with silicone glob top to make a chamber. The ITO coated glass is positioned on top of the chamber to act as a counter electrode; (b) Zoomed optical image of post-processed CMOS microelectrode array with exposed gold capping for bio-sensing; and (c) Cross-sectional scanning electron micrograph of a 22-m wide microelectrode with 6 stacks of metal layers. A 0.1-m thick Ti adhesion layer is sandwich between Au and Al (not shown).

A software interface for control unit was designed to locate and activate the working electrodes. An HP 4284 LCR meter was connected to a PCB control unit through SMA connectors. Impedance measurement of the working electrode over a wide frequency and voltage range was realized by an LCR meter controlled by a program developed in LabVIEW.

3.4.2.2 Sample Preparation

Breast cancer cell, MCF-7 (American Type Culture Collection, MD, USA), derived from breast adenocarcinoma, is a popular cell model to study the spreading of cancer. The cells were cultured in minimum essential media (MEM) (Gibco, cat# 11095-080) supplemented with 10% fetal bovine serum (FBS) (Gibco, cat# 0270106), 1 mM sodium pyruvate (Gibco, cat# 11360-070), 0.1 mM MEM nonessential amino acids (Gibco, cat# 11140-050), and grown at 37 °C under a 5% CO_2 atmosphere in a T75 flask.

3.4.3 Results

With a 20-μl phosphate buffered saline (PBS) solution on top of the chip, electrode impedance was monitored at alternative current (AC) potential of 25 mV peak to peak and frequencies ranging from 100 Hz to 1 MHz using an LCR meter. EIS recording for electrodes was done in a sequential manner in a two electrode measurement system. Then, a 20 μl of the MCF-7 cells ($5 \times 10_5$ cell/ml) solution in PBS was injected and incubated for 15 min to allow the cells to settle on the electrodes. The barrier from 1 μm height silicone nitrate passivation along the side of each electrode pixel makes a small chamber on each electrode and helps to occupy only a single cell. The cell started to flatten on the surface and covered the electrode more compactly over time. Optical image of the sensing area was taken and electrodes covered with cells were identified to correlate with the impedance reading. After incubation, impedance measurements were recorded and the impedance change of electrodes with and without cells was calculated. For basic electrical characterization of the chip, the impedance spectra of electrodes were recorded with 25 mV peak-to-peak sinusoidal voltage at 200 kHz across 6500 electrodes in PBS. All recordings were performed at room temperature.

3.4.3.1 Data Fitting for Single Cell Impedance Measurement

The impedance of cells cultured over microelectrodes has been investigated extensively [18,21–23]. The characteristic frequency response of cell-covered microelectrodes shows a significant dependence on electrode size [11], cell adhesion, and spreading on the electrode [19]. To investigate the frequency-dependent characteristics of the CMOS-based electrode, we have recorded impedance spectrum of electrode with and without cells attached under two different measuring buffer conditions, in pure PBS and in PBS spiked with cells (called cell buffer). Figure 3.9(a) shows the plot of the impedance measured in pure PBS in the absence of any cell (black circle) and that measured with a single cell occupying the electrode (red triangle) in the cell buffer. From the figure, it is clear that there is an increase in the impedance at intermediate frequency (50–500 kHz), which is attributed to cells obstructing the current flow. At the low-frequency end of the spectrum (f < 10 kHz), the impedance of the system is dominated by the rather high resistance of the electrode/electrolyte interface. Looking at the high-frequency end (>500 kHz), the resistance seems to remain constant due to the current spreading from localized electrode to a distant counter electrode into the solution. This is the spreading resistance dominated regime. Figure 3.9(b) is a control experiment where changing of measuring buffer conditions shows negligible change in the impedance spectrum of electrode without cell capturing.

Using the circuit model presented in Figure 3.2, the data from the experiment were fitted and the values of electrode impedance, cell impedance, sealing resistance, and spreading resistance were derived. The solid lines in Figure 3.9(a) show a good fit to the measured impedance. Table 3.1 reveals the model parameter values extracted from the fitted results.

Although, in Figure 3.9(a), measured impedance change due to cell is significant at the intermediate frequency in Bode magnitude plot, an alternate way of plotting the same data, that is, normalized impedance change (Figure 3.9(c)) using Equation (3.4), can be used to better observe the effect of the cell on the electrode:

$$r = \frac{Z_{cell} - Z_{nocell}}{Z_{nocell}} \tag{3.4}$$

where Z_{cell} is impedance with the cell covered electrode, and Z_{nocell} is impedance without the cell on the electrode. The normalized impedance change is represented as a percentage (%) value.

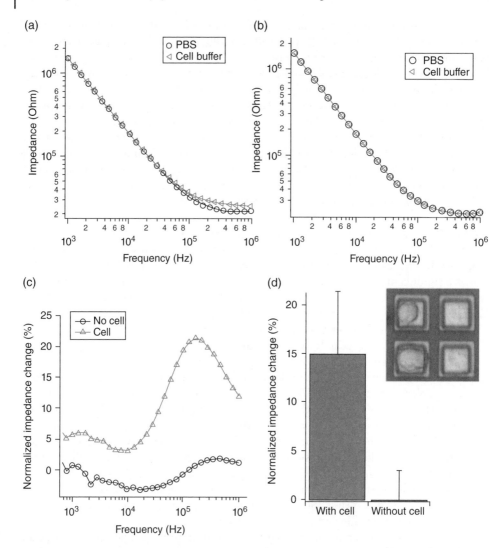

Figure 3.9 (a) Impedance spectroscopy of electrode with cell attached in cell buffer; (b) Impedance spectroscopy of electrode without cell attached in cell buffer. The black circles represent impedance spectrum of electrode without cell in pure PBS; (c) Percentage of normalized impedance change as a function of measured frequency; (d) Statistical normalized impedance changes with the presence and absence of cell on microelectrode (n = 45 over three chip with cell, n = 47 over three chip without cell). The inset shows an optical image of microelectrodes with presence of cells (left column) and absence of cell (right column).

Compared to an empty electrode, a distinct peak of 21% impedance change was observed due to a single cell on the electrode measured at a frequency of 200 kHz (Figure 3.9(c)). The results reveal that impedance measurement on the CMOS electrode enables distinguishing the presence of the cell on the electrode and a single frequency point measurement can be used for cell detection and counting. Figure 3.9(d) shows the statistic of the normalized impedance changes when electrode impedance is recorded

Table 3.1 Extracted parameter from equivalent circuit model.

Parameter	Values
Z_{elec}	$k/(i\omega)m$; $k = 3.89 \times 10^9$; $m = 0.9$
R_{sp}	Without cell 20.79 kΩ; With cell 22.90 kΩ
Z_{cell}	$C_m = 7.67$ pF, $R_m = 32.5$ MΩ
R_{seal}	0.14 MΩ

at 200 kHz. All plotted bars are mean values of three data series measured in three CMOS chips. As shown in Figure 3.9(d), the averaged normalized impedance change due to a single cell on an electrode is $14.9 \pm 6.4\%$, whereas the highest change of the electrode without the cell is around 5%. Therefore, we are confident to use the 7% normalized impedance change as a cut-off point for determining the "on" and "off" states of the working electrode. Each "on" state of the working electrode is counted as a single cell occupying the electrode and the "off-state" is represented as an empty electrode.

3.4.3.2 Cell and Electrode Impedance Analysis
The value of the normalized impedance change calculated from experimental data is significant to reveal the presence of the cell on the electrode. However, it is worth noting that Narayana *et al.* reported more than 50% normalized impedance change due to the cell on the electrode [24]. The difference can be attributed to the 24 hours of incubation used by other works, which causes the flattening of cells on the electrode surface to cover more area and decreases the cell separation distance from the electrode on longer incubation. However, longer incubation increases the testing time. In contrast, in this study, electrode impedance was recorded after 15 minutes of cell incubation and clear differentiation was observed in the presence or absence of the cell on the electrode. Thus, the present system shortens the testing time with a high confidence level in determining cell presence.

Furthermore, to understand how the cell adhesion affects the electrode impedance, cell modeling and simulation were performed for varying sealing resistance. The values for modeling parameters were obtained from the experiment data. Figure 3.10(a) shows the impedance spectrum of the electrode covered with a single cell. The impedance of the cell covered electrode shows an increase at intermediate frequency with sealing resistance. The results agree well with the lumped equivalent circuit models proposed by Huang *et al.* [18]. As shown in Figure 3.10(b), a distinct peak value can also be observed in the spectrum of normalized impedance change. It is clear that a sealing resistance of 0.84 MΩ results in more than 100% normalized impedance change. Thus, the simulation results suggest that sealing resistance (determine by the cell electrode separation distance) becomes a dominant component in measured signals for cells tightly adhered onto the electrode surface.

3.4.3.3 EIS for Single-Cell Impedance Enumeration
Experiments to assess the correlation between the impedance signals and the cell occupancy on the electrode array were also conducted. Figure 3.11(a) depicts the optical

(a)

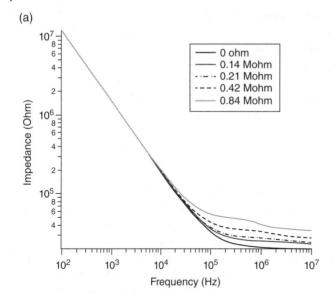

(b)

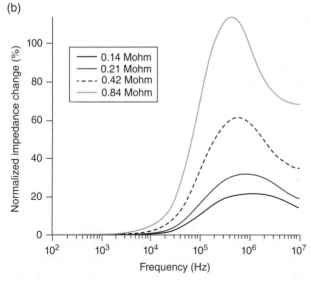

Figure 3.10 Calculated impedance magnitude as a function of frequency for 22 μm² electrode covered with cells: (a) Impedance evolution when R_{seal} increases for cell covered electrode, and (b) Normalized impedance change as a function of frequency. Each line corresponds to values of R_{seal} in the range of 0.14–0.84 MΩ.

image of electrode array with and without cells present. The membrane giving the cell shape is clearly seen on the electrode occupied by a cell. To correlate with impedance signals, each electrode was associated with a binary color (black and gray), depending on cell presence on the electrode. The black square indicates an electrode covered with cells on top, whereas the gray square indicates an empty electrode. EIS recording was performed at 200 kHz with an excitation AC voltage of 25 mV to obtain the electrode

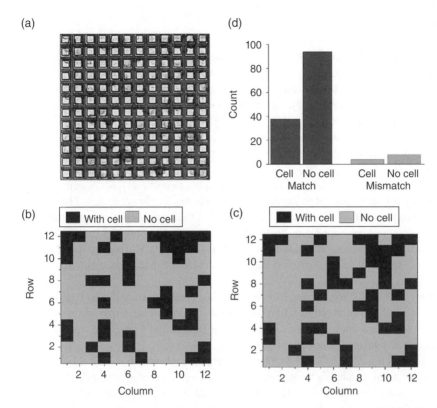

Figure 3.11 (a) Optical image of cells seeded on a 12×12 microelectrode array; (b) Optical mapping; and (c) Impedance mapping of cells on the microelectrode array. The dark and gray square denote the status of an individual electrode; (d) The categories plot shows the accuracy of impedance mapping from an array of 144 pixels. A mapping accuracy of 90% was achieved.

impedance. The "on" states of the working electrode are recorded when normalized impedance change is above 7%. Figures 3.11(b) and (c) are the comparison between optical mapping and the impedance spectroscopy measurement on the 12×12 electrode array. In the maps, most of the electrode pixels are a good match, indicating good agreement between impedance spectroscopy and optical measurement.

Figure 3.11(d) presents a detailed matching statistic from 144 working electrodes. The best match of electrode pixels with cells and without cells are 38 and 94 electrodes respectively. The mismatch of electrode pixels with cells and without cells is with a small number electrodes, which are 4 and 8 electrodes respectively. A mapping accuracy is calculated by dividing the total number of matched electrodes to the total working electrodes and found to be more than 90%. We also study the impedance percentage change over a large number of working electrodes (46 by 46) by incubating with a large number of cells. The results indicated clearly that the impedance change of the electrode covered by cells is more than 7%, whereas the impedance change in the control experiment by changing the PBS solution is negligible. As a result, the present device has clearly shown digitized cell counting capability and results are not subjected to operator variance.

References

1 S.B. Prakash and P. Abshire (2008) Tracking cancer cell proliferation on a CMOS capacitance sensor chip. *Biosensors and Bioelectronics*, 23, 1449–1457.

2 F. Xie, Y. Xu, L. Wang, K. Mitchelson, W. Xing, *et al.* (2012) Use of cellular electrical impedance sensing to assess *in vitro* cytotoxicity of anticancer drugs in a human kidney cell nephrotoxicity model. *Analyst*, 137, 1343–1350.

3 T. Li, Q. Fan, T. Liu, X. Zhu, J. Zhao and G. Li (2010) Detection of breast cancer cells specially and accurately by an electrochemical method. *Biosensors and Bioelectronics*, 25, 2686–2689.

4 T.S. Pui, A. Agarwal, F. Ye, N. Balasubramanian and P. Chen (2009) CMOS-compatible nanowire sensor arrays for detection of cellular bioelectricity. *Small*, 5, 208–212.

5 A. Han, L. Yang and A.B. Frazier (2007) Quantification of the heterogeneity in breast cancer cell lines using whole-cell impedance spectroscopy. *Clinical Cancer Research*, 13, 139–143.

6 R. de la Rica, S. Thompson, A. Baldi, C. Fernandez-Sanchez, C.M. Drain and H. Matsui (2009) Label-free cancer cell detection with impedimetric transducers. *Analytical Chemistry*, 81, 10167–10171.

7 A.A. Adams, P.I. Okagbare, J. Feng, M.L. Hupert, D. Patterson, *et al.* (2008) Highly efficient circulating tumor cell isolation from whole blood and label-free enumeration using polymer-based microfluidics with an integrated conductivity sensor. *Journal of the American Chemical Society*, 130, 8633–8641.

8 Y.K. Chung, J. Reboud, K.C. Lee, H.M. Lim, P.Y. Lim, *et al.* (2011) An electrical biosensor for the detection of circulating tumor cells. *Biosensors and Bioelectronics*, 26, 2520–2526.

9 A. Manickam, A. Chevalier, M. McDermott, *et al.* (2010) A CMOS Electrochemical Impedance Spectroscopy (EIS) biosensor array. *IEEE Transactions on Biomedical Circuits and Systems*, 4(6), 379–390.

10 G.T. Budd, M. Cristofanilli, M.J. Ellis, A. Stopeck, E. Borden, *et al.* (2006) Circulating tumor cells versus imaging – predicting overall survival in metastatic breast cancer. *Clinical Cancer Research*, 12, 6403–6409.

11 S.K. Arya, K.C. Lee, D.B. Dah'alan and A.R. Rahman (2012) Breast tumor cell detection at single cell resolution using an electrochemical impedance technique. *Lab Chip*, 12, 2362–2368.

12 X. Jiang and M.G. Spencer (2010) Electrochemical impedance biosensor with electrode pixels for precise counting of CD4+ cells: A microchip for quantitative diagnosis of HIV infection status of AIDS patients. *Biosensors and Bioelectronics*, 25, 1622–1628.

13 Q. Bai and K.D. Wise (2001) Single-unit neural recording with active microelectrode arrays. *IEEE Transactions on Biomedical Engineering.* 48, 911–920.

14 F. Heer, W. Franks, A. Blau, S. Taschini, C. Ziegler, *et al.* (2004) CMOS microelectrode array for the monitoring of electrogenic cells. *Biosensors and Bioelectronics*, 20, 358–366.

15 L. Berdondini, P.D. van der Wal, O. Guenat, N.F. de Rooij, M. Koudelka-Hep, *et al.* (2005) High-density electrode array for imaging *in vitro* electrophysiological activity. *Biosensors and Bioelectronics*, 21, 167–174.

16 F. Heer, S. Hafizovic, T. Ugniwenko, U. Frey, W. Franks, *et al.* (2007) Single-chip microelectronic system to interface with living cells. *Biosensors and Bioelectronics*, 22, 2546–2553.

17 Y. Chen, C.C. Wong, T.S. Pui, R. Nadipalli, R. Weerasekera, *et al.* (2012) CMOS high density electrical impedance biosensor array for tumor cell detection. *Sensors and Actuators B: Chemical*, 173, 903–907.

18 X. Huang, N. Duc, D.W. Greve and M.M. Domach (2004) Simulation of microelectrode impedance changes due to cell growth. *IEEE Sensors Journal*, 4, 576–583.

19 N. Goda, Y. Yamamoto, T. Nakamura, T. Kusuhara, S. Mohri, *et al.* (2006) Quantitative evaluation of micro-motion of vascular endothelial cells in electrical cell-substrate impedance sensing (ECIS) method using a precision mathematical model. In: *International Conference on Microtechnologies in Medicine and Biology*, pp. 23–26.

20 R.W. Wiertz, W.L. Rutten and E. Marani (2010) Impedance sensing for monitoring neuronal coverage and comparison with microscopy. *IEEE Transactions on Biomedical Engineering*, 57, 2379–2385.

21 W. Franks, I. Schenker, P. Schmutz and A. Hierlemann (2005) Impedance characterization and modeling of electrodes for biomedical applications. *IEEE Transactions on Biomedical Engineering*, 52, 1295–1302.

22 R.W. Wiertz, E. Marani and W.L. Rutten (2010) Inhibition of neuronal cell–cell adhesion measured by the microscopic aggregation assay and impedance sensing. *Journal of Neural Engineering*, 7, 1.

23 M. Thein, F. Asphahani, A. Cheng, R. Buckmaster, M. Zhang and J. Xu (2010) Response characteristics of single-cell impedance sensors employed with surface-modified microelectrodes. *Biosensors and Bioelectronics*, 25, 1963–1969.

24 S. Narayanan, M. Nikkhah, J.S. Strobl and M. Agah (2010) Analysis of the passivation layer by testing and modeling a cell impedance micro-sensor. *Sensors and Actuators A: Physical*, 159, 241–247.

4

CMOS Terahertz Sensor

4.1 Introduction

The terahertz (THz) radiation (0.1–30 THz) is categorized between millimeter-wave (mm-wave) and infrared light wave [1]. Recently, a great deal of attention has been paid to the THz spectroscopy and imaging system due to the moderate wavelength of THz wave that can leverage the advantages of both millimeter-waves (mm-waves) and light waves [1–3]. As with the mm-wave, the THz wave has deep penetration to dielectric substances such as ceramics, plastics, powders, and food; like light waves, THz images with high spatial resolution can be obtained by two-dimensional (2-D) detection with a THz sensor array [4].

THz imaging has been used in many applications, as shown in Figure 4.1. It has several distinct advantages when compared to other imaging techniques, such as ultrasound scan, magnetic resonance imaging (MRI), confocal microscopy (CM), and optical coherence tomography (OCT). First, THz imaging has higher resolution than ultrasound scan or MRI, due to its much shorter wavelength. It is also more sensitive to thin tissues due to a stronger reflection and attenuation in the water content. Second, compared to existing optics-based imaging methods such as CM and OCT, even though THz imaging system has a lower resolution, it has much higher penetration depth due to its much longer wavelength. Recently, remarkable contrast in skin and breast cancer has been demonstrated in THz images [7,8]. The THz imaging system has been used as an intra-operative tool during breast cancer surgery at Guys Hospital in London [9].

4.2 CMOS THz Pixel

4.2.1 Differential TL-SRR Resonator Design

4.2.1.1 Stacked SRR Layout

The on-chip split ring resonator (SRR) can be implemented in a stacked fashion with on-chip multi-layer interconnection [10]. As shown in Figure 4.2(a), one SRR unit-cell is realized by the top two metal layers stacked alternately, considering a trade-off among resonant frequency, area, and loss. When its size is fixed, S21 of the T-line SRR (TL-SRR) with different stacked layers is shown as in Figure 4.2(b). It is found that more stacked layers result in lower resonant frequency, but suffer from lower Q at the same time.

CMOS Integrated Lab-on-a-Chip System for Personalized Biomedical Diagnosis,
First Edition. Hao Yu, Mei Yan, and Xiwei Huang.
© 2018 John Wiley & Sons Singapore Pte. Ltd. Published 2018 by John Wiley & Sons Singapore Pte. Ltd.

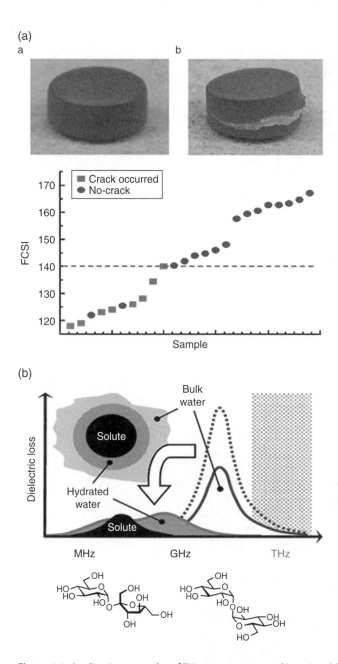

Figure 4.1 Application examples of THz spectroscopy and imaging: (a) Nondestructive detection of crack initiation in a film-coated layer on a swelling tablet [5]; (b) Hydration state characterization in solution [6];

(c)

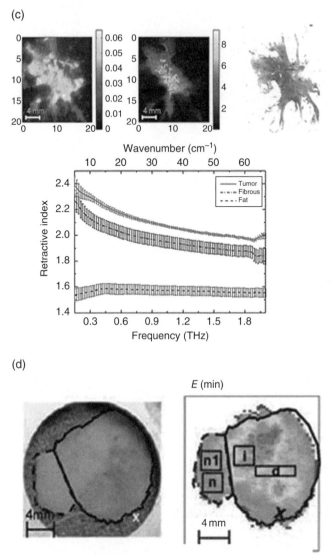

(d)

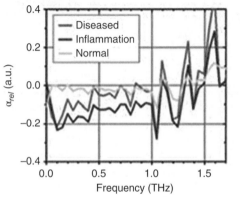

Figure 4.1 (Continued) (c) *In-vitro* breast cancer diagnosis [7]; and (d) *In-vivo* skin cancer diagnosis [8].

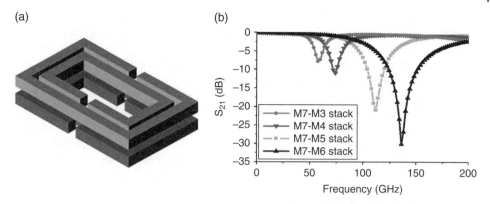

Figure 4.2 (a) Stacked SRR unit-cell designed by metal layers of M7 and M6; and (b) S21 simulation results with different stacking methods.

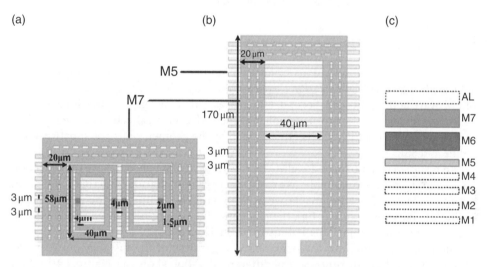

Figure 4.3 Geometries of resonators with slow-wave shielding: (a) Differential T-line loaded with stacked SRR; (b) T-line based standing-wave resonator; and (c) Cross-section of BEOL.

With the increased resonant frequency, TL-SRR reveals a steeper and higher rejection property, which means a higher Q. Thus, TL-SRR shows potential application for on-chip MMIC designs.

Figure 4.3(a) shows a differential T-line with stacked on-chip SRR (DTL-SRR) in the CMOS process, of which the cross-section is illustrated in Figure 4.3(c). A T-line-based standing-wave resonator is also shown here as a comparison in Figure 4.3(b). The two loaded SRR unit-cells are excited by the axial magnetic field generated by the host T-line. It has the following advantages in Q improvement. First, as the SRR-load is metamaterial with stop-band properties, it results in large impedance with the open circuit condition formed. Thus, electromagnetic (EM) energy can be perfectly reflected in the host T-line. Second, the differential design provides local ground to reduce EM loss and enhance the EM-energy coupling.

For example, the magnetic field generated by the differential T-line is equidirectional and superimposed when applied to the two SRR unit-cells. Therefore, a stronger coupling between T-line and SRR is achieved with larger mutual capacitance and mutual inductance, which can store more EM-energy with less EM-energy leakage into the substrate. Due to the stronger EM coupling, the DTL-SRR needs less SRR unit-cells than STL-SRR when the same rejection property is achieved. This makes the DTL-SRR achieve higher area efficiency as well. To strengthen the coupling between the T-line and SRRs, the shortest distance (or gap) between the T-line and SRRS is selected with the consideration of the process limitation (1.5 μm in STM 65 nm CMOS). Lastly, floating metal shielding is also employed in this design to further reduce substrate loss.

4.2.1.2 Comparison with Single-ended TL-SRR Resonator

In the following, we show a detailed analysis of the enhancement of the Q factor with a comparison between the DTL-SRR and STL-SRR. Assuming both terminals of SRR unit-cell observe the same characteristic impedance (Z_0)

$$\Gamma = \frac{R'_s}{R'_s + 2Z_0} = \frac{k^2}{k^2 + 2Z_0 L_s / R_s L} \tag{4.1}$$

We can make two observations from Equation (4.1). First, if the Q factor of SRR is sufficiently high that $k^2 \gg 2Z_0 L_s / R_s L$ Γ approaches unity, which means a perfect reflection of EM-wave at the SRR-load. Second, Γ increases with k for a given SRR with a finite Q. Thus, improving k is the means to enhance the EM-energy reflection efficiency. Note that the coupling coefficient k is often limited by the geometry mismatch between the T-line and SSR.

As a result, in order to have a high-Q DTL-SRR design, we need to have the reflection coefficient Γ as high as possible. We can observe from Equation (4.1) that Γ increases with the coupling coefficient between SSRs and the T-line. In the single-ended T-line, as shown in Figure 4.4(a), the magnetic flux cannot be fully covered between the SRR and the T-line. This is illustrated in Figure 4.4(c), as there is part of the magnetic flux leaking into the open space, regardless of the distance between the SRR and the T-line. In contrast, the differential T-line shown in Figure 4.4(b) does not have this limitation. As we can see from Figure 4.4(d), it is possible to have the SRR fully covering the magnetic flux generated by the differential T-line. Thus, a high EM coupling coeffcient can be achieved with a higher Γ for the DTL-SRR structure than the STL-SRR structure.

To further validate the high-Q of DTL-SRR, EM simulation (Agilent ADS momentum) is performed for STL-SRR and DTL-SRR structures, as shown in Figures 4.4(a) and (b). The conductivity of the top-most metal layers M6 and M7 are 4.6 × 107 S/m, the metal layers M1 ~ M5 are 4.1 × 107 S/m, and the silicon substrate is 10 S/m according to the 65-nm CMOS process files. The simulation results of Γ are plotted against the different gap size in Figure 4.5. We can observe that the reflection coefficient of DTL-SRR is much higher than STL-SRR. Moreover, the reflection coefficient is increased for a smaller gap size. For example, at the minimum gap of 2 μm that is allowed by the design rule, the reflection coefficient of the differential T-line is 10.6% higher than that of the single-ended T-line. Since the minimum gap size is limited by the design rule, the maximum reflection coefficient we can obtain is around 0.9. The Q factor

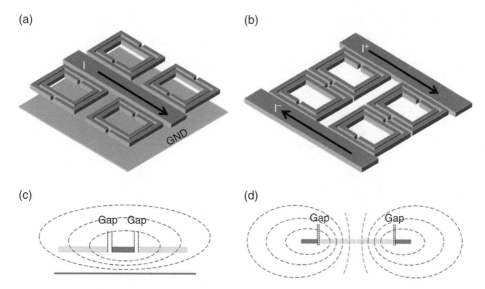

Figure 4.4 T-line-based SRR excitation: (a) Single-ended approach; (b) Differential approach; (c) Magnetic field distribution of single-ended approach; and (d) Magnetic field distribution of differential approach.

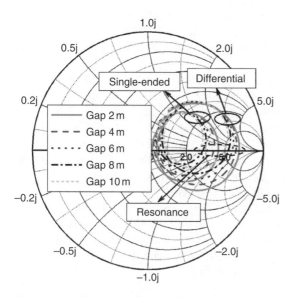

Figure 4.5 Reflection coefficients of both single ended and differential resonators.

for both resonators is also comparable to the reflection coefficient, as shown in Figure 4.6. As discussed, a high reflection coefficient of DTL-SRR can be directly transferred into a high Q. We can observe that the Q of DTL-SRR is around 20 ~ 40% higher than that of STL-SRR with the same gap size.

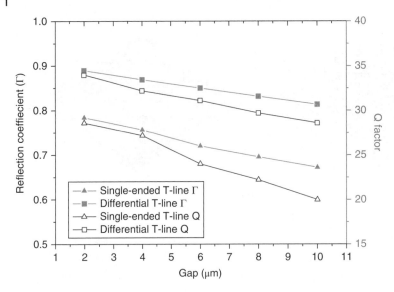

Figure 4.6 Simulated Γ and quality factor (Q) of SRR/T-line unit cell at resonance.

4.2.1.3 Comparison with Standing-Wave Resonator

We further compare the proposed DTL-SRR resonator with the standing-wave resonator using a coplanar stripline (CPS). As shown in Figure 4.3, they are both designed under the same resonance frequency and are also provided with floating metal shielding to reduce substrate loss.

The optimization of the two structures is conducted with the full-wave EM simulator (Agilent Momentum). As with the DTL-SRR-based metamaterial resonator, the stacked SRR unit-cell is designed with the top two metal layers (M7, M6). M7 and M5 are used for the design of the host T-line and the floating metal strips for shielding of the two resonators, respectively. The sizes of the T-line, the SRR, and floating metal strips are carefully selected to obtain the desired frequency. Moreover, for the CPS-based standing-wave resonator, its Q factor also depends on the width and the separation of the T-line, the width of the floating metal strip, and the spacing between two adjacent floating metal strips. Due to the parasitic capacitance of the cross-coupled NMOS transistors and the layout-dependent parasitic effect, the physical length of CPS is shorter than the ideal length of λ/4. The detailed physical sizes are shown in Figure 4.3) and we can observe that the use of SRR has a 40% area reduction than with the use of CPS.

Note that the Q of one resonator can be described by:

$$Q = \omega \frac{\text{Average\_energy\_stored}}{\text{Energy\_loss / second}} \tag{4.2}$$

As such, we can now compare the Q factors of the DTL-SRR with the standing-wave resonator. First, the smaller size of the DTL-SRR leads to a lower substrate loss, and hence the denominator above decreases. Second, for the DTL-SRR, the strong EM-energy coupling between the SRR and T-line with perfect reflection can enhance the energy storage capability with the nominator in Equation (4.2) increasing. Thereby, we can expect that a higher quality factor can be achieved by DTL-SRR than with the standing-wave resonator, which is further validated by the measured experiment results.

4.2.2 Differential TL-CSRR Resonator Design

It is not feasible to directly deploy the etched CSRR from the ground on-chip due to the lossy substrate in CMOS process [11]. To realize a low-loss and high-Q implementation for on-chip CSRR, we now show that the CSRR can be etched directly onto the metal layer using signal lines. Compared with the previous method [11], CSRRs on the metal layer can form a much stronger coupling between the T-line and CSRR, because they are on the same metal layer. More EM-energy can thereby be stored in the resonator and the n-turn results in a higher Q-factor.

A differential CSRR structure is proposed in Figure 4.7 to provide a compact area. Both inputs are designed on the same side to provide an ac-ground for easy dc-supply, which further reduces the potential coupling to the lossy substrate. Note that the metamaterial property of the proposed differential T-line loaded CSRR and its high-Q feature can be illustrated through simulation as follows.

For example, the metamaterial property can be calculated from S-parameters by [12,13]:

$$\cos(nkd) = \frac{1 - S_{11}^2 + S_{21}^2}{2S_{21}},$$

$$z = \pm\sqrt{\frac{(1 + S_{11})^2 - S_{21}^2}{(1 - S_{11})^2 - S_{21}^2}}, \tag{4.3}$$

$$\varepsilon = \frac{n}{z}, \ \mu = nz.$$

where n is the refractive index, z is the wave-impedance, k is wave-factor, and d is the physical length. Because the metamaterial is considered as a passive medium, n and z in

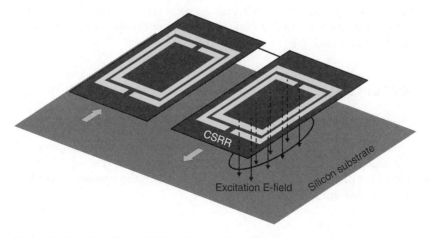

Figure 4.7 On-chip differential T-line loaded with CSRR.

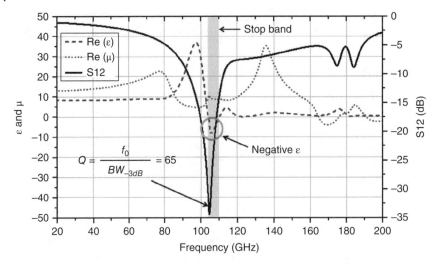

Figure 4.8 EM characterization of the proposed differential CSRR resonator.

Equation (4.3) can be determined by two requirements: $\mathcal{J}(n) \geq 0$ and $\mathcal{R}(z) \geq 0$, where $\mathcal{J}(n)$ and $\mathcal{R}(z)$ denote the imaginary part and real part of n and z, respectively.

Based on Equation (4.3), we can characterize the metamaterial resonator. The proposed DTL-CSRR structure in Figure 4.7 is implemented on-chip with resonance frequency biased around 100 GHz. ADS Momentum is used for the EM simulation to obtain the S-parameters. As shown in Figure 4.8, a negative μ can be observed within a narrow band near the resonance frequency. As stated earlier, the negative μ and positive ε create the electric plasma, where the propagating EM wave becomes an evanescent wave and is largely reflected backwards. The deep rejection frequency band with a sharp cut-off can be viewed from the S12 plot in Figure 4.8, which corresponds to a high-Q performance.

The Q-factor can be estimated from the simulation by $Q = f_0 / BW_{-3dB}$, where f_0 is the resonance frequency and BW_{3dB} is the bandwidth. As such, the obtained Q-factor is 65, which is much higher than the normal Q value by a resonator composed of an LC-tank at similar frequency, of around 30 as indicated in [14].

4.3 Readout Circuit

4.3.1 Super-regenerative Amplification

Generally, an SRX consists of a quench-controlled oscillator injected by an external signal and an envelope detector. The process of injecting an external signal into a quench-controlled oscillator is first reviewed to understand the operation of SRX, called super-regenerative amplification (SRA).

4.3.1.1 Equivalent Circuit of SRA

A simplified circuit model of SRA is shown in Figure 4.9. The resonator is modeled by the RLC block, and its oscillation is quench-controlled by a time-dependent negative

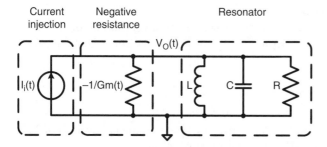

Figure 4.9 Simplified equivalent circuit model of super-regenerative amplifier.

resistance $-1/G_m(t)$, where G_m is the equivalent conductance determined by the associated active devices. The external signal injected is modeled as a time-dependent current source where $I_i(t)$. $V_O(t)$ is the output voltage. The resonance frequency is $\omega_0 = \dfrac{1}{\sqrt{LC}}$; the quality factor is $Q_0 = R/Z_0 = 0.5\zeta_0^{-1}$ and Z_0 and ζ_0 are the characteristic impedance and quiescent damping factor, respectively.

Assume $G_m(t)$ varies much slower than ω_0, such that a quasi-static condition holds in the system to have a time-varying transfer function in s-domain by:

$$\frac{V_o(s,\,t)}{I_i(s)} = \frac{Z_0\omega_0 s}{s^2 + 2\zeta(t)\omega_0 s + \omega_0^2} \tag{4.4}$$

where $\zeta(t) = \zeta_0\big[1 - G_m(t)R\big]$ is the instantaneous damping factor.

A second-order linear time variant system can be observed from Equation (4.4). By varying $\zeta(t)$ the pole can be shifted between the left and right sides of the s-plane periodically. In other words, the oscillation starts in SRA when $\zeta(t)$ is negative, and stops when $\zeta(t)$ is positive. Note that Equation (4.4) is only valid when SRA works in linear mode, such that $V_O(s,t)$ is small enough to prevent significant distortion in each quench cycle. Generally, SRA working in linear mode is preferred in the application of THz imaging, since it has a better sensitivity than that in the logarithmic mode [15,16].

After Laplace transform, Equation (4.4) can be written as a second-order differential equation in the time domain:

$$v_o''(t) + 2\zeta(t)\omega_0 v_o'(t) + \omega_0^2 v_o(t) = Z_0\omega_0 I_i'(t) \tag{4.5}$$

Assume the oscillation is fully quenched in each cycle, such that $v_o(t)$ is independent of the previous ones. For a particular quench cycle $t \in (t_a, t_b]$ with $t_a < 0 < t_b$, if $\zeta(t)$ is positive for $t \in (t_a, 0]$ and negative for $t \in (0, t_b]$, then Equation (4.5) can be written as [16]:

$$v_o(t) = \frac{Z_0}{s(t)} \int_{t_a}^{t} I_i'(\tau)\, s(\tau) \sin\big[\omega_0(t-\tau)\big]\, d\tau \tag{4.6}$$

where $s(t) = e^{\omega_0 \int_0^t \zeta(\lambda)\, d\lambda}$ is called the sensitivity function, and reaches its maximum when $t = 0$; and decays rapidly with t. As a result, the SRA is only sensitive to the input $I_i'(t)$ in the time window centered at $t = 0$ when $\zeta(t)$ turns from positive to negative.

4.3.1.2 Frequency Response of SRA

The frequency response of SRA can be analyzed with the convolution model [17]. For an AC current input with $I_i(t) = I_0 \sin(\omega_i t + \varnothing_i)$, the output waveform can be approximated by:

$$v_o(t) \approx \frac{Z_0 \omega_i I_0}{2s(t)} |S(\Delta\omega)| \sin(\omega_0 t + \phi_i) \qquad (4.7)$$

where $\Delta\omega = \omega_0 - \omega_i$ and S(ω) is the Fourier transform of s(t). In the application of THz imaging, we are more interested in the envelope of v_o, which is:

$$Env[v_o(t)] = \frac{Z_0 \omega_i I_0}{2s(t)} |S(\Delta\omega)| \qquad (4.8)$$

Assuming that ω_i is close to $\omega_0 (\Delta\omega \ll \omega_i)$, a quasi-static condition holds in Equation (4.8) that the frequency response of $Env(v_o(t))$ is determined by $|S(\Delta\omega)|$. For a typical ramping quench signal with time variant conductance $G_m = \frac{1}{R}(kt + 1)$, where k is the normalized ramping slope of G_m with the unit of 1/s, the instantaneous damping factor is $\zeta(t) = -\frac{k}{2Q_0}t$. Thus the envelope of $v_o(t)$ can be solved by:

$$Env[v_o(t)]_{ramp} = \frac{\sqrt{\pi} Z_0 \omega_i I_0}{\Omega_0} e^{\frac{\Omega_0^2}{4}t^2} e^{-\frac{\Delta\omega^2}{\Omega_0^2}} \qquad (4.9)$$

where $\Omega_0 = \sqrt{k\omega_0/Q_0}$ is a constant that determines the frequency response of SRA, for example the 3-dB bandwidth of SRA equals 1.177 Ω_0 As such, we can observe that for the given k and ω_0, the bandwidth is inversely proportional to Q_0.

4.3.1.3 Sensitivity of SRA

The sensitivity of SRA is defined as the minimum detected power, which means the induced output signal power is the same as its variance:

$$S_{SRA} = P_{min}|_{I_x^2 = \sigma_x^2} = \frac{I_0^2 R}{2} \Big|_{I_x^2 = \sigma_x^2} \qquad (4.10)$$

where I_x is the equivalent induced current in SRA in response to the ac input I_i and σ_x^2 is the variance of I_x. As discussed in [17], for a typical ramp-damping function with a normalized ramping slope of k, we have:

$$I_x = \frac{I_0 \omega_0 \sigma_s}{2}, \quad \sigma_x^2 = \frac{N\omega_0^2 E_g}{2} \qquad (4.11)$$

where $\sigma_s = \sqrt{2Q_0/\omega_0 k}$ is the SRA time constant with a unit of $s/\sqrt{rad} E_g = \sigma_s \sqrt{\pi}$ is the energy of density function, and N is the noise power density with $N = 4K \cdot T \cdot F/R$. Note that K and F denote the Boltzmann constant and noise factor of SRA contributed by active devices, respectively.

As such, the sensitivity of SRX can be found by substituting Equation (4.11) into Equation (4.10):

$$S = 2KTF \sqrt{\frac{k\omega_0}{\pi Q_0}}$$ (4.12)

Note that the receiver noise figure (NF) can be approximated as [18]:

$$NF = \frac{S}{K \cdot T \cdot B}$$ (4.13)

Note that the NF of a SRX is independent of quench signal. For a typical 3-dB bandwidth of the SRX (B = 1.177 Ω_0), the NF becomes 0.958 F. In addition, the noise equivalent power (NEP) can be calculated by $S / \sqrt{B}$:

$$NEP = 1.38KTF \sqrt[4]{\frac{k\omega_0}{\pi Q_0}}$$ (4.14)

Note that k is usually determined by the frequency of the quench signal and the sampling rate of SRA. Therefore, it can be observed from Equation (4.12) and Equation (4.14) that, for a given ω_0 and k, the sensitivity and NEP is inversely proportional to the square-root and the fourth-root of Q_0. Therefore, the resonator with higher Q will significantly improve the sensitivity within the bandwidth of interest for imaging applications.

4.3.2 Super-regenerative Receivers

Two SRXs working at 96 GHz and 135 GHz are implemented into the CMOS process to demonstrate the advantages of applying quench-controlled oscillators with metamaterial resonators in super-regenerative receivers (SRX). The fundamentals of quench-controlled oscillator design are introduced first.

4.3.2.1 Quench-controlled Oscillation

High-Q Resonance with Standing Wave: In the practical on-chip resonator design with finite Q of SRR or CSRR, the reflection coefficient ($|\Gamma|$) depends on the number of cascading TL-SRR or TL-CSRR unit-cells. Figure 4.10 shows the circuit level simulation of TL-CSRR at 96-GHz resonance frequency with following observations. First, the reflection coefficient $|\Gamma|$ is more sensitive to the cells number when Q is below 200. Second, $|\Gamma|$ can be improved by cascading more unit-cells.

Voltage Controlled Negative Resistance: The oscillation can be sustained by compensating the reflection loss ($|\Gamma| < 1$) with a negative resistance. Similarly, a quench-controlled oscillating can be achieved by controlling voltage controlled negative resistance (VCNR), which determines the instantaneous damping factor ($\zeta(t)$). Equation (4.4), as discussed above. The sensitivity of SRX is also a function of ($\zeta(t)$) that is determined by VCNR. Usually a cross-coupled NMOS pair is applied for the differential negative resistance design as depicted in Figure 4.11, where the tail current of the cross-coupled NMOS pair (I_D) can be quench-controlled by another NMOS biased in the saturation region.

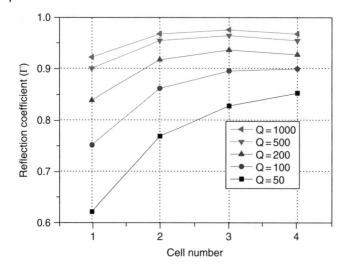

Figure 4.10 Reflection coefficient of T-line loaded with CSRR unit-cells.

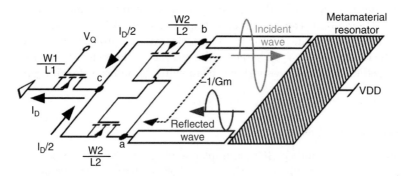

Figure 4.11 Reflection loss compensation by cross-coupled NMOS pair with controlled tail current.

The equivalent differential negative conductance between nodes "a" and "b" can be expressed as Equation 4.15, by neglecting the channel-length modulation:

$$G_m = \frac{gm_2}{2} = \frac{I_D}{2V_{od2}} \tag{4.15}$$

where gm_2 and V_{od2} are the transconductance and overdrive voltage of cross-coupled NMOS FETs, respectively. Note that I_D can be obtained by:

$$I_D = \frac{W_1}{2L_1}\mu_n C_{ox} V_{od1}^2 = \frac{W_2}{2L_2}\mu_n C_{ox} V_{od2}^2 \tag{4.16}$$

where W_1, L_1 and $V_{od1} = V_Q - V_T$ are the channel width, length, and overdrive voltage of tail NMOS; W_2, L_2 and V_{od2} are the channel width, length, and overdrive voltage of the cross-coupled NMOS pair; $\mu_n C_{ox}$ and V_T are the process related parameters. As such, Equation (4.15) can be written as a function of V_{QY}:

$$G_m = \frac{\mu_n C_{ox}\left(V_Q - V_T\right)}{4}\sqrt{\frac{2W_1 W_2}{L_1 L_2}} \tag{4.17}$$

We can observe from Equation (4.17) that G_m is linearly controlled by V_Q of which the slope is determined by the product of W_1/L_1 and W_2/L_2. Note that the oscillation starts when $1/G_m < R$ and stops when $1/Gm > R$. As such, $(W_1/L_1)(W_2/L_2)$ is just be large enough to satisfy the oscillation start condition $(1/Gm < R)$. However, large W_2/L_2 will introduce additional parasitic capacitance, which will be counted into the resonator rank and reduce the oscillation frequency. Moreover, in order to provide sufficient head room for the cross-coupled NMOS pair, W_1/L_1 is selected several times larger than W_2/L_2.

4.3.2.2   SRX Design by TL-CSRR

Folded Differential T-line Loaded with CSRR: TL-CSRR structure cannot be directly employed for the SRX design. First, the single-ended approach will bring large common-mode noise in the oscillator; second, cascading more unit cells will increase area overhead. A folded differential T-line loaded with CSRR (DTL-CSRR) structure is proposed to reduce the area by half, while doubling the number of the unit cells [19]. As shown in Figure 4.12, two cascaded TL-CSRR unit cells (with CSRR size of $60 \times 60\,\mu m^2$) are folded in the two top-most metal layers (M6 and M7).

The S-parameters of the proposed DTL-CSRR structure is verified by an EM simulation tool EMX with a parasitic capacitance of 40 fF from transistors. Both ε and μ of DTL-CSRR are extracted from the simulation results according to Equation (4.3), which both become complex numbers due to the existence of loss factor induced imaginary parts. The metamaterial property is illustrated by the real parts of ε and μ in Figure 4.13. At the vicinity of 105 GHz resonance frequency, an electric plasmonic medium is formed with ε < 0 and μ > 0. A stop-band is thereby formed within a narrow bandwidth of 1.8 GHz, where the Q factor is found to be 58 by $Q = \omega_0/\omega_{3dB}$ from the differential impedance (Z_{diff}) between P1 and P2.

96 GHz DTL-CSRR-based SRX: Figure 4.14 depicts the schematic of DTL-CSRR-based SRX. DTL-CSRR is first connected to a differential negative resistance formed by cross-coupled NMOS (M2 and M3). To further improve the detection efficiency,

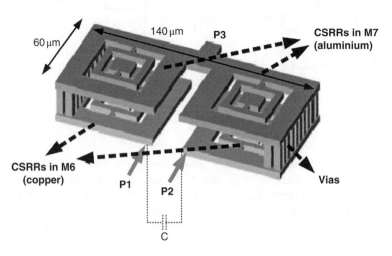

Figure 4.12 Layout for CMOS on-chip implementation of DTL-CSRR for 96 GHz SRX.

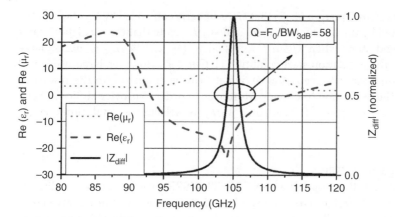

Figure 4.13 EM-simulation based comparison of DTL-CSRR and LC-tank resonator for CMOS 96 GHz SRX design.

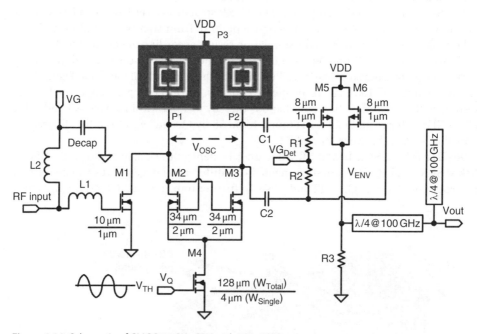

Figure 4.14 Schematic of CMOS 96 GHz SRX with DTL-CSRR.

a virtual ground at 96 GHz is formed by two $\lambda/4$ stubs. The size of M4 is designed as four times that of M2 and M3. Note that W_{Total} and W_{Single} are the total and individual finger width of transistors in Figure 4.14, respectively, and the channel length of every active device is 60 nm. The remaining circuit consists of a common source input buffer (M1) for current injection and an envelope detector formed by M5 and M6.

The common source stage (M1) is designed for input signal injection and also reverse isolation from the oscillator to the input. The size of M1 is optimized with consideration of minimized parasitic capacitance, as well as the input matching. Similarly, M5 and M6 also need to be minimized, but doing so will reduce the detection efficiency. To solve this problem, a capacitance coupling by C1 and C2 is introduced between the outputs of oscillator tank and the envelope detection. First, the capacitance loading from M5 and M6 are reduced by series connection of the coupling capacitors; second, M5 and M6 are biased externally by large resistors (R1, R2) to optimize the detection; third, 1/f noise from M5 and M6 is also isolated.

4.3.2.3 SRX Design by TL-SRR

Differential T-line Loaded with SRR: The TL-SRR structure with horizontal placement of SRRs is also unsuitable for the practical implementation for SRX, mainly due to the large area overhead. Compared to TL-CSRR, TL-SRR inherently has better layout flexibility, because SRRs can be vertically stacked within a compact area. One differential T-line loaded with stacked SRRs (DTL-SRR) is proposed in this work, for the application of 135 GHz SRX design in the 65 nm CMOS RF process.

As shown in Figure 4.15(a), the DTL-SRR is designed by stacking SRRs with the same dimensions of $24 \times 24\,\mu m^2$ in four metal layers (M5–M8). All SRRs are closely coupled to the same host T-line implemented in the topmost metal layer (M8). The overall size of the proposed DTL-SRR is $35 \times 34\,\mu m^2$. For the purpose of comparison, a traditional LC-tank resonator is designed in the M8 metal layer, as shown in Figure 4.15(b), which has the same resonance frequency of 135 GHz. The S-parameters of both structures are also verified by EMX, with the same parasitic capacitance of 18 fF.

As shown in Figure 4.16, at the vicinity of 142-GHz resonance, $\varepsilon > 0$ and $\mu < 0$, and a magnetic plasmonic medium is formed. As a result, a stop-band is formed with deep rejection of -33 dB within a narrow bandwidth of 1 GHz. The Q factor of the DTL-SRR

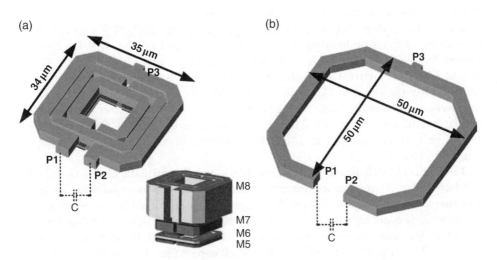

Figure 4.15 Layout for CMOS on-chip implementation of DTL-SRR for 135 GHz SRX.

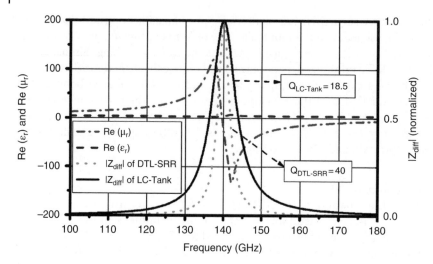

Figure 4.16 EM-simulation-based comparison of DTL-SRR and LC-tank resonator for CMOS 135 GHz SRX design.

resonator is 142, which is nearly four times of the Q of the LC-tank resonator. Moreover, the DTL-SRR resonator layout area ($1190\,\mu m^2$) is less than half of the LC-tank resonator ($2500\,\mu m^2$). Such a Q-factor enhancement effect can also be explained by the strong phase non-linearity in the frequency range close to SRRs resonance. Note that the Q factor can also be obtained by the phase-based method:

$$Q = \frac{\omega_0}{2} \cdot \left| \frac{d\angle Z(j\omega)}{d\omega} \right| \tag{4.18}$$

where $\angle Z(j\omega)$ is the phase of resonator impedance.

Figure 4.17(a) shows the impedance diagram of both DTL-SRR and LC-Tank without any capacitor loading. A resonance generated by the SRR loadings is observed at 167 GHz for DTL-SRR. Such resonance causes a non-linear phase shift at 140 GHz. Figure 4.17(b) shows that DTL-SRR has a much stronger phase non-linearity than that of LC-Tank around 140 GHz. As shown in Figure 4.17(c), both structures have the same resonance frequency of 140 GHz after including the ideal capacitance ($C = 16$ fF). The phase non-linearity in DTL-SRRs increases the phase gradient of Z_{diff} at 140 GHz, resulting in a higher Q, according to Equation (4.18).

135-GHz DTL-SRR-based SRX: Figure 4.18 depicts a schematic of 135-GHz DTL-SRR-based SRX. First, transformer-based matching network is applied to the input matching for M1 for the electrostatic discharge (ESD) protection when integrating with the antenna; second, the virtual ground formed by two $\lambda/4$ T-lines is replaced by the high-Q MOM capacitor to further reduce the chip area; third, the detected envelope signal VENV is directly averaged by an on-chip low-pass filter formed by R3 and C3 at the output.

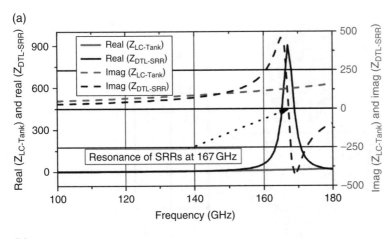

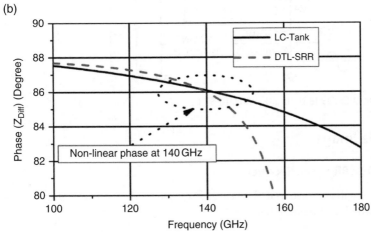

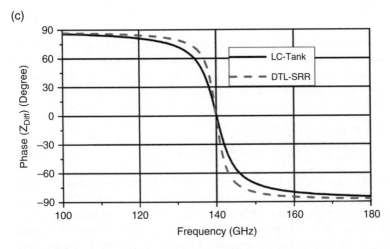

Figure 4.17 Impedance diagram of DTL-SRR and LC-Tank in Globalfoundries 65-nm CMOS process: (a) Real and imaginary parts of Z_{Diff}; (b) Phase of Z_{Diff}; and (c) Phase of Z_{Diff} when the ideal 16-fF capacitor is included.

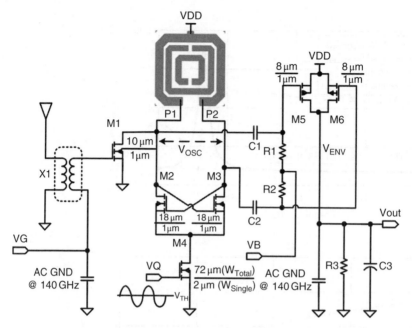

Figure 4.18 Schematic of CMOS 135 GHz SRX with DTL-SRR.

4.4 A 135 GHz Imager

4.4.1 135 GHz DTL-SRR-based Receiver

THz radiation is usually attenuated due to absorption and scattering during the propagation [20], which can be modeled by:

$$I_{\gamma_1} = I_{\gamma_0} e^{-\int_{\gamma_0}^{\gamma_1} \alpha_e(z)dz} \tag{4.19}$$

where $I_{\gamma 0}$ and I_{γ_1} are the incoming and outgoing radiance intensity along path (γ_0, γ_1) and $\alpha_e(Z)$ is the extinction coefficient, which is the summation of absorption α_a and scattering α_s coefficients. For a homogeneous material placed between (γ_0, γ_1), α_a is a constant. The scattering only occurs at the interface with scattering coefficients of $\alpha_s(\gamma_0)$ and $\alpha_s(\gamma_1)$. The received power (P_R) in a transmissive-type THz imaging system is [2]:

$$P_R\left(\text{dBm}\right) = P_T\left(\text{dBm}\right) + G_R\left(\text{dBi}\right) - L\left(\text{dB}\right)$$
$$-8.686\left[\Delta\gamma\alpha_a + \alpha_s\left(\gamma_0\right) + \alpha_s\left(\gamma_1\right)\right]\left(\text{dB}\right) \tag{4.20}$$

where P_T is the effective isotropic radiated power (EIRP) of the transmitter, G_R is the receiver antenna gain, and L is the path loss without any objects placed in the propagation path, including both the free space path loss (FSPL) and atmosphere absorption.

The envelope of receiver output is proportional to the injected current or the square root of input power. A DC output can be obtained by averaging $E_{nv}(v_0(t))$ in each periodic quenching cycle.

$$V_{DC} = \frac{\omega_i Z_0 |S(\Delta\omega)| \sqrt{P_R}}{\sqrt{2R}(t_b - t_a)} \int_0^{t_b} \frac{1}{s(t)} dt \qquad (4.21)$$

As such, the received power could be detected by measuring V_{DC} from the SRA output. As a result, the THz image of an object can be further obtained by the 2-D scanning of V_{DC} with fixed P_T, G_R and L. Moreover, by analyzing V_{DC} as well as P_R with various object thickness $\Delta\gamma$, we can further find the absorption coefficient of the object under test.

4.4.2 System Implementation

The SRX can be integrated with the THz imaging system by replacing the GSG probe with bonding wires connected to a 135-GHz antenna. It is demonstrated by wires bonding from the input of the proposed 135-GHz SRX to a 2 × 4 antenna array with hybrid series/parallel feeding network, as show in Figure 4.19(a). The receiver and antenna must be well aligned to minimize the connection loss, which is estimated to be 3 ~ 5 dB according to the EM simulation in Ansoft HFSS. The entire THz imaging setup is also shown in Figure 4.19(b). The 135 GHz radiation from a VDI source (0 dBm output power) is received by the proposed SRX after propagating through the objects under test, which is held by an X-Y moving stage (STANDA) placed in the middle. Although a substantial portion of the object is illuminated due to the divergent beam from the source antenna, only the power propagating to the direction of receiver is detected. As such, a high resolution image can be obtained without focus lens. The resulting V_{out} at each X-Y stage position is recorded in a 2-D matrix, which can be plotted in a colored image by Matlab with JET colormap.

4.4.3 Results

Figures 4.20 and 4.21 show the imaging results by the proposed CMOS THz image system. Figure 4.20 shows that we can differentiate the moisturized animal skin or Panadol pill from the corresponding dry sample. Due to the strong water absorption at THz frequencies, a moisturized sample (skin or Panadol) has higher absorption than the dry one. Figure 4.21 shows the imaging of various types of edible oil, including sunflower, olive, fresh soybean, and soybean that has been used once. Note that four Petri dishes are used to hold the oil samples.

The imaging system can also be applied in transmission analysis to characterize the material in the propagation path. The absorption ratio of each oil type can be identified by comparing the received power under different sample volumes with the help of Equation (4.20), and is depicted in the box chart in Figure 4.22. It is interesting to observe that the soybean oil that has been used once has higher absorption to the 135 GHz energy than the fresh one. With the significantly improved receiver sensitivity, the proposed CMOS THz imager results in high contrast images and can be further utilized in the analysis of moisture levels as well as the identification of a particular liquid content.

(a)

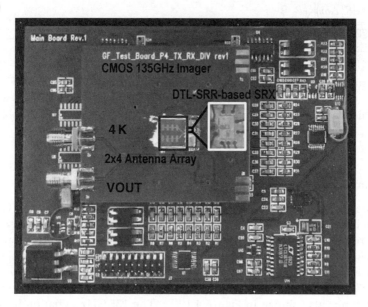

(b)

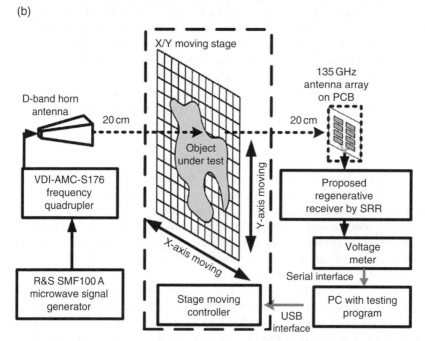

Figure 4.19 (a) PCB integration of CMOS 135-GHz SRX with antenna; and (b) THz imaging measurement setup with the proposed receiver chip integrated on PCB and object under test fixed on an X-Y moving stage.

Moisturized skin   Dry skin

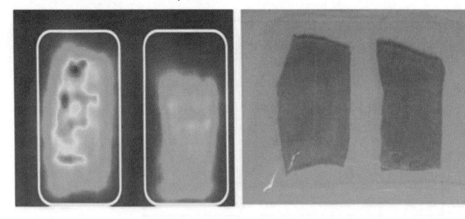

Moisturized   Normal

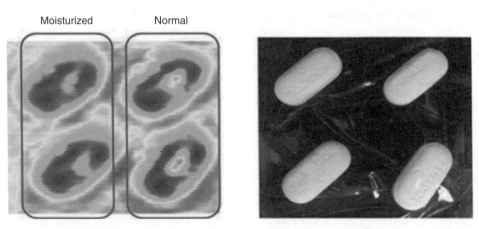

Figure 4.20 Images captured by imaging system with the proposed 135-GHz SRX receiver: animal skin samples and Panadol pills.

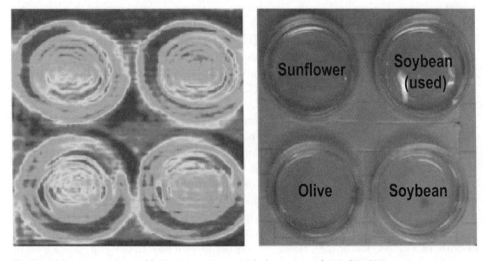

Figure 4.21 Images captured by imaging system with the proposed 135-GHz SRX receiver: various types of oil.

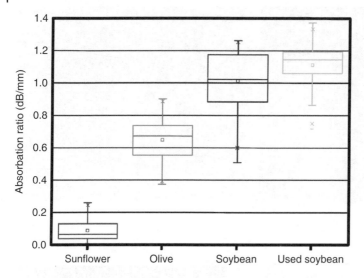

Figure 4.22 Absorption ratio of various types of oil detected at 135 GHz.

4.5 Plasmonic Sensor for Circulating Tumor Cell Detection

4.5.1 Introduction of CTC Detection

Cell testing has attracted intensive attention recently due to the need for early detection of diseases such as cancer [22,23]. As a typical example, circulating tumor cells (CTCs), which are tumor cells shed into the circulatory system, such as blood or lymph from the primary tumor region, have become an important target to monitor tumor growth. Current CTC detection is usually based on the so-called fluorescent-labeled method, that is, cells are labeled with fluorescent molecules and investigated under fluorescence microscopy [22]. However, this method has limitations of low specificity, high cost, and complicated operation when using labels. In recent years, another detection method based on the cell's electrical properties obtains considerable development in a label-free fashion [24,25]. However, previous cell electrical measurement works [25] are mainly based on dc or low-frequency studies. It is still an invasive method with electrode contact. Moreover, it lacks spectrometrical information that can be largely observed at high frequencies. In addition, the readout circuit suffers from low-frequency noise.

Instead, the dielectric properties of CTCs at high frequency can be of great significance [26–28]. The mm-wave or sub-THz dielectric measurement may reveal the fingerprint features of cells due to the interaction between water and biological molecules. Besides, the miniaturized devices have a higher spatial resolution if integrated into an array. As shown in Figure 4.23, the detection principle is based on the fact that the resonance frequency of a device-under-test is a function of the dielectric constant of the loaded sensing objective. The frequency-dependent of the extracted dielectric parameters thereby can distinguish between the cell types. However, the direct dielectric measurement at sub-THz is difficult, due to high loss and poor sensitivity [26].

A surface-plasmonic device-based biosensor has shown a high detection sensitivity, because of a high Q factor [28]. However, it is not known how to develop such a kind of

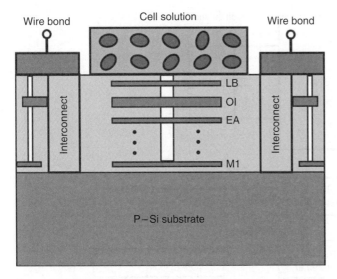

Figure 4.23 CMOS sub-THz cell impedance detection system.

surface-plasmonic sensor in the CMOS process for CTC impedance measurements. In this work, we investigate split-ring resonator (SRR)-based plasmonic sensors with layout designs in the standard 65-nm CMOS process at sub-THz.

4.5.2 SRR-based Oscillator for CTC Detection

SRR can be modeled as a series of *RLC* circuits [29], and hence its resonant frequency ω_0 can be expressed by the effective inductance L_0 and capacitance C_0 as:

$$\omega_0 = \frac{1}{\sqrt{L_0 C_0}} \tag{4.22}$$

Figure 4.24 shows the simplified equivalent circuit and the route to extract the cell dielectric parameters using an SRR biosensor loaded with CTC solutions. When CTC solution with a permittivity of $\varepsilon = \varepsilon_r + i\,\varepsilon_i$, is loaded onto the SRR biosensor, it is equivalent to adding a parallel capacitance C and a resistance R [26]. Here, $C = A\varepsilon_0\varepsilon_r$, $R = 1/\omega\varepsilon_0\varepsilon_i$, and A is a geometric parameter. The resulted resonant frequency ($\omega = f(L_0, C_0, C(\varepsilon_r))$) will shift due to the additional capacitance C, which depends on the type and also the concentration of cells. From the amount of frequency shift, we can infer the cell electrical property by extracting impedance from the frequency response. Note that the above discussion does not consider the frequency dispersion. The frequency dependent complex permittivity of one solution with cells can be extracted from the measured S parameters.

The Y-parameter of the cell solution can be obtained by subtracting the Y-parameter of SRR (denoted as Y) from the total Y-parameter of SRR and cell (Y'), that is:

$$\left(j\omega C + \frac{1}{R}\right)\begin{bmatrix} 1 & -1 \\ -1 & 1 \end{bmatrix} = \begin{bmatrix} Y'_{11} & Y'_{12} \\ Y'_{21} & Y'_{22} \end{bmatrix} - \begin{bmatrix} Y_{11} & Y_{12} \\ Y_{21} & Y_{22} \end{bmatrix} \tag{4.23}$$

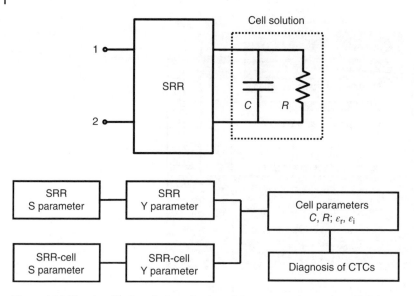

Figure 4.24 The simplified equivalent circuit and the route to extract the cell dielectric parameters using a SRR biosensor loaded with CTCs solutions.

For the case of the SRR and the case of the SRR + cell, the measured S parameters are denoted as S and S' respectively. In this case, ε_r and ε_i can be extracted from cells using Equations (4.24) and (4.25) respectively:

$$\varepsilon_r(\omega) = \frac{1}{\omega A \varepsilon_0} \mathrm{Im}\left\{ \begin{bmatrix} \dfrac{1}{Z_0}\dfrac{-2S_{12}}{(1+S_{11})(1+S_{22})} - S_{12}S_{21} \end{bmatrix} \\ -\begin{bmatrix} \dfrac{1}{Z_0}\dfrac{-2S'_{12}}{(1+S'_{11})(1+S'_{22})} - S'_{12}S'_{21} \end{bmatrix} \right\} \tag{4.24}$$

$$\varepsilon_i(\omega) = \frac{1}{\omega A \varepsilon_0} \mathrm{Re}\left\{ \begin{bmatrix} \dfrac{1}{Z_0}\dfrac{-2S_{12}}{(1+S_{11})(1+S_{22})} - S_{12}S_{21} \end{bmatrix} \\ -\begin{bmatrix} \dfrac{1}{Z_0}\dfrac{-2S'_{12}}{(1+S'_{11})(1+S'_{22})} - S'_{12}S'_{21} \end{bmatrix} \right\} \tag{4.25}$$

Based on the resonant frequency shift of SRR, a new kind of 135-GHz oscillator has been designed for label-free and non-invasive electrical CTC detection. Instead of using the sophisticated frequency division circuit to enable low frequency detection, the change in frequency of the oscillator is directly converted into a different output voltage through charging the load capacitor. Also the voltage sensitivity is enhanced by the use of the charge accumulation technique. Figure 4.25 shows the schematic of the unit-cell of the sensor that comprises of oscillator, envelope detector, current mirror, and its charge accumulation circuit. The oscillator consists of a high Q resonator, which is a stacked SRR structure, as shown in Figure 4.15, and cross-coupled NMOS (M1&M2).

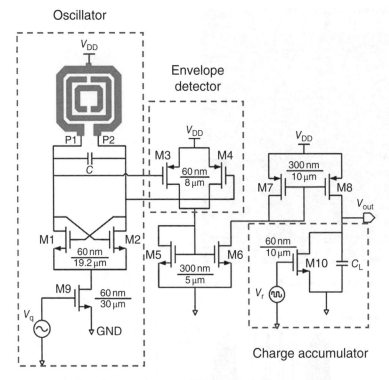

Figure 4.25 The schematic diagram of SRR-based-oscillator sensor.

The differential outputs of the oscillator are fed into the envelope detector circuit, which is formed by M3 and M4. The PMOS transistors M3 and M4 detect the peak negative value of the oscillation output signal and produce transient output current. The raising time of the output current of M3 and M4 depends on the build-up time of the oscillation, which is affected by the frequency. The current of the output detector will be copied by the current mirror circuit that is formed by M5–M8 transistors. This transient current will charge the load capacitor C_L to produce the output voltage. The rise time of output voltage level is dependent on the oscillation frequency of the oscillator.

4.5.3 Sensitivity of SRR-based Oscillator

As shown in Figure 4.26, a THz sensor was fabricated in the 65-nm Global Foundries process. It occupies an area of $1\,mm \times 1\,mm$ with a 10^*3 SRR-based oscillator array. CTCs can be loaded onto the chip surface for detection.

Figure 4.27 shows the simulation results at various points of the circuit, as given by Figure 4.25. The black curve is the output of the oscillator that is formed by cross-coupled NMOS (M1 and M2). In this case, the oscillator will produce its sinusoidal response if the transistor M9 is activated by the quench signal V_q. So, only when the peak of the sinusoidal signal V_q is greater than the required threshold voltage of tail transistor M9, will the oscillator produce its sine wave output. The output of the oscillator is fed into the envelop detector that is formed by M3 and M4. The output of the envelop detector is given by the blue saw-like curve. In this case, M3 and M4 will produce current when the peak

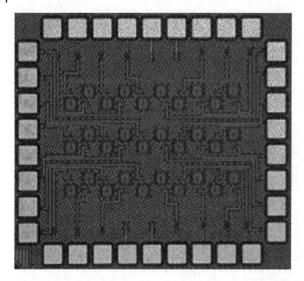

Figure 4.26 THz chip in the 65 nm process for CTC detection.

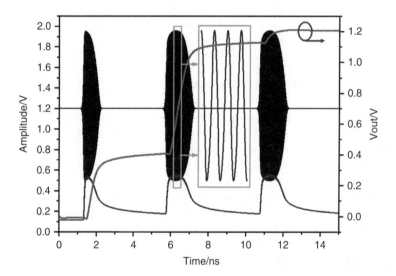

Figure 4.27 The outputs of oscillator and charge accumulator based on circuit simulation.

negative value of oscillation output frequency is larger than the threshold voltage of PMOS M3 and M4. Otherwise, M3 and M4 will remain off, which results in the saw-like output response in the envelop detector output. The current mirrors M5–M8 will copy the current produced by the envelop detector and use it to charge the output capacitor C_L.

Note that capacitor C_L will be discharged first during the initial cycle by transistor M10. When M10 is activated, the load capacitor will be discharged by M10 and the initial cycle can begin. During the detection process, M10 will remain off after initialization. This will allow load capacitance C_L to be charged by the output current of the current mirror. Depending on the number of cycles of the oscillator, the voltage of C_L

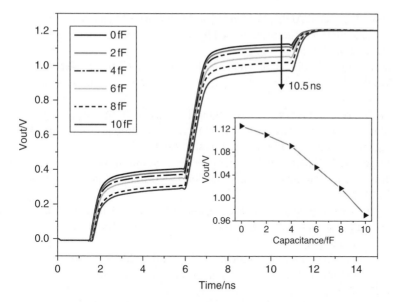

Figure 4.28 The voltage outputs under various capacitance values of loaded CTC solution. The inset shows the relationship between voltage output and loaded capacitance.

will increase due to the charge accumulation effect. In Figure 4.27, the load capacitor C_L is charged by three oscillation output cycle and the voltage of C_L is raised from 0 V to 1.2 V, as shown by the red curve.

Figure 4.28 presents the voltage output under different capacitances. CTC solutions with different concentrations have different equivalent dielectric constants, which will produce different capacitance values. Hence, different CTC concentrations will result in different oscillation frequencies of the oscillator. At the output of sensor, different oscillation frequencies will produce different output voltages. As shown by Figure 4.28, various CTC concentrations have different output voltages due to their associated equivalent capacitances. Thus, CTC concentration can be detected based on the output voltage produced by the sensor.

As can be seen, the voltage level decreases remarkably at the first and second charge periods, as the capacitance increases from 0 fF to 10 fF. The inset of Figure 4.28 shows the relationship between the voltage output and capacitance value when 10.5 ns is selected as the voltage monitoring time. For the oscillator with no CTC solution (reference), the voltage output is 1.125 V; as the capacitance of the loaded CTC solution increases to 10 fF, the output will be reduced to 0.971 V. Thus, the average voltage difference with unit capacitance (sensitivity) reaches ~15.4 mV/fF. This plasmonic biosensor has shown high detection sensitivity, as a charge accumulation circuit is employed.

References

1 M. Tonouchi (2007) Cutting-edge terahertz technology. *Nature Photonics*, 1, 97–105.
2 D. Arnone, C. Ciesla and M. Pepper (2000) Terahertz imaging comes into view. *Physics World*, 13(4), 35–40.

3 Y. Sun, M.Y. Sy, Y.X. Wang, A.T. Ahuja, Y.T. Zhang and E. Pickwell-Macpherson (2011) A promising diagnostic method: Terahertz pulsed imaging and spectroscopy. *World Journal of Radiology*, 3(3), 55–65.

4 R. Han, Y. Zhang, Y. Kim, D.Y. Kim, H. Shichijo and K. Kenneth (2012) Terahertz image sensors using CMOS Schottky barrier diodes. In: *International SoC Design Conference*, pp. 254–257.

5 W. Momose, H. Yoshino, Y. Katakawa, K. Yamashita, K. Imai, *et al.* (2012) Applying terahertz technology for non-destructive detection of crack initiation in a film-coated layer on a swelling tablet. *Results in Pharma Sciences*, 2, 29–37.

6 T. Arikawa, M. Nagai and K. Tanaka (2008) Characterizing hydration state in solution using terahertz time-domain attenuated total reflection spectroscopy. *Chemical Physics Letters*, 457(1–3), 12–17.

7 P.C. Ashworth, E. Pickwell-MacPherson, E. Provenzano, S.E. Pinder, A.D. Purushotham, *et al.* (2009) Terahertz pulsed spectroscopy of freshly excised human breast cancer. *Optics Express*, 17(15), 12444–12454.

8 R. Woodward, V. Wallace, D. Arnone, E. Linfield and M. Pepper (2003) Terahertz pulsed imaging of skin cancer in the time and frequency domain. *Journal of Biological Physics*, 29(2–3), 257–261.

9 *Terahertz Detection of Skin, Mouth and Epithelial Cancers* [Online]. Available at: http://www.teraview.com/applications/medical/oncology.html

10 A. Tsuchiya and H. Onodera (2009) On-chip Metamaterial Transmission-line based on stacked split-ring resonator for millimeter-wave LSIs. In: *Asia Pacific Microwave Conference*, pp. 1458–1461.

11 F. Falcone, T. Lopetegi, J. Baena, R. Marques, F. Martin and M. Sorolla (2004) Effective negative-ε topband microstrip lines based on complementary split ring resonators. *IEEE Microwave and Wireless Components Letters*, 14(6), 280–282.

12 D.R. Smith, S. Schultz, P. Markoš and C.M. Soukoulis (2002) Determination of effective permittivity and permeability of metamaterials from reflection and transmission coefficients, *Physics. Review B*, 65, 195104.

13 X. Chen, T.M. Grzegorczyk, B.-I. Wu, J. Pacheco and J.A. Kong (2004) Robust method to retrieve the constitutive effective parameters of metamaterials. *Physics Review E*, 70, 016608.

14 K.-H. Tsai and S.-I. Liu (2012) A 104-GHz phase-locked loop using a VCO at second pole frequency. *IEEE Transactions on VLSI Systems*, 20(1), 80–88.

15 L. Franca-Neto, R. Bishop and B. Bloechel (2004) 64 GHz and 100 GHz VCOs in 90 nm CMOS using Optimum Pumping Method. In: *IEEE International Solid State Circuits Conference*, pp. 444–538.

16 J.R. Whitehead (1950) *Super-Regenerative Receivers*, 1st edition. Cambridge University Press: Cambridge UK.

17 J. Bohorquez, A. Chandrakasan and J. Dawson (2009) Frequency-domain analysis of super-regenerative amplifiers. *IEEE Transactions on Microwave Theory and Techniques*, 57(12), 2882–2894.

18 A. Tang, Z. Xu, Q. Gu, Y.-C. Wu and M. Chang (2011) A 144 GHz 2.5 mW multistage regenerative receiver for mm-wave imaging in 65 nm CMOS. In: *IEEE Radio Frequency Integrated Circuits Symposium*, pp. 1–4.

19 Y. Shang, H. Yu, D. Cai, J. Ren and K.S. Yeo (2013) Design of high-Q millimeter wave oscillator by differential transmission line loaded with metamaterial resonator in 65 nm CMOS. *IEEE Transactions on Microwave Theory and Techniques*, 61(5), 1892–1902.

20 M.C. Wanke, M.A. Mangan and R.J. Foltynowicz (2005) *Atmospheric Propagation of THz Radiation*. OSTI.

21 T. Schneider, A. Wiatrek, S. Preussler, M. Grigat and R.-P. Braun, (2012) Link budget analysis for terahertz fixed wireless links. *IEEE Transactions on Terahertz Science and Technology*, 2(2), 250–256.

22 H.B. Hsieh, D. Marrinucci, K. Bethel, D.N. Curry, M. Humphrey, *et al.* (2006) High speed detection of circulating tumor cells. *Biosens. Bioelectron.*, 21, 1893–1899.

23 H.W. Wu (2016) Label-free and antibody-free wideband microwave biosensor for identifying the cancer cells. *IEEE T. Microwave Theory*, 64, 982–990.

24 C. Jin, S.M. McFaul, S.P. Duffy, X. Deng, P. Tavassoli, *et al.* (2014) Technologies for label-free separation of circulating tumor cells: From historical foundations to recent developments. *Lab Chip*, 14, 32–44.

25 Y. Chen, C.C. Wong, T.S. Pui, R. Nadipalli, R. Weerasekera, *et al.* (2012) CMOS high density electrical impedance biosensor array for tumor cell detection. *Sensor. Actuat. B-Chem.*, 173, 903–907.

26 T. Mitsunaka, N. Ashida, A. Saito, K. Iizuka, T. Suzuki, *et al.* (2016) 28.3 CMOS biosensor IC focusing on dielectric relaxations of biological water with 120 GHz and 60 GHz oscillator arrays. *In: IEEE International Solid-State Circuits Conference (ISSCC)*.

27 H. Wang, A. Mahdavi, J. Park, T. Chi, J. Butts, *et al.* (2014) Cell culture and cell-based sensor on CMOS. In: *IEEE Biomedical Circuits and Systems Conference (BioCAS)*, pp. 468–471.

28 Y.F. Xiao, C.L. Zou, B.B. Li, Y. Li, C.H. Dong, *et al.* (2010) High-Q exterior whispering-gallery modes in a metal-coated micro-resonator. *Physics Review Letters*, 105, 153902.

29 T. Okamoto, T. Otsuka, S. Sato, T. Fukuta and M. Haraguchi (2012) Dependence of LC resonance wavelength on size of silver split-ring resonator fabricated by nanosphere lithography. *Optics Express*, 20, 24059–24067.

5

CMOS Ultrasound Sensor

5.1 Introduction

Ultrasound Imaging is a widely-used biomedical image sensing modality, which employs high-frequency sound waves to image internal structures [1]. The basic principle is that when a beam of sound waves is projected onto objects and bounces back from the interface between those structures, the differing reflection signals produce the ultrasound images. Due to its harmless characteristic to the human body, lower cost, higher penetration depth, and real-time imaging capability compared with existing medical imaging modalities such as magnetic resonance imaging (MRI) [2], computed tomography (CT) [3], and X-rays [4], the research and development of ultrasound image sensing systems has gained much attention [5].

The overall architecture of a typical ultrasound sensing system is shown in Figure 5.1, which includes the CMUT transducers and analog front-end (AFE), followed by signal conditioning and processing blocks. One key part of the ultrasound imaging is the transducer. Tradition ultrasound imaging systems mostly employ high-cost piezoelectric transducers. The development of the CMUT [6] provides the advantages of low-cost CMOS compatible fabrication capability, superior frequency characteristics, ease of fabrication into dense arrays, and integration with the front-end transmitting and receiving integrated circuits [7], which has increased ultrasound applications in biomedical imaging. Until now, different types of CMUT devices have been designed and fabricated using surface micro-machining [8,9] and wafer-bonding technologies [10,11]. Most of the application developments for CMUTs have focused on 2-D and 3-D medical imaging [12,13], non-destructive testing [14], and high density focused ultrasound therapy [15].

Ultrasound systems usually operate at sub-10 MHz frequencies with a 1-D CMUT array for 2-D diagnostic imaging applications. However, to obtain better image resolution, higher sensitivity, and signal-to-noise ratio (SNR), advanced 3-D ultrasound imaging at even higher frequency operation is required. High frequency 3-D ultrasound imaging requires:

1) 2-D transducer array configuration with an increased number of elements to transmit acoustic waves at various angles; and
2) high bandwidth AFE interfacing to read out the reflected signals [16,17].

CMOS Integrated Lab-on-a-Chip System for Personalized Biomedical Diagnosis,
First Edition. Hao Yu, Mei Yan, and Xiwei Huang.
© 2018 John Wiley & Sons Singapore Pte. Ltd. Published 2018 by John Wiley & Sons Singapore Pte. Ltd.

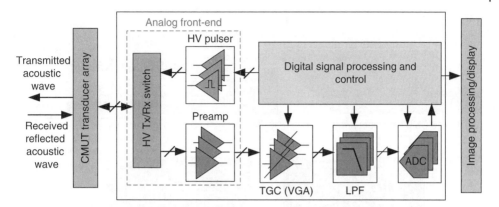

Figure 5.1 Overall system diagram of an ultrasound imaging system with an AFE receiver integrating with the capacitive micro-machined ultrasound transducer (CMUT).

In this chapter, a two-channel ultrasound sensor unit cell as the AFE for 320×320 CMUT array towards high-frequency 3-D ultrasound medical imaging applications is presented. The AFE ultrasound sensor unit cell consists of two high-voltage (HV) pulsers in the transmit path to drive the transducers to generate ultrasound waves, and a shared low-noise preamplifier with HV protection switches to receive the reflected echo signals. The acoustic functionality of the proposed ultrasound sensor has also been verified through the pulse-echo measurement in an oil-immersed environment using our in-house developed CMUT device sample.

5.2 CMUT Pixel

CMUT is basically a transducer that converts ultrasound acoustic waves into electrical signals and vice versa [18]. It is operated upon electrostatic forces. A DC bias voltage V_{Bias} is applied to one of the CMUT electrodes, which causes the membrane to deflect towards the substrate; while an AC pulse is imposed on the device, which causes the membrane to vibrate, and emit acoustic power to the surrounding medium. When deployed for reception, the incident acoustic wave with pressure causes a change in the device capacitance, which will be detected by the receiving circuit. This variation in capacitance generates an AC current signal by:

$$I_{CMUT} = V_{Bias} \frac{\partial(\Delta C)}{\partial t} = \frac{\partial(\Delta Q)}{\partial t} \tag{5.1}$$

where ΔC is the change in capacitance, and ΔQ is the proportional change in the amount of charge. And when deployed for transmission, the principle is similar.

For proof of concept demonstration, the CMUT device array was in-house fabricated. The CMUT element consists of a 16×16 identical cell array, where each cell (its cross-section is schematically shown in Figure 5.2) was designed to be a square shape with $28\,\mu m$ side length and $31\,\mu m$ pitch size. A 3-μm thick silicon membrane with a 500-nm Al layer deposited on top acted as the top electrode, while the whole silicon substrate

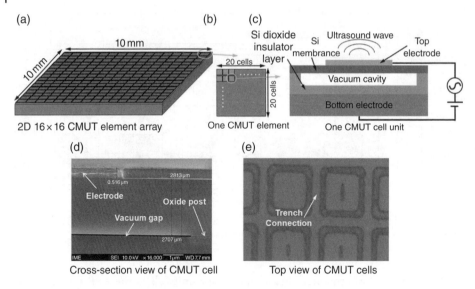

Figure 5.2 (a) Diagram of 2-D CMUT array; (b) One CMUT element; (c) One CMUT cell; (d) Cross-section view of CMUT cell; and (e) Top view of CMUT cells.

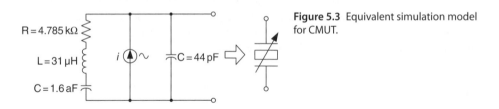

Figure 5.3 Equivalent simulation model for CMUT.

was used as the bottom electrode. The vacuum gap between the electrodes was selected to be 100 nm for lowering the operation voltage and improving receiving sensitivity. The center frequency in immersion is 35 MHz with a fractional bandwidth of 100%, while the target focal depth is 12 mm for bio-microscope application. The capacitance variation of the CMUT element due to the acoustic pressure is 2.12 aF/Pa.

The maximum acoustic pressure at the surface is calculated to be 3.31 e4 Pa, while the returning minimum echo pressure is calculated to be 1.23 e2 Pa from the specified focal depth with the attenuation rate of −1 dB/MHz/cm. The corresponding minimal capacitance variation calculated is 2.62 e2 aF. During fabrication, the thermal oxide layer was first deposited onto a polished silicon substrate via thermal oxidation process and patterned to define the vacuum cavity. The cavity patterned wafer was then bonded to another silicon-on-insulator (SOI) wafer using a direct fusion bonding process. The handle substrate and the buried oxide layer of the SOI wafer were subsequently removed, leaving its device layer as the membrane. After depositing and patterning an Al layer for electrical connection, the device was fabricated, as shown in Figure 5.2(e). The equivalent circuit model of CMUT calculated from the device parameters are shown in Figure 5.3, and the design parameters are summarized in Table 5.1.

5.3 Readout Circuit

For CMUT readout, the AFE of the ultrasound imaging system typically consists of an HV pulser, a TX/RX protection switch, and a readout preamplifier (i.e. transimpedance amplifier, TIA, in our system), as shown in Figure 5.1. For 3-D ultrasound image sensing with a 2-D CMUT array, the overall system consists of the multi-channel AFE integrated with a CMUT transducer array through flip-chip bonding [12], in order to minimize the connection parasitics. For the transmitter side, the HV pulsers in the AFE IC are driven by low-voltage trigger signals generated by the digital signal processor (DSP) with controlled delays for beamforming [19]. The HV pulses from the pulser output excite the CMUT elements, generating acoustic waves into the acoustic medium.

While these acoustic signals propagate through the medium, some of them are reflected back as echo signals, due to the difference in the acoustic impedance levels of tissue layers, which are converted back into electrical signals by the CMUT elements, and processed by the receiver front-end. For the receiver side, the low-noise preamplifiers in the AFE are followed by time-to-gain compensation (TGC) amplifiers [20], which typically consist of variable gain amplifiers (VGA) and a digital-to-analog converter (DAC) to control the gain according to the depth of the received echo signal. The anti-aliasing filters follow the TGC, with analog-to-digital converters (ADC) to digitize the signals and connect to the DSP for signal processing and ultimately construct an image from the pulse-echo signal information.

In this chapter, a two-channel AFE unit cell as the CMOS ultrasound sensor is implemented, as shown in Figure 5.4. It consists of two HV pulsers in the transmitter path and a single low-noise preamplifier in the receiver path shared by the two CMUT elements. This is to ultimately minimize the area per channel on the IC chip, as the specified layout area per CMUT element on the IC chip underneath the CMUT wafer for flip-chip bonding is 600 μm by 600 μm, decided by the CMUT device, and it is difficult to integrate one preamplifier per one channel. Between the pulser and the

Table 5.1 Design Parameters for CMUT.

Parameter		Values
CMUT array (elements)		16×16
CMUT cells per element		20×20
CMUT cell geometrical profile	Width	$28\,\mu m$
	Depth	$28\,\mu m$
	Thickness	$3\,\mu m$
	Gap size	$0.1\,\mu m$
CMUT element dimension		$600\,\mu m \times 600\,\mu m$
CMUT excitation voltage (V_{P-P})		$20\,V$
Bandwidth		17.5–$52.5\,MHz$
Capacitance variation		$2.12\,aF/Pa$
Capacitance per element (deflated)		$44\,pF$

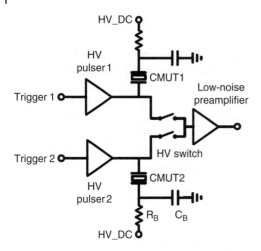

Figure 5.4 Two-channel analog front-end IC unit cell consisting of two HV pulsers, two HV protection switches, and a shared low-noise preamplifier.

preamplifier, an HV protection switch using an HV double-diffused lateral MOS (DMOS) transistor is placed in order to isolate the preamplifier circuit to avoid possible break-down in the transmit mode and also to select the individual CMUT element during the echo receive mode. Among several DC biasing schemes for the CMUT, the HV DC biasing for the CMUTs is done through a large external resistor RB and a shunt capacitor C_B is added for AC ground for the CMUT [17].

5.4 A 320 × 320 CMUT-based Ultrasound Imaging System

5.4.1 Top Architecture

In this chapter, the overall system is ultimately targeted for 3-D ultrasound bio-micro-scope application to obtain a high-resolution image of a patient's eye to diagnose glau-coma with high frame rate while minimizing the discomfort given to the patient. Considering flip-chip bond integration between the AFE and CMUT using post-wafer processing, the overall die floor plan of the 2-D multi-channel AFE IC system is pre-sented in Figure 5.5. The AFE IC consists of identical AFE unit cells in a 2-D array, along with digital multiplexer and demultiplexer blocks for column/row address and enables control for transmission and reception modes, pulser trigger controls, bias circuits, and output buffers to drive the following external components in the receive path. The size of the array and the allocated unit cell area for flip-chip bond integration is decided by the CMUT device characteristics.

The system specifications can be obtained as follows. Based on the previous discus-sion on the CMUT device and readout architecture, the gain of the receiver front-end preamplifier is specified so that the output of the preamplifier is to produce a maximum of a 1 VP-P voltage signal to input into the following TGC block when the maximum acoustic pressure signal is received by the CMUT. Therefore, the maximum fixed gain of the preamplifier is 61 dBΩ. As the input signal to the preamplifier is a current signal, the input-referred current noise is important. In the case where the minimum acoustic pressure echo signal is received, the required input-referred current noise of the pream-plifier is calculated to be less than 1.15 µArms integrated over 35 MHz of bandwidth.

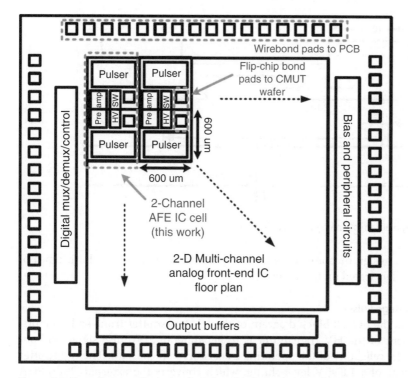

Figure 5.5 Overall system floor plan for 2-D multi-channel analog front-end IC.

For the transmitter front-end, the HV pulse has a pulse width of 30 ns with a repetition rate at around 30–35 kHz, while generating a 30 V_{P-P} unipolar HV signal to drive the CMUT in order to produce a large enough acoustic pressure signal to travel to the specified focal depth. The simplified timing diagram for the two-channel AFE operation in transmission and reception mode is shown in Figure 5.6.

5.4.2 System Implementation

5.4.2.1 Process Selection
In order to radiate a large acoustic pressure from the transducer surface, the CMUT needs to be biased at a high DC voltage and driven with an HV pulse signal. In this work, the Global Foundry HV 0.18 μm Bipolar/CMOS/DMOS (BCD) process is selected, which provides a maximum of 30-VP-P drain-to-source voltage (VDS) for HV asymmetrical and symmetrical DNMOS and DPMOS transistors with 0.74 and 0.79 threshold voltages (VTH), respectively. In order to avoid channel hot carrier effects and eventual avalanche breakdown, the method of extending the vertical length and doping concentration of the n-well at the drain region of an HV DMOS transistor is used. As a result, DMOS transistors occupy layout areas that are orders of magnitude larger than nominal transistors. The main limitation of these devices is the low gate-to-source breakdown voltage of 6 V compared to an over 30 V breakdown between drain and source, which has to be taken into account in the design stage of HV circuits. In addition to the HV DMOS transistors, 1.8-V, 5/6-V standard NMOS/PMOS transistors are

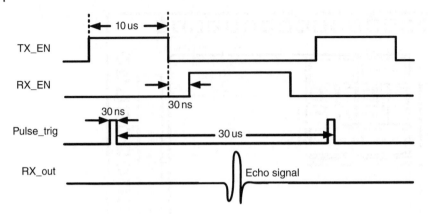

Figure 5.6 Timing diagram of analog front-end operation.

provided for the design of nominal voltage core blocks and allows for both types of transistors to be fabricated on the same die.

5.4.2.2 High Voltage Pulser

Figure 5.7 shows the overall block diagram of the HV transmitter front-end. The primary requirement of the HV transmitter is to generate an HV pulse signal without compromising the reliability of the operating transistors in the circuit. The transmitter front-end consists of a 1.8–5 V level-shifter, which converts the external DSP/FPGA generated 1.8 Vp-p trigger signal to swing between 0 and 5 V at the output. Then the 5-Vp-p signal is divided into two separate paths. The upper path contains a second level-shifter to convert the signal to swing between 25 V and 30 V in order to drive the gate of the DPMOS transistor of the output driver. However, the lower path goes through inverter-based delay buffers to drive the gate of the DNMOS transistor of the output driver. The output driver is followed by the corresponding CMUT element where the CMUT is driven with a 30-Vp-p HV pulse so that an ultrasound signal with sufficient acoustic pressure is generated for propagation through the acoustic medium.

Figure 5.8 shows a schematic diagram of a 1.8–5 V level-shifter. The circuit consists of cross-coupled PMOS transistors and two NMOS transistors driven by two complementary input signals noted as IN and IN_B. When the input voltages IN and IN_B are low

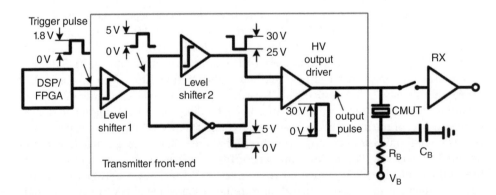

Figure 5.7 Block diagram of transmitter front-end IC.

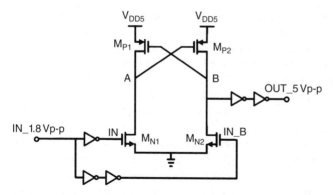

Figure 5.8 Schematic of 1.8-to-5 V level-shifter.

and high, then M_{N1} and M_{N2} are OFF and ON, respectively. Then M_{N2} pulls down node B and M_{P1} is turned ON, so this will pull up node A. This will turn OFF M_{P2} and OUT_5Vp-p will pull down to GND. On the other hand, when the input voltages IN and IN_B are high and low, then M_{N1} and M_{N2} are ON and OFF, respectively. Then M_{N1} pulls down node A and M_{P2} is turned ON, so this will pull up node B resulting in OUT_5Vp-p to be at 5 V.

Figure 5.9 shows a schematic of the second level-shifter and the HV output driver to generate 30 V_{P-P} unipolar pulses to excite the transducer. As the DMOS transistors can only sustain 5-V gate-to-source voltage, a second level-shifter is needed to produce a pulse that swings between 25 V and 30 V to drive the DPMOS transistor of the output driver. In order to prevent junction breakdown of the regular MOS transistors during

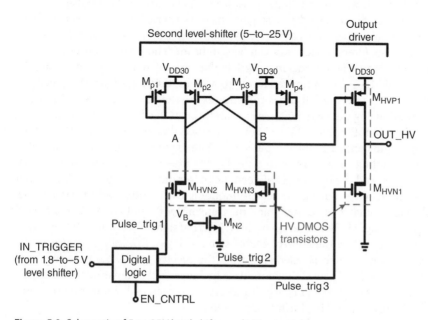

Figure 5.9 Schematic of 5-to-25 V level-shifter and HV output driver.

HV operation, DMOS transistors are used in both the level-shifter and output driver, so that reliability in the circuit operation is maintained. However, the disadvantage of these DMOS transistors is the added process cost, increased layout size, and parasitic capacitance. In addition, the device on-resistance of these transistors is larger than regular CMOS transistors and the sizing has to be sufficiently large in order to drive the following CMUT element to an HV at megahertz frequencies. Therefore, for the proposed work, standard CMOS transistors are used wherever possible in order to minimize the overall area of the transmitter front-end.

The output driver stage consists of DMOS transistors M_{HVP1} and M_{HVN1}, in which the gates are driven by two signals created from the regular voltage triggering logic. The gate of M_{HVN1} is controlled by Pulse_trig3, which swings between ground and 5-V. However, the control signal at node B driving the gate of M_{HVP1} needs a level shift to operate between V_{DD30} (30 V) and V_{DD30}-5 V, which is made possible by the transistors M_{HVN2}-M_{HVN3} and M_{P1}-M_{P5}. 5-V_{P-P} trigger signals go through a digital logic block consisting of delay cells to create non-overlapping trigger signals Pulse_trig1 and Pulse_trig2. Pulse_trig1 is used to control the unipolar HV pulse applied across the transducer element, while Pulse_trig2 with phase delay is used to completely turn OFF M_{HVP1} during the pulse repetition time. These two signals are used to drive the gate of M_{HVN2} and M_{HVN3}, which will have the A and B nodes to swing between 25 and 30 V due to the diode-connected transistors M_{P1} and M_{P4} connected in parallel to the M_{P2} and M_{P3} transistors. The signal at the B node will then switch M_{HVP1} ON and OFF to apply the 30 V to the output, which excites the CMUT.

The triggering pulse duration is equal to 28.5 ns, which is equal to 35 MHz of the resonating frequency of the transducer element. In order to avoid M_{HVP1} and M_{HVN1} turning on simultaneously and to decrease the power consumption of the driver, the timing of the Pulse_trig1, Pulse_trig2, and Pulse_trig3 signals are carefully adjusted through sizing of the internal digital logic.

As the transmitter has to drive a large transducer capacitance in short pulse duration, the correct sizing of the output driver stage transistors is critical. The sizes cannot be designed too large as the parasitic capacitances associated with the transistors M_{HVP1} and M_{HVN1} as well as the interconnect lines can be significant. Those large capacitances can reduce the output signal amplitude and degrade the element sensitivity. Therefore, the sizes of M_{HVP1} and M_{HVN1} are optimized through careful simulation so that the generated pulse can have steep rise and fall times to better excite the ultrasound transducer elements while minimizing the high dynamic current through the driver transistors.

The transmitter output is 30 V, 0 V, or high impedance, depending on the values of the triggering input and control enabled input signal. The high impedance state is adopted so that no AC coupling capacitors are required at the preamplifier input when the HV switch is turned on and the bias level between the pulser output and preamplifier input is decided by the receiver during the reception mode. During the transmission mode, the control enable signal is logic "high" and the transmitter output voltage is controlled by input triggering signal. The duration of this triggering signal determines the duration of the output pulse. When the control enable signal is logic "low", the output is at the high impedance state, which is selected during the receive mode. Considering large array implementation, the power-down mode is included in the transmitter to save the static power so that non-selected transmit pulsers are powered-down during transmit mode, while all pulsers are OFF during receive mode.

5.4.2.3 Low-Noise Preamplifier and High Voltage Switch

Among several choices for the low-noise preamplifier, such as resistive feedback type TIA [7,12,13,21] and capacitive feedback charge amplifier [22,23], the chosen preamplifier circuit is a TIA due to the ease of biasing, composed of a single-ended amplifier and a feedback resistor RF. The single-ended amplifier consists of a common-source amplifier followed by a source follower, as shown in Figure 5.10. A TIA acts as a current-to-voltage converter, which has a low input impedance, making it well-suited for high-impedance sources, so that the received input current is maximized.

For the design, an equivalent circuit to represent the CMUT is used, as shown in Figure 5.3, together with an additional parasitic capacitance of 1 pF at the preamplifier input to consider the addition due to the flip-chip bonding [12]. As mentioned in the previous section, no AC coupling capacitors are adopted at the preamplifier input in order to minimize the area and at the same time to reduce bandwidth degradation.

Considering the maximum output voltage swing of 1 V_{P-P} at the maximum received acoustic pressure condition already specified, 6 V CMOS transistors are used for the design. In order to maximize the input current, the input impedance of the closed-loop preamplifier R_{IN} must be minimized. R_{IN} is shown to be $R_{IN} = R_f/(A + 1)$, where A is the open-loop gain of the preamplifier. The value of the feedback resistor R_f and the sizing of the main input transistor MN1 is critical in deciding the gain, bandwidth, and the noise performance of the preamplifier. The closed-loop gain of the TIA is set by R_f, which has a value of 1.15 kΩ, and the translated gain results as 61.2 dBΩ, meeting the required specifications. The −3-dB bandwidth of the preamplifier is dominated by the large CMUT capacitance at the input of the preamplifier, which is approximated by:

$$\omega_{TIA,-3dB} = \frac{1}{R_{IN}\left(C_{CMUT} + C_p\right)} \tag{5.2}$$

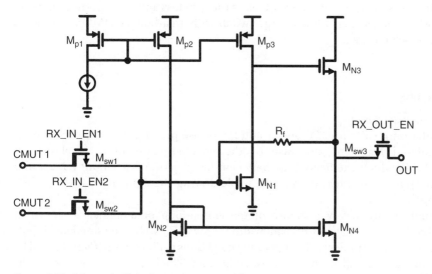

Figure 5.10 Schematic of the low-noise preamplifier.

where C_p is the parasitic capacitance in parallel with the CMUT capacitor. With the dominant pole at the input and additional poles at the drain nodes of the transistors MN1 and MP3 and at the output, the phase margin in the open-loop configuration is simulated to be over 55° with a load of around 4 pF representing the input impedance of the following external TGC.

The input-referred noise current of the TIA can be represented as:

$$\overline{i^2_{N\_in\_total}} = \overline{i^2_{N\_amp}} + \overline{i^2_{R_f}} + \overline{v^2_{N\_amp}} \times \left(\frac{1}{R_{in\_amp}} + \omega C_{in} + \frac{1}{R_f}\right)^2 \tag{5.3}$$

where $\overline{i^2_{N\_amp}}$ and $\overline{v^2_{N\_amp}}$ are the input-referred current and voltage noise of the core amplifier, $\overline{i^2_{R_f}}$ is the noise of the feedback resistor, R_{in_amp} is the input resistance of the core amplifier, and C_{in} is the total input capacitance including the CMUT capacitance and the input parasitic capacitance. Note that $\overline{i^2_{N\_amp}}, \overline{v^2_{N\_amp}}$ and $\overline{i^2_{R_f}}$ are determined by:

$$\overline{i^2_{N\_amp}} \approx \left(\omega C_{in}\right)^2 \frac{4kT\gamma}{g_{m1}}, \quad \overline{v^2_{N\_amp}} \approx \frac{4kT\gamma}{g_{m1}}, \quad \overline{i^2_{R_f}} = \frac{4kT}{R_f} \tag{5.4}$$

The primary noise sources of the TIA are the noise of the main transistor MN1, which dominates the noise of the core amplifier, and R_f. The transconductance gm_1 of MN1 and the value of R_f must therefore be maximized to suppress the noise while considering the bandwidth requirement. Due to the area constraint of the CMUT element described before, one preamplifier is shared by two CMUT elements, and thus two HV DNMOS switches are connected to the input of the preamplifier so that a selection can be achieved between the two while isolating the preamplifier from the HV pulser output during the transmitting mode. The sizing of the switches are done by considering the switch-on resistance RON, as the gain loss and noise performance are affected with small sizing, while a large switch with area-hungry DMOS transistors consumes much die area.

5.4.3 Results

5.4.3.1 Simulation Results

The simulation results for HV pulser and low-noise preamplifier are shown first. The simulated transient response of the enabled transmitter is shown in Figure 5.11, in which the delay time between the 30-ns 1.8-V_{P-P} input trigger and 30-V_{P-P} output pulse is less than 14 ns, while driving the equivalent CMUT electrical model.

The simulated frequency response of the closed-loop preamplifier is shown in Figure 5.12(a). The simulated 3-dB bandwidth is around 75 MHz. The simulated input-referred current noise under typical operating conditions is 17.5 pA/sqrt(Hz) at 35 MHz, as shown in Figure 5.12(b), which corresponds to a 0.09 µArms integrated over a 35-MHz bandwidth. The total power consumption of the preamplifier is 13 mA at 6-V

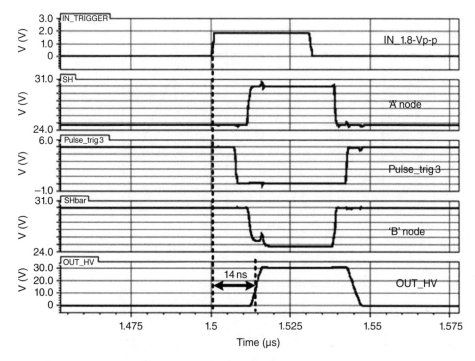

Figure 5.11 Simulated timing response of the HV transmitter front-end.

supply voltage. Due to the existence of a large CMUT capacitance at the input of around 44 pF, a sufficient amount of current has been used to meet the bandwidth and output swing requirement.

5.4.3.2 Two-channel AFE IC Measurement Results

The 320 × 320 CMUT cell array-based ultrasound sensor array and the two-channel ultrasound sensor unit cell are both fabricated in the one-poly six-metal (1P6M) HV 30-V 0.18-µm BCD process. The micro-photograph of the ultrasound sensor array chip is shown in Figure 5.13(a). The chip microphotograph for a two-channel sensor unit cell is shown in Figure 5.13(b). In order to support large dynamic current consumption for the HV pulser during transmit mode operation, multiple wide top metal paths stacked from metal-1 to metal-6 layers are used for the 30-V HV supply and ground routing lines. In addition, an excessive number of custom-made pads located at the top and right side of the chip is used for the 30-V HV supply and ground pins. The total chip area of the core is 1.2 mm × 0.6 mm including the two HV pulsers, one preamplifier, two HV protection switches, and all the routing paths for the control/trigger signals and power/ground lines.

The two inputs of the shared preamplifier and the two outputs of the pulsers are placed as close as possible to the two input/output bonding test pads (mimicking the 100 µm × 100 µm flip-chip bonding pads for CMUT element connection) to minimize the parasitic along the interconnection. The die is housed in a QFP32

(a)

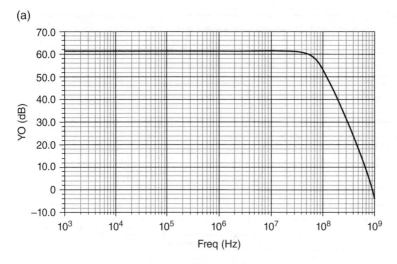

(b)

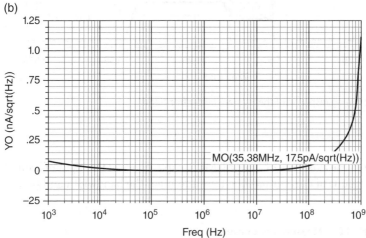

Figure 5.12 Simulated: (a) closed-loop frequency response; and (b) Input referred noise current.

package for measurement on an FR4 PCB. For the ultrasound sensor IC-only characterization without the CMUT, the equivalent CMUT model is assembled on the PCB using surface mounted type passive components, which can sustain an HV of up to 50 V.

First, the HV transmitter is tested using an external arbitrary waveform generator as the input trigger. Figure 5.14 presents the 1.8-Vp-p input signal versus HV output pulse measurement capture. A pulse width of 33 ns and repetition rate of 500 ns for the 1.8 V input trigger pulse is used in this measurement example. A delay of 16.2 ns is measured between the input trigger pulse and the 30 $V_{P\text{-}P}$ HV output pulse, while driving the total load capacitance of 43 pF at the pulser output that meets the specification.

Figure 5.15(a) shows the measured frequency response of the preamplifier. In order to measure the transimpedance gain, an off-chip resistor is placed in series on the PCB at

(a)   (b)

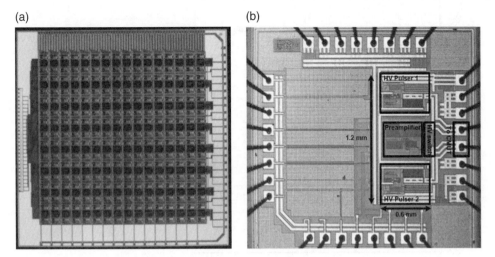

Figure 5.13 Chip microphotograph of: (a) AFE array; and (b) 2-channel AFE IC cell.

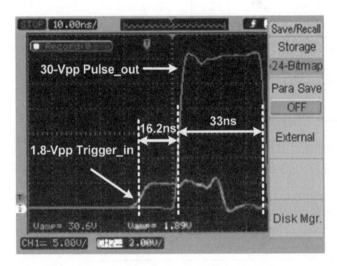

Figure 5.14 Measured transient response of the HV pulser.

the preamplifier input and the voltage across it is measured by using an active probe to calculate the input AC current. Over 62 dBΩ of transimpedance gain is observed while the 3-dB bandwidth is 75 MHz, which closely follows the post-layout simulation results. The offline calculated input noise current density from the measured output noise voltage density is plotted in Figure 5.15(b). The measured results closely follow the simulation results and satisfy the required specifications. The measured transceiver front-end IC performance is summarized in Table 5.2.

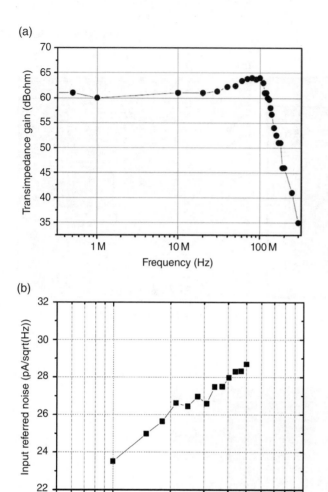

(a)

(b)

Figure 5.15 Measured: (a) Frequency response; and (b) Input noise current of the preamplifier.

Table 5.2 Measured transceiver front-end IC performance.

Parameter	Values
Blocks	Preamplifier + HV pulser
Preamplifier Gain	62 dBΩ
Preamplifier input noise current	27.5 pA/√Hz
Preamplifier bandwidth	100 MHz
Preamplifier current consumption	13 mA @ 6 V
HV Pulser output voltage	30 Vpp unipolar
HV Pulser current consumption	300 mA dynamic, 28 mA static
HV Pulser input trigger pulse width	28–35 ns
Area	0.7 mm^2
Technology	30-V HV 0.18 mm BCD

(a)

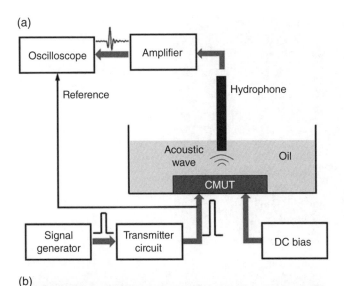

(b)

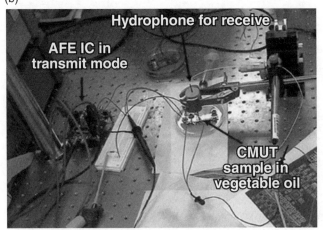

Figure 5.16 Acoustic transmission testing setup for the implemented ultrasound sensor and fabricated CMUT sample.

5.4.3.3 Acoustic Transmission Testing with AFE IC and CMUT

The acoustic transmission experiment is carried out with the AFE IC and in-house developed high-frequency CMUT elements. CMUT samples with center frequency at 10 MHz are used for testing instead of 35 MHz CMUT samples due to fabrication yield problems. The block diagram and photo of the acoustic transmit testing setup is shown in Figures 5.16(a) and (b). The CMUT sample is mounted on a separate PCB and is connected to the transmitted IC through a board-to-board wire connection. The CMUT-mounted PCB is placed in a glass container filled with vegetable oil to mimic an underwater environment, while the IC mounted board is placed outside. A hydrophone is placed at a close distance away from the CMUT in oil to measure the resulting transmitted

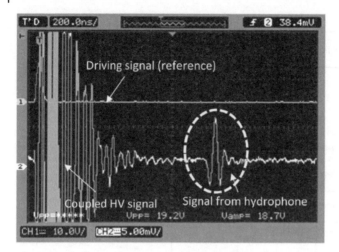

Figure 5.17 Measured hydrophone output voltage signal.

acoustic pressure and convert it to a voltage signal. The external arbitrary waveform generator is again used to generate a 10 MHz 1.8-Vp-p input pulse and is amplified to a 30-Vp-p pulse signal by the AFE IC in transmission mode to drive the CMUT at the output. The CMUT converts the electrical signal to an acoustic pressure signal corresponding to the amount of applied voltage. A 20-V DC bias voltage is applied to the top electrode of the CMUT for testing. Figure 5.17 shows the measured acoustic pressure-to-converted voltage at the hydrophone output. The results show a successful transmission demonstration of the proposed AFE ultrasound sensor while driving a CMUT in an acoustic environment.

5.4.3.4 Acoustic Pulse-echo Testing with AFE IC and CMUT

The acoustic pulse-echo experiment is carried out with the developed AFE IC and CMUT sample. The basic idea is to transmit an acoustic pressure signal from the transmitting CMUT in oil and receive the echo signal resulting from the reflection due to the oil–air layer interface using the receiving CMUT. The block diagram and photo of the acoustic transmit testing setup is shown in Figure 5.18. In this setup, two AFE ICs are used for the testing. The first AFE IC is used to drive the transmitting CMUT with an HV signal, while the second AFE IC is placed close to the receiving CMUT in oil to amplify the weak current signal resulting from the echo signal. The pulse-echo measurements are plotted in Figure 5.19, where the first and second echo reflections are measured. The change in the depth of the oil inside the water tank results in a longer distance between the immersed CMUT and the oil–air surface, resulting in an increased delay of the received echo as shown.

This confirms a successful demonstration of the proposed HV, high-frequency two-channel AFE IC cell for CMUT interface, and can be utilized as a unit cell for future 2-D multi-array AFE IC development for 3-D high-resolution ultrasound systems.

(a)

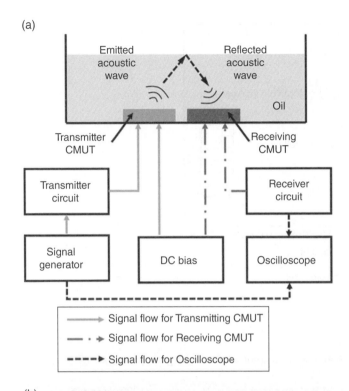

- ——► Signal flow for Transmitting CMUT
- — · ► Signal flow for Receiving CMUT
- ----► Signal flow for Oscilloscope

(b)

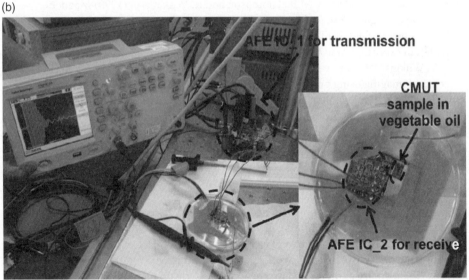

Figure 5.18 Acoustic pulse-echo testing setup for implemented AFE IC and fabricated CMUT sample.

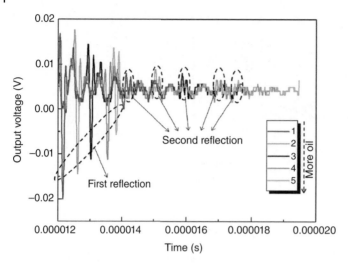

Figure 5.19 Measured pulse-echo response.

References

1 B.T. Khuri-Yakub, Ö. Oralkan and M. Kupnik (2009) Next-gen ultrasound. *IEEE Spectrum*, 46(5), 44–54.
2 E.M. Haacke, R.W. Brown, M.R. Thompson and R. Venkatesan (1999) Magnetic resonance imaging. *Physical Principles and Sequence Design*.
3 D.J. Brenner and E.J. Hall (2007) Computed tomography – an increasing source of radiation exposure. *New England Journal of Medicine*, 357(22), 2277–2284.
4 S.W. Wilkins, T.E. Gureyev, D. Gao, A. Pogan and A.W. Stevenson (1996) Phase-contrast imaging using polychromatic hard X-ray. *Nature*, 384(6607), 335–338.
5 M.I. Fuller, K. Ranganathan, S. Zhou, T.N. Blalock, J.A. Hossack and W.F. Walker (2008) Experimental system prototype of a portable, low-cost, C-scan ultrasound imaging device. *IEEE Trans. Biomedical Engineering*, 55(1), 519–530.
6 B.T. Khuri-Yakub and O. Oralkan (2011) Capacitive micromachined ultrasound transducers for medical imaging and therapy. *Journal of Micromechanics and Microengineering*, 21, 054004.
7 O. Oralkan (2004) Acoustical imaging using capacitive micromachined ultrasonic transducer arrays: devices, circuits, and systems, PhD dissertation, Department of Electrical Engineering, Stanford University, Stanford, CA.
8 N. Lamberti, G. Caliano, A. Iula and A.S. Savoia (2011) A high frequency CMUT probe for ultrasound imaging of fingerprints. *Sensors and Actuators A: Physical*, 172(2), 561–569.
9 R.O. Guldiken, J. Zahorian, F. Yamaner and F. Degertekin (2009) Dual-electrode CMUT with non-uniform membranes for high electromechanical coupling coefficient and high bandwidth operation. *IEEE Transactions on Ultrasonics, Ferroelectrics and Frequency Control (TUFFC)*, 56(6), 1270–1276.
10 P. Kwan Kyu, L. Hyunjoo, M. Kupnik and B.T. Khuri-Yakub (2011) Fabrication of capacitive micromachined ultrasonic transducers via local oxidation and direct wafer bonding. *Journal of Microelectromechanical Systems*, 20(1), 95–103.

11 A.S. Logan, L.L.P. Wong and J.T.W. Yeow (2011) A 1-D capacitive micromachined ultrasonic transducer imaging array fabricated with a silicon-nitride-based fusion process. *IEEE/ASME Transactions on Mechatronics*, 16(5), pp. 861–865.

12 I.O. Wygant, N. Jamal, H. Lee, A. Nikoozadeh, O. Oralkan, *et al.* (2009) An integrated circuit with transmit beamforming flip-chip bonded to a 2-D CMUT array for 3-D ultrasound imaging. *IEEE Transactions on Ultrasonics, Ferroelectrics and Frequency Control (TUFFC)*, 56(10), 2145–2156.

13 G. Gurun, P. Hasler and F.L. Degertekin (2011) Front-end receiver electronics for high-frequency monolithic CMUT-on-CMOS imaging arrays. *IEEE Transactions on Ultrasonics, Ferroelectrics and Frequency Control (TUFFC)*, 58(8), 1658–1668.

14 K.K. Park, H.J. Lee, G.G. Yaralioglu, A.S. Ergun, Ö. Oralkan, *et al.* (2007| Capacitive micromachined ultrasonic transducers for chemical detection in nitrogen. *Applied Physics Letters*, 91(9), 094102.

15 S.H. Wong, M. Kupnik, R.D. Watkins, K. Butts-Pauly and B.T. Khuri-Yakub, (2010) Capacitive micromachined ultrasonic transducers for therapeutic ultrasound applications. *IEEE Transactions on Biomedical Engineering (TBME)*, 57(1), 114–123.

16 K.K. Shung, J. Cannata, Z. Qifa and L. Jungwoo (2009) High frequency ultrasound: A new frontier for ultrasound. *International Conference of the IEEE Engineering in Medicine and Biology Society (EMBC)*, 1953–1955.

17 I.O. Wygant, Z. Xuefeng, D.T. Yeh, O. Oralkan, A.S. Ergun, *et al.* (2008) Integration of 2-D CMUT arrays with front-end electronics for volumetric ultrasound imaging. *IEEE Transactions on Ultrasonics, Ferroelectrics and Frequency Control (TUFFC)*, 55(2), 327–342.

18 X. Huang, J.H. Cheong, H.-K. Cha, H. Yu, M. Je and H. Yu (2013) A high-frequency transimpedance amplifier for CMOS integrated 2-D CMUT array towards 3-D ultrasound imaging. *International Conference of the IEEE Engineering in Medicine and Biology Society (EMBC)*, pp. 101–104.

19 G.I. Athanosopoulos, S.J. Carey and J.V. Hatfield (2011) Circuit design and simulation of a transmit beamforming ASIC for high-frequency ultrasound imaging systems. *IEEE Trans. Ultrason. Ferroelectr. Freq. Control*, 58(7), 1320–1331.

20 Y. Wang, M. Koen and D. Ma (2011) Low-noise CMOS TGC amplifier with adaptive gain control for ultrasound imaging receivers. *IEEE Trans. Circuits and Systems II*, 58(1), 26–30.

21 A. Sharma, M.F. Zaman and F. Ayazi (2007) A 104-dB dynamic range transimpedance-based CMOS ASIC for tuning fork microgyroscopes. *IEEE Journal of Solid-State Circuits*, 42(8), 1790–1802.

22 S.-Y. Peng, M.S. Quresh, P. Hasler, A. Basu and F.L. Degertekin, (2008) A charge-based low-power high-SNR capacitive sensing interface circuit. *IEEE Trans. Circuits and Systems I*, 55(7), 1863–1872.

23 L.R. Cenkeramaddi, A. Bozkurt, F.Y. Yamaner and T. Ytterdal (2007) A low noise capacitive feedback analog front-end for CMUTs in intra vascular ultrasound imaging. In: *IEEE Ultrasonics Symposium*, pp. 2143–2146.

6

CMOS 3-D-Integrated MEMS Sensor

6.1 Introduction

Three-dimensional integration has been widely recognized as the next generation of technology for integrated microsystems with small form factor, high bandwidth, and low power consumption, and enables heterogeneous More-than-Moore integration [1–4]. Hence, it is one promising technique for the future LOC personalized diagnosis applications, since LOC systems need to integrate CMOS sensor chips, micro-electro-mechanical system (MEMS), and microfluidic channels, etc., for multi-modal sensing. Among them, the MEMS-CMOS integration is critical for the future development of multi-sensor data fusion in a low-cost chip size system. However, until recently, the primary methods for MEMS/CMOS integration were still monolithic and hybrid/package approaches, where chip-to-chip wire bonding was required [5–8].

Towards this issue, the 3-D CMOS-on-MEMS integration technique is of great importance. Previous studies have demonstrated low-temperature (300 °C) Cu–Cu thermo-compression bonding to obtain hermetic packaging of 3-D microsystems in accordance with the MIL-STD-883E standard [9]. Three-dimensional integration of MEMS and CMOS via low temperature (300 °C) Cu–Cu thermos-compression bonding has also been proposed [10]. However, it is difficult to produce silicon-on-insulator (SOI) MEMS dies with Cu pads as the insulator release process will also strip away common Cu barrier materials. This chapter presents one TSV-less 3-D CMOS-on-MEMS integration technique using direct (i.e. solder-less) metal bonding. The CMOS-on-MEMS integration leads to a simultaneous formation of electrical, mechanical, and hermetic bonds, eliminates chip-to-chip wire-bonding, and hence presents competitive advantages over hybrid or monolithic solutions. The CMOS die also serves as a capping medium to isolate the MEMS from the ambient, removing the need of hermetic packaging, thus reducing the thickness of the overall package. Al–Au thermo-compression bonding is used to simultaneously form a hermetic seal and connections. Au is chosen as it is a common pad material for MEMS dies and Al–Au bonding is commonly found in wire-bonding. Al–Au thermo-compression bonding is evaluated according to MIL-STD 883 for shear strength [11] and leak test [12].

CMOS Integrated Lab-on-a-Chip System for Personalized Biomedical Diagnosis,
First Edition. Hao Yu, Mei Yan, and Xiwei Huang.
© 2018 John Wiley & Sons Singapore Pte. Ltd. Published 2018 by John Wiley & Sons Singapore Pte. Ltd.

6.2   MEMS Sensor

The MEMS sensor is a capacitive accelerometer. The basic working principle of the MEMS accelerometer is the displacement of a small proof mass etched into the silicon surface of the integrated circuit and suspended by small beams. As acceleration is applied to the device, a force develops which displaces the mass. The support beams act as a spring, and the fluid (usually air) trapped inside the device acts as a damper, which results in a second-order lumped physical system [13]. This is the source of the limited operational bandwidth and non-uniform frequency response of accelerometers. Capacitive accelerometers output a voltage dependent on the distance between two planar surfaces. One or both of these "plates" are charged with an electrical current. Changing the gap between the plates changes the electrical capacity of the system, which can be measured as a voltage output. Compared with piezoelectric accelerometers, capacitive accelerometers are also less prone to noise and variation with temperature, typically dissipating less power, and can have larger bandwidths due to internal feedback circuitry [14].

Our capacitive accelerometer is fabricated using bulk micromachining technology with SOI substrate (resistivity ~0.002 Ω/cm). The sensitivity is approximately 4.88 fF/g. It is designed and fabricated by deep reactive ion etching (DRIE), as shown in Figure 6.1. A metal layer is patterned onto the MEMS prior to etching for electrical contact and hermetic seal. The resonant frequency is approximately 136 kHz.

6.3   Readout Circuit

The CMOS readout circuit for MEMS consists of a low-noise, band-pass gain stage, a fully differential synchronous demodulator, and an off-chip, low-pass filter. The block diagram for the readout circuit is shown in Figure 6.2. The low noise, band-pass gain stage is realized by using two identical single-ended output amplifiers, as shown in Figure 6.3. These single-ended output amplifiers are based on folded-cascode topology, which offers the advantages of a much improved common-mode input range and an increased output swing. This allows more flexibility in selecting the gain factor, which can be conveniently set externally via tunable feedback capacitance C_f. The flexibility in selecting the gain factor enables the same readout circuit design to work well with a wider range of accelerometer designs, in terms of output capacitance and sensitivity.

It is also desirable to have a large feedback resistance R_f since the lower corner of the band-pass gain stage is determined by $1/2\pi R_f C_f$. However, using a large feedback resistor means an inefficient utilization of on-chip space. This can be taken care of by using pseudo-resistors in place of real resistors, which can provide high feedback resistance, of the order of MΩ, while consuming minimal space. The unity gain bandwidth of the folded-cascode single-ended output amplifiers determines the upper corner frequency of the band-pass gain stage. The lower and the upper corner frequency limits of the gain stage thus determine the working carrier frequency range, which are 10 kHz and 18 MHz respectively for the reported readout design. The first amplifier of the gain stage boosts

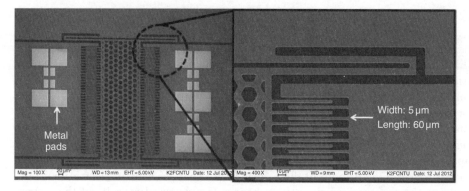

Figure 6.1 The MEMS capacitive accelerator is fabricated on an SOI wafer using DRIE and release. The single layer of patterned metal consists of an electrical contact pad and a hermetic seal is used. Electrical feed-through is routed through the on-chip interconnect in the CMOS chip.

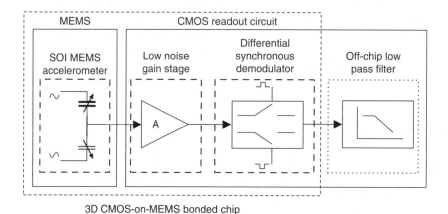

Figure 6.2 System block diagram for the readout circuit.

up the MEMS sensor's input, while the second amplifier works as an inverting stage to generate a second differential input for the synchronous demodulator.

A fully differential synchronous demodulator is the second building block of the readout circuit. Demodulation is done through envelope detection, by implementing a four-switch full-wave rectifier. The demodulator helps in easing the filtering requirements and reduces the second-order harmonic distortion at the same time. The fully differential synchronous demodulator makes it possible to move the low-pass filter off-chip, which greatly helps in saving on-chip space. Moreover, as a result of ease in filtering requirements, there is no longer any need to use an active filter and this minimizes the overall circuit's power consumption. The implemented filter is a passive, second-order low-pass filter with a cut-off frequency of 200 Hz. The die diagram is shown in Figure 6.4. Key components are highlighted and specific ones are seal ring, mechanical support, and alignment marks to assist the MEMS-CMOS bonding. The CMOS readout chip is implemented in a 0.35 μm (2-Poly 4-Metal) process.

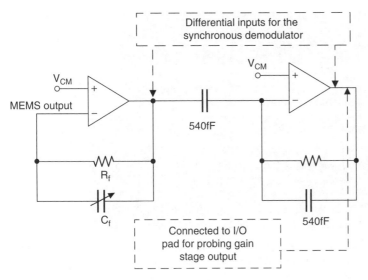

Figure 6.3 Schematic diagram of the low noise, band-pass gain stage, which consists of two single-ended output amplifiers based on folded-cascode architecture. Pseudo-resistors are used in the feedback path of the amplifiers. Tunable feedback capacitance allows variable gain.

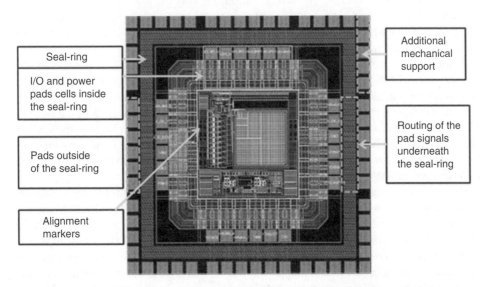

Figure 6.4 Die micrograph of the readout circuit fabricated through MPW (0.35 μm, 2P4M process).

6.4 A 3-D TSV-less Accelerometer

6.4.1 CMOS-on-MEMS Stacking

The Heterogeneous 3-D TSV-less accelerometer structure is shown in Figure 6.5. The CMOS readout circuit is stacked on the MEMS accelerometer using face-to-face (F2F) direct metal bonding, which provides smaller form factor, latency, and power

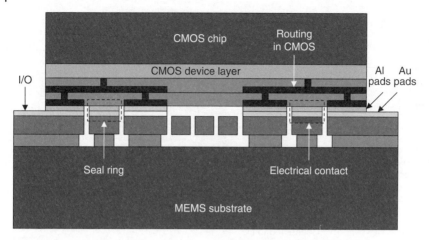

Figure 6.5 Heterogeneous 3-D CMOS-on-MEMS stacking with face-to-face direct metal bonding (no solder) that realizes electrical, mechanical, and hermetic bonds simultaneously.

consumption. In the stacking process, to ensure proper operation, the delicate micro-structures (MEMS) should be protected from the environment. In this approach, a hermetic seal ring is formed simultaneously during stacking of CMOS on MEMS and hence eliminating the need for post-processing hermetic encapsulation. Effectively, the CMOS layer acts as an "active cap" that encapsulates and provides interconnect routing to the MEMS chip.

In addition, I/Os to the MEMS chip are routed through the CMOS metal layers to simplify the MEMS process. Since the I/O count is low, TSV is not used and electrical feed-through is achieved by peripheral pads. A standard CMOS chip has a passivation layer that is typically over 2 μm thick, which can pose problems with thick metal deposition on the MEMS side. As no solder is applied, the top passivation layer of the CMOS chip is partially etched in a depth controlled manner to expose the CMOS metal layer for ease of direct bonding with the MEMS metal layer, as shown in Figure 6.6. Bonding is performed at 300 °C for 10 min under a force of 50 N.

The cross-sectional view of the bonded layer and elemental mapping from dummy structure is shown in Figure 6.7, which is inspected with TEM and EDX. The TEM images of the Al–Au interface of the sample with increasing magnifications are shown in Figures 6.7(a) and (b). There is no distinct interface observable. An EDX line scan is performed in the location shown in Figure 6.7(a) and the result of the line scan is shown in Figure 6.7(c). The EDX elemental mapping of the bonded layer is shown in Figure 6.7(d). It is observed that Al and Au are evenly distributed throughout the original Au and Al layer. This shows that all the original Al and Au layers have mixed and formed intermetallically.

The stacking process is illustrated in Figure 6.8. Alignment marks on the dies aid in orienting the dies properly before stacking. This TSV-less approach of stacking CMOS on top of MEMS results in a simultaneous formation of the hermetic seal-ring and thereby eliminates any need for post-stacking hermetic encapsulation. The vertically stacked CMOS and MEMS chip has a thickness of 1155 μm. The bonded MEMS/CMOS dies are then packed inside 44 pin J-leaded surface mount ceramic chip packages for verifying the functionality of the bonded chips, as shown in Figure 6.9.

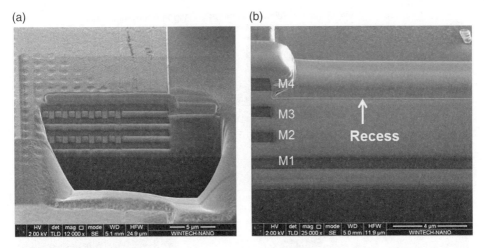

Figure 6.6 (a) FIB/SEM image showing the on-chip metal layers in the CMOS chip; and (b) Since no solder bumping is applied, the top passivation layer is intentionally recessed to create a standoff gap for the metal pads to facilitate direct metal bonding (thermo-compression) with the matching pads on the MEMS chip.

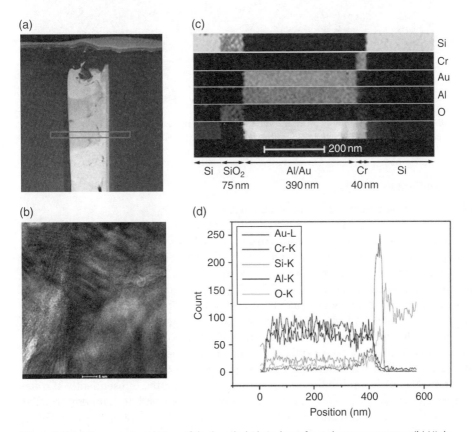

Figure 6.7 (a) Cross-sectional view of the bonded Al–Au layer from dummy structure; (b) High resolution TEM view; (c) EDX elemental mapping of the bonded layer; and (d) EDX line scan results.

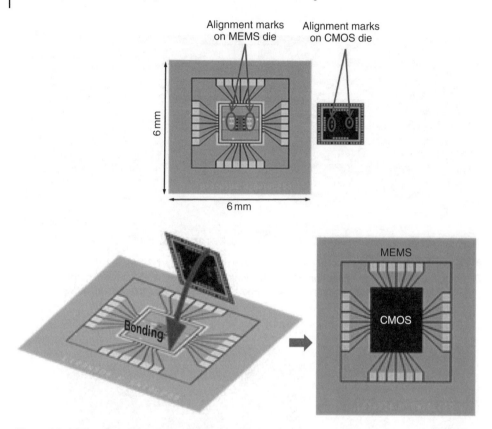

Figure 6.8 (a) The alignment marks on MEMS and CMOS die are used for orienting the dies before stacking; and (b) The CMOS die is vertically stacked on top of the MEMS die.

6.4.2 Bonding Reliability

6.4.2.1 Al–Au Thermo-compression Shear Strength

The metal bonding quality is investigated using shear and helium leak tests, following the requirements in MIL-STD-883E, 1014.9. Au–Al die level thermos-compression bondings are produced and tested for die shear strength. Silicon wafers (600 μm thick) are used in the thermo-compression bonding experiment. The wafer is deposited with 50 nm of Cr followed by 150 nm of Au. The Cr is deposited to ameliorate the adhesion between Au and Si. Dicing of the wafer is done to produce 5 mm × 5 mm size dies. A second blank wafer is PECVD deposited with 500 nm of SiO_2 and sputtered with a layer of Al of 150 nm thickness. This wafer is diced into 10 mm × 10 mm dies.

The 5 mm × 5 mm die with Au and the 10 mm × 10 mm die with Al are placed with the metal layers facing each other. They are bonded with a die bonder with an applied force of 210 N at different bonding temperatures for 10 minutes. Subsequently, the dies are annealed at the same temperature as the respective bonding temperature. The bonding temperatures and annealing temperature used are 350, 300, 290, and 280 °C, respectively. The dies are shear strength tested and the results are shown in Figure 6.10. The points in Figure 6.10 are the mean values (sample size of 5) of the shear strength

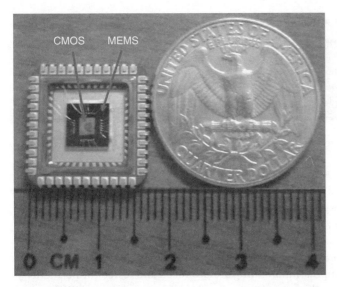

Figure 6.9 The face-to-face bonded CMOS chip on MEMS chip. The bonded chip is then wire bonded to the package for electrical testing.

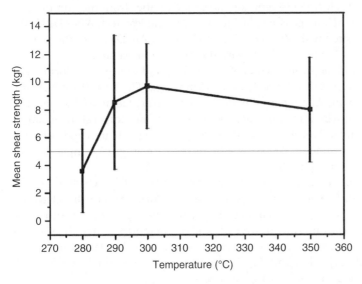

Figure 6.10 Shear strength test results with varying bonding temperature.

at the corresponding bonding temperature, while the standard deviations are depicted in the bars. The requirement of shear strength indicated in the MILSTD-883E standard is 5 kg of force.

Figure 6.10 shows that with a bonding temperature at 290 °C and above, the bonding strength produced is acceptable. When the samples are bonded with a 280 °C bonding temperature, the average shear strength of the dies is below 5 kgf. Figure 6.11 shows the C-SAM image of the samples bonded at 290 °C. The C-SAM shows that well bonded

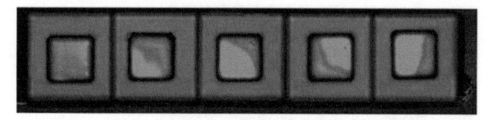

Figure 6.11 Shear strength test results with varying bonding temperature C-SAM image of samples bonded at 290 °C.

areas are presented in only half of the dies. This non-uniformity of bonding is due to the non-uniform application of force from the die bonder.

6.4.2.2 Al–Au Thermo-compression Hermeticity

Au–Al die level thermo-compression bonding are produced and tested for hermeticity. Silicon wafers are used in the thermo-compression bonding experiment. DRIE is used to form the cavities and the seal rings to a depth of 120 μm using photo-resist as an etching mask. All cavities are designed and etched to a volume of 1.4×10^{-3} cm^3. The surrounding air channel is formed to separate the sealed cavities from the dummy area and to provide a path for helium gas flow during bombing and leak test. After DRIE, the patterned wafer is deposited with 50 nm of Cr and 150 nm of Au. Dicing of the wafer is done to produce 10 mm × 10 mm sized dies with the cavity in the center.

A blank wafer is PECVD deposited with 500 nm of SiO$_2$ and sputtered to form an Al layer of 150 nm. This wafer is diced into 15 mm × 15 mm dies. The 10 × 10 mm die with Au and 15 × 15 mm die with Al are placed with the metal layers facing each other. The samples are bonded using a bonding force of 2100 N and bonding temperature of 300 °C. The samples are held under 2100 N and bonding temperature for 10 min and annealed at 300 °C for 1 h in wafer bonder. The schematic of the formation of sample dies for hermetic testing is shown in Figure 6.12.

After the dies are bonded, they are tested for hermeticity according to the MILSTD-883E standard. The helium leak test has been performed on the bonded dies. The bonded samples are placed in a chamber filled with helium gas at a pressure of 75 Psi (~0.52 MPa) for an exposure time of over 2 h (helium bombing). Then the samples are tested for helium leak using a mass spectrometer within 1 h. The leak rates for the samples are less than the rejection limit (5×10^{-8} atm-cc/s) stated in the MILSTD-883E standard, with a mean leak rate of 2.7×10^{-8} atm-cc/s.

Subsequently, the perfluorocarbon gross leak test is performed by submerging the dies in fluorocarbon FC-72 (C6F14) in a pressurized chamber of 75 Psi for 3 h. The dies are taken out and allowed to dry for 2 min. The dried dies are placed in a beaker of fluorocarbon FC-43 (C12F27N) at 125 °C. If a stream of small bubbles or a single large bubble is observed, the sample will fail the gross leak test. The samples have to pass both the helium fine leak test and the gross leak test. Only the samples that passed the gross leak test are considered in the mean fine leak rate calculated in the previous paragraph. Figure 6.13 shows the C-SAM image of a few samples, where the sealing rings are visible and continuous.

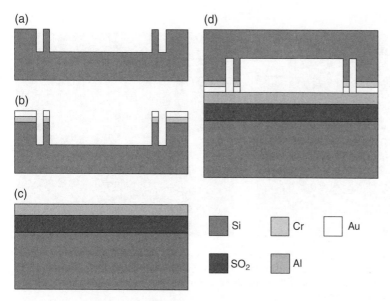

Figure 6.12 Schematics of the formation of a sealed cavity for helium leak rate detection: (a) Forming of cavities, seal rings, and air channel using DRIE; (b) Sequential deposition of Cr layer and Au bonding layer; (c) Deposition of SiO_2 isolation and Al bonding layer; and (d) Au–Al thermo-compression bonding of the cavity wafer to the capping wafer.

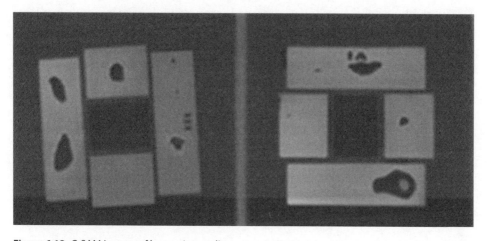

Figure 6.13 C-SAM images of hermetic test dies.

6.4.3 Results

6.4.3.1 Standalone Validation of the Readout Circuit

The working of the readout circuit was verified with a commercial MEMS accelerometer chip. The accelerometer is driven by differential sinusoid excitation carriers and its corresponding output, based on change in differential capacitance, drives the CMOS readout. The results shown in Figure 6.14 are obtained when the MEMS chip is excited

(a)

(b)

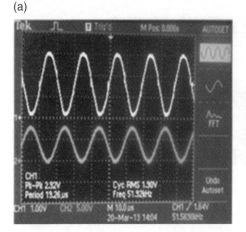
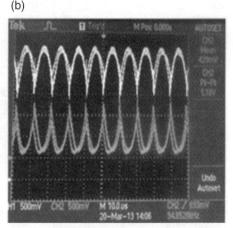

Figure 6.14 (a) The band-pass gain stage output (upper trace) during the standalone testing of the CMOS readout, when one of the carrier amplitude is 7.5 Vpp (lower trace) at 50 kHz frequency and 0 g acceleration; and (b) Fully rectified sinusoids at the synchronous demodulator outputs, verifying that the readout is working as intended.

by anti-phase but unequal amplitude excitation carriers, 5 Vpp and 7.5 Vpp, at 50 kHz carrier frequency and 0 g acceleration. Using sinusoid carriers gives a sinusoid gain stage output. The peak-to-peak amplitude of this output is dependent on:

1) *The amplitude of the excitation carriers*: Large amplitude carriers result in a large amplitude gain stage output.
2) *The frequency of the excitation carriers*: Attenuation at carrier frequencies near the corners or outside the flat-band region of the band-pass gain stage significantly diminishes the output.
3) *The gain factor of the gain stage*: Using smaller feedback capacitance Cf gives a larger gain factor.
4) *The tilt angle of the accelerometer axis with respect to the horizontal*: Larger tilt results in a larger change in capacitance and hence an enhanced input to the gain stage.

Differential sinusoid inputs to the synchronous demodulator from the gain stage, along with an externally supplied clock input, generates fully-rectified sinusoids at its outputs.

6.4.3.2 Functionality Testing of CMOS-on-MEMS Chip

The functionality of the bonded MEMS/CMOS microsystem is verified by conducting the −1 g/+1 g flip test. The results presented in Figure 6.15 are obtained using fully differential sinusoid carriers of 1 Vpp amplitude and 50 kHz frequency. The peak-to-peak amplitude of the band-pass gain stage output shows a variation that is proportional to the sine of the tilt angle between the accelerometer axis and the horizontal. Using a single-axis accelerometer restricts the total rotation to 180° (tilt angles between −90° and +90°) that corresponds to an acceleration range of −1 g to +1 g.

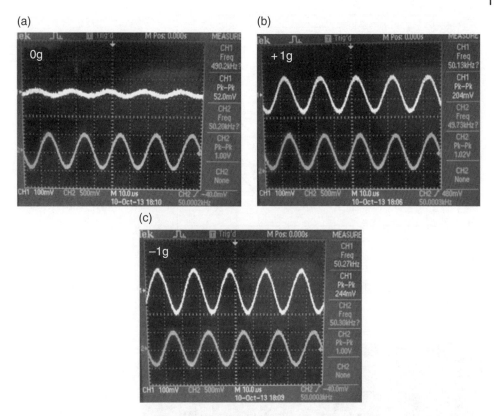

Figure 6.15 The gain stage output (yellow, upper trace) when the excitation carrier amplitude is 1 Vpp (blue, lower trace) at 50 kHz frequency and the bonded chip is tilted at: (a) 0 g; (b) +1 g; and (c) –1 g orientation. Acceleration at a tilt angle θ is given by g sin(θ).

The minimum amplitude case in Figure 6.15(a) is when the chip is at 0 g orientation. The peak-to-peak amplitude of the gain stage grows out-of-phase and in-phase with respect to carrier in –g and + g flip directions respectively. The mean of the positive rectified sinusoid at the demodulator output is plotted against g at various carrier frequencies in Figure 6.16. The maximum peak-to-peak amplitudes observed in the two flip directions are roughly equal, thereby implying an approximately symmetrical behavior of the accelerometer.

Noise performance of the bonded MEMS/CMOS microsystem was assessed using a spectrum analyzer. The analyzer output at 50 kHz carrier frequency and +1 g acceleration is shown in Figure 6.17, when the carrier amplitude is 1 Vpp. Likewise, the FFT spectrum at other carrier frequencies and flip orientations was used for computing the signal-to-noise ratio (SNR) and output voltage noise. Reduction in SNR at increasing carrier frequencies is due to an increase in the noise floor level and a simultaneous gradual reduction in the gain stage output at higher frequencies (refer to Figure 6.18). Other specifications are listed in Table 6.1.

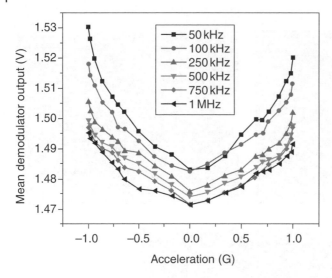

Figure 6.16 Variation in the mean demodulator output with g at various carrier frequencies for the bonded chip.

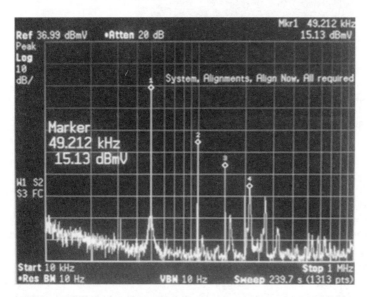

Figure 6.17 FFT spectrum showing fundamental peak at the carrier frequency and higher-order harmonics at integer multiples of carrier frequency.

6.4.3.3 Reliability Testing of CMOS-on-MEMS Chip

The bonded MEMS/CMOS chip was subjected to 500 g mechanical shock test for testing the reliability of the metal–metal contact at the MEMS–CMOS interface. The setup for this test is shown in Figure 6.19. Under this setup, the bonded chip experiences 10 repetitive vertical vibrations, where each vibration lasts for a short period of

(a)

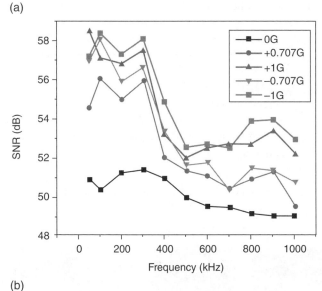

(b)

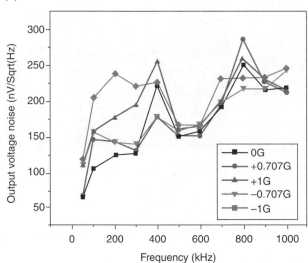

Figure 6.18 (a) SNR as a function of carrier frequency at various g orientations, when the carrier amplitude is 1 Vpp; and (b) Output voltage noise as a function of carrier frequency at various g orientations, when the carrier amplitude is 1 Vpp.

1.03 m and exerts a maximum vertical acceleration of 503.55 g on the chip, as shown in Figure 6.20. This test is in accordance with the industrial standard JESD22-B104C.

The working of the bonded chip was again checked by conducting the −1 g/+1 g flip test and the chip was still functional after going through the shock test. It can thus be concluded that the low temperature Al–Au contact at the MEMS–CMOS interface remained intact and successfully survived the shock test.

Table 6.1 Specifications summary of the vertically bonded MEMS/CMOS chip.

Parameters	Measured Values
Supply Voltage	3.3 V
Power Consumption	1.491 mW
Input Referred Noise of the readout circuit	32.663 nV/√Hz
Total Harmonic Distortion	0.380% at 50 kHz carrier frequency and +1 g acceleration
Minimum Detection Signal	±0.139 g
Resonant Frequency	136 kHz
Technology	SOI bulk micromachining for MEMS and AMS 0.35 μm (2 P4M) for the CMOS readout

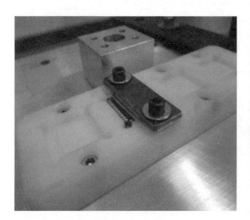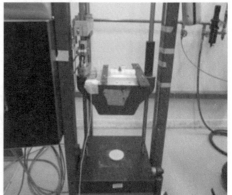

Figure 6.19 Setup for the 500 g shock test. The chip is subjected to a maximum vertical acceleration of 503.55 g for a short duration of 1.03 m for a total number of 10 times.

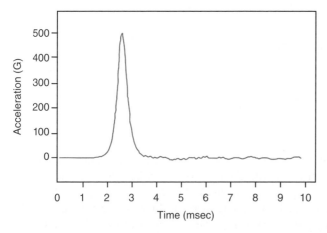

Figure 6.20 General control profile during the 500 g and 1 ms mechanical shock test.

References

1 W.R. Davis, J. Wilson, S. Mick, J. Xu, H. Hua, *et al.* (2005) Demystifying 3-D ICs: The pros and cons of going vertical. *IEEE Design & Test of Computers*, 22(60), 498–510.

2 H. Qian, X. Huang, H. Yu and C.-H. Chang (2011) Cyber-physical thermal management of 3-D multi-core cache-processor system with microfluidic cooling. *Journal of Low Power Electronics*, 7(1), 110–121.

3 K. Banerjee, S.J. Souri, P. Kapur and K.C. Saraswat (2001) 3-D ICs: A novel chip design for improving deep-submicrometer interconnect performance and systems-on-chip integration. *Proceedings of the IEEE*, 89(5), 602–633.

4 P.A. Thadesar, A. Dembla, D. Brown and M.S. Bakir (2013) Novel through-silicon via technologies for 3-D system integration. *IEEE International Interconnect Technology Conference – IITC*, pp. 1–3.

5 A. Witvrouw (2008) CMOS–MEMS integration today and tomorrow. *Scripta Materialia*, 59(9), 945–949.

6 A. Witvrouw (2006) CMOS-MEMS integration: Why, how and what? *International Conference on Computer Aided Design*, pp. 826–827.

7 J.H. Smith, S. Montague, J.J. Sniegowski, J.R. Murray and P.J. McWhorter (1995) Embedded micromechanical devices for the monolithic integration of MEMS with CMOS. *Proceedings of the IEEE International Electron Devices Meeting*, pp. 609–612.

8 G.K. Fedder, *et al.* (2008) Technologies for cofabricating MEMS and electronics. *Proceedings of the IEEE*, 96(2).

9 J. Fan, *et al.* (2012) Wafer-level hermetic packaging of 3-D microsystems with low-temperature Cu-to-Cu thermo-compression bonding and its reliability. *Journal of Micromechical Microengeering*, 22(10).

10 R. Nadipalli, *et al.* (2012) 3-D integration of MEMS and CMOS via Cu–Cu bonding with simultaneous formation of electrical, mechanical and hermetic bonds. *Proceedings of the IEEE International 3-D Systems Integration Conference*, pp. 1–5.

11 MIL-STD-883E, METHOD 2019.5, 1996.

12 MIL-STD-883E, METHOD 1014.9, 1996.

13 M. Elwenspoek and R. Wiegerink (1993) *Mechanical Microsensors*. New York: Springer, pp. 132–145.

14 N. Yazdi, F. Ayazi and K. Najafi (1998) Micromachined inertial sensors. *Proceedings of the IEEE*, 86(8), 1640–1659.

7

CMOS Image Sensor

7.1 Introduction

The solid-state image sensor is the critical component of photo-electronic devices such as mobile phones, digital video cameras, automotive imaging, surveillance, and biometrics, etc. Two types of solid-state image sensor technologies have been developed: Charged Coupled Devices (CCD) and CMOS Image Sensors (CIS). CCD image sensor technology [1,2] has been the dominant electronic imaging technology since the 1970s. A CCD sensor is composed of a photo detector and a series of metal oxide semiconductor (MOS) capacitors. The charge generated by the photosensitive detector is transferred out through the capacitors. A special manufacturing process is needed to create the ability to transport charge across the chip without distortion. This special process leads to high-quality sensors in terms of fidelity and light sensitivity, but the cost is high.

The CCD read-out architecture performs the following three basic functions, as shown in Figure 7.1:

1) *Charge collection*: When the light is incident on a photo-detector (photo-gate or photo-diode), an absorbed photon creates an electron-hole pair, which is collected and stored in a capacitor. The amount of charge stored is proportional to the number of photons absorbed. Applying a positive voltage to the CCD gate causes the generated positive holes in the P-type silicon to migrate towards the ground, and the electrons to be collected by the gate.
2) *Charge transfer*: The CCD register consists of a series of gates. Manipulation of the gate voltage in a systematic and sequential manner transfers the electrons from one gate to the next. The charge transfer from one gate to the next is illustrated in Figure 7.2.
3) *Conversion into a voltage*: When the charge reaches the end of the array, it is converted to a voltage by a floating diffusion (FD) node, that acts as a capacitor to transfer the charge to a measurable voltage: $V = Q/C$.

CCD technology has delivered superior image performance, such as high quantum efficiency (QE) and low dark current; however, this required a specialized and expensive fabrication process. In additional, the largest disadvantage is the requirement for a high drive voltage to maintain charge transfer efficiency and sufficient dynamic range. It leads to high power consumption, which is a major concern for mobile devices.

CMOS Integrated Lab-on-a-Chip System for Personalized Biomedical Diagnosis,
First Edition. Hao Yu, Mei Yan, and Xiwei Huang.
© 2018 John Wiley & Sons Singapore Pte. Ltd. Published 2018 by John Wiley & Sons Singapore Pte. Ltd.

Charge collection

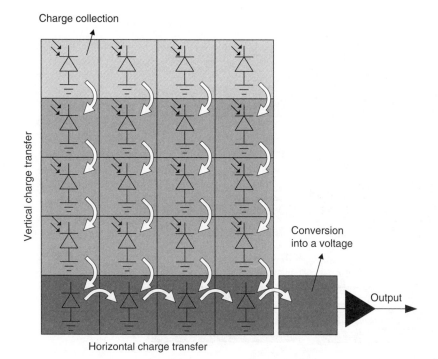

Vertical charge transfer

Conversion into a voltage

Output

Horizontal charge transfer

Figure 7.1 CCD read out architecture.

CIS technology is based on the most common and highest yielding semiconductor process, Complementary Metal Oxide Semiconductor (CMOS). The first-to-market CMOS image sensors were based on the Passive Pixel Structure (PPS) architecture (Figure 7.3(a)) invented in 1968 by Weckler and Dyck at the University of Edinburgh (later becoming VLSI Vision Ltd) [3]. The PPS pixel contains a photodiode and one transistor that operate as a switch to connect the signal to a common read-out structure. The working principle is based on the fact that a reverse biased p-n junction behaves as a capacitor charged by a photocurrent proportional to the incident light intensity. The PPS pixel has a high fill factor (ratio of photosensitive area to total pixel area). However, it suffers from low data rate and high noise due to the large capacitor connected to the photo-detector, thus PPS did not succeed commercially because of poor image quality.

A 3 T APS structure (Figure 7.3(b)) is then proposed by integrating amplifier (source follower, SF) within the pixel, thus the pixel output signal will be driven to the column output signal line. However, the photodiode is normally a p-n junction based in the reverse region. After applying an incident light, the photo-generated carriers within the depletion region are separated by the junction electric field, then electrons are collected in the n+ region and the holes in the p region. Almost all charges that are generated inside the depletion region are collected. However, photo-charges generated too close to the surface in the n-diffusion region do not diffuse to the space charge region (or depletion region) but recombine at surface states. Since the blue light is absorbed close to the surface, the surface recombination leads to a loss of blue

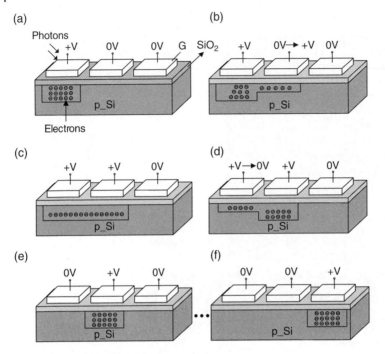

Figure 7.2 CCD charge transfer operations.

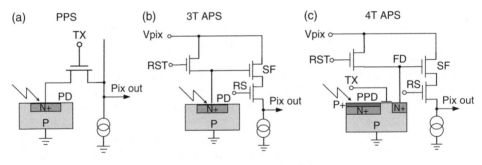

Figure 7.3 Passive and active pixel schematic and potential well diagram.

light sensitivity. The large junction capacitance at the photodiode node results in a smaller conversion gain, and thus a lower sensitivity.

To address dark current issues of photodiode, Teranishi invented the buried p-n junction PPD in 1982 [4]. This buried structure added a heavily doped p+ thin layer on the top of the n layer of the p-n junction, making a vertical p+/n/p structure. This device consists of an extremely lower dark current compared to p-n junctions [5], and also with enhancement of photo QE through the reduction of the p+ layer thickness. In 1992, the 4T APS structure (Figure 7.3(c)) was invented by Eric Forsum at the US Jet Propulsion Laboratory (JPL) [6]. By integrating an active buffer within the pixel and additional charge transfer gate (TX) separating the PPD from sensing node, the readout is faster, also achieving much higher signal-to-noise ratio (SNR) because the charge integration area is connected to the gate of the active buffer isolated from the column bus. With economy scaling of CMOS process, the cost of fabricating a CMOS wafer is lower than the cost of fabricating through more specialized CCD processes, thus the 4 T APS technology enabled the CIS to compete commercially with CCD technology.

The market for the solid-state image sensors has been experiencing explosive growth due to the increasing demands of mobile devices, therefore CIS technology has overtaken CCD in most of the fields based on reduced power (the high-voltage clock of the CCD, to control charge transfer, is no longer needed), lower cost (use standard process instead of the special CCD technology), decreased size (system-on-chip integration), and addressable readout (good for image functions such as auto-focus and motion tracking). Although CCDs had an excellent imaging performance, their fabrication processes are dedicated to making photo-sensing elements instead of transistors and hence it is difficult to implement good performance transistors using CCD fabrication processes. Therefore, it is very challenging to integrate circuitry blocks on a CCD chip. However, if the similar imaging performance can be achieved using CMOS imagers, it is even possible to implement all the required functional blocks together with the sensor, such as a camera-on-a-chip, which may significantly improve the sensor performance and lower the cost. For example, the architecture of a typical CCD digital imaging system is shown in Figure 7.4(a). Because the CCD image sensor uses a special fabrication process, the discrete blocks are implemented on separate chips. Depending on the manufacturer, several of these blocks may be integrated into a single chip. The fewest number of chips in a modern CCD system is three, and some manufacturers require as many as five chips. While CIS use a standard manufacturing process, all of the required circuits can be integrated on a single chip (Figure 7.4(b)).

In this chapter, the low-noise CIS sensor design for biomedical application is introduced. In Section 7.2, the key sensor design block pixel and associated noise sources are analyzed in detail. In Section 7.3, the different sensor readout architectures are also discussed. In Section 7.4, a 3 Meg pixel CIS design is introduced, and sensor performance is also evaluated for a lensless imaging system.

7.2 CMOS Image Pixel

7.2.1 Structure

The pinned photodiode is a key photo-detector structure used in CIS due to its low noise, high QE, and low dark current. Over the past 10 years, the steady growth of the mobile phone market has been the primary driver for CIS technology revolution, by shrinking pixel size and continuously lowering the sensor cost [7]. Here we will introduce three generations of pixel technology: FSI pixel, BSI pixel, and stack pixel.

7.2.1.1 FSI 4 T Pixel
Figure 7.5(a) shows the schematic of a conventional FSI 4 T active pixel sensor based on the pinned diode (p+/n+/p), where the n+ region is pulled away from the silicon surface in order to reduce the surface defect noise (such as due to dark current) [8]. The cross-section of a PPD shows not only the stacked n and p+ layers, but also the shallow trench

(a)

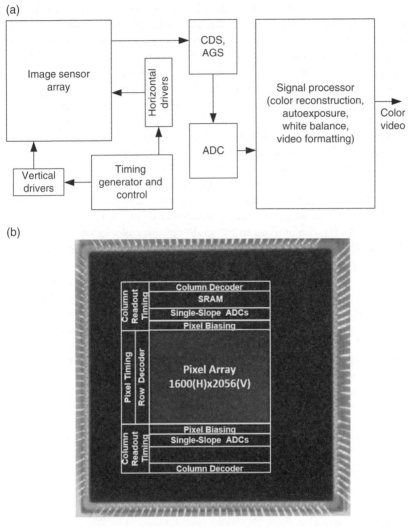

(b)

Figure 7.4 (a) Architecture of a typical digital imaging system with CCD sensor; and (b) CIS chip integrates pixel, analog readout and digital control.

insulator (STI) used to isolate the PPD. A heavily doped p + area separates the STI oxide from the PPD n well and p epitaxial layer, in order to reduce the impact of interface imperfections. Besides the pinned photodiode, the pixel consists of four transistors (4 T) that include a TX, reset transistor (RST), source follower (SF), and row-select (RS) transistor. Unlike the photodiode APS 3T structure, the pinned photodiode architecture has the FD node separated from the photodiode by the TX, so the capacitance of the FD node can be optimized. It needs to be large enough to hold all charges transferred from the photodiode; meanwhile it needs to be minimized to increase the conversion gain in order to lower the readout noise floor. Figure 7.5(b) shows the cross-section of the APS pixel structure, where the color filter separates Red, Green, and Blue light, therefore converting the scene to a color image. The micro-lens directly

(a)

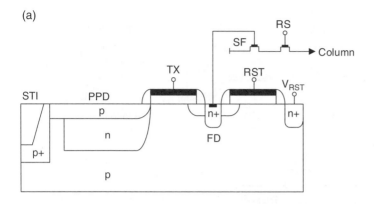

(b)

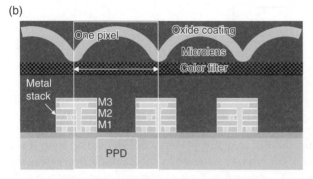

Figure 7.5 FSI 4T pinned PD pixel structure: (a) Pixel Schematic; and (b) CIS chip cross-section (Samsung NX200).

integrated above the pixel will direct the light signal passing through several metal layers and reach to the PD at the bottom of the silicon.

The pixel operation with different readout steps and timing diagram is shown in Figure 7.6. During integration phase, the photon was collected and converted to charge in a PD N well. Typical values of the TX low voltage range is slightly negative to reduce dark current, and the potential under the TX is lower enough than the pin voltage of the PPD in order to keep the integrated charge in the PPD N well. During the readout phase, after the photon is collected, the charge will be transferred from PD to FD then converted to voltage output. The readout operation is known as correlated double sampling (CDS). The FD node is first reset to V_{RST}, then the reset voltage is read out. Next the TX is turned on, and the complete photo-generated charges are transferred to the FD node, which ensures lag-free operation, then the voltage V_{SIG} is sampled again. The difference between V_{RST} and V_{SIG} is the final readout signal value. The advantage of CDS technology is to suppress the noise that is correlated between the reset time and the transfer time such as the flicker noise.

7.2.1.2 Back Side Illumination Pixel

Driven by the mobile phone market, the architecture of pixels was changed to improve resolution by shrinking pixel size, because more pixels could be arranged in designated areas to lower the sensor cost. Shared structure was first proposed by keeping some

(a)

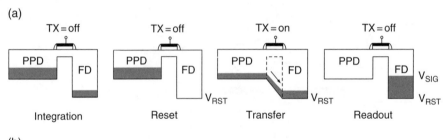

(b)

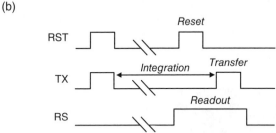

Figure 7.6 (a) Potential well diagram during pixel readout; and (b) Timing diagram during pixel readout.

transistors in common to retain the PD area and preserve image quality, even if the pixel size shrank [9]. A pixel size of 0.9 um was achieved by substantially decreasing the number of transistors from 4 to 1.37, where 8 pixels kept transistors in common [10]. When the pixel share structure reaches the limit, backside illumination pixel structure mimicking CCD technology was proposed to continuously support pixel shrinkage. As CCDs do not have any metal layers in the pixel area, the distance from the on chip lens (OCL) to the PD is shorter, and so easier to gather relatively high light and achieve better sensitivity. However, FSI CISs had several metal layers between the OCL and PD to build a transistor connection for the purpose of data readout, drive circuits, and supply voltage, meaning that it is difficult to gather light and has lower sensitivity than CCDs. Back-illuminated CISs (BI-CISs) have been developed to resolve this problem [11].

Figure 7.7 shows the structure of backside illuminated (BSI) pixel, illuminated through the back of a silicon wafer. It does not have any metal layer above the PD light sensing area, and the window of the PD is even larger than that of the CCD. Therefore, BSI CISs has almost double the sensitivity of FSI CISs, and the pixel pitch is able to shrink even below the 1-um pitch.

7.2.1.3 Stack Pixel

The stack image sensor separates chips for the pixel array and analog/digital circuitry and connects the signal through a through-silicon vias (TSV) connection. The motivations for stacked chip CIS development are optimizing process for circuitry, isolating noise, reducing area, adding functionality, enabling flexible manufacturing options, and facilitating optimization for each die in a 3-D stack. Although one of the advantages of CIS is incorporating transistor and basic signal processing circuits into CISs, because of similarities in their technologies, the required characteristics of transistors and the

(a)

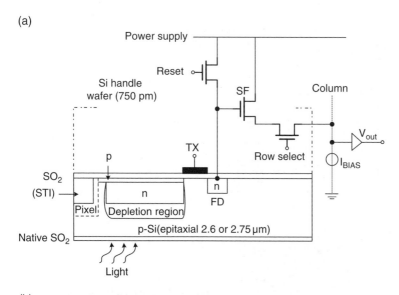

(b)

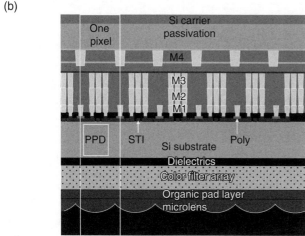

Figure 7.7 Backside illuminated (BSI) 4T CIS pixel structure: (a) Schematic; and (b) Cross-section of CIS chip (OmniVision).

number of wiring layers for pixels and peripheral circuits are essentially different. Transistors in the pixel region need relatively high voltage for accurate analog signals, and also low noise technology. However, transistors in the peripheral circuit region need high drivability at low voltage to achieve high-speed operation and low-power consumption. The difference in technologies for pixel transistors and peripheral transistors increases with the advancing generation of technology, so that it has become difficult to fabricate these high-performance pixels and peripheral circuits in one chip.

Three-dimensional stack integration is a method of electrically connecting chips that consist of different kinds of devices, which effectively resolves this problem [12]. Stacked CISs were manufactured by connecting pixel chips and peripheral circuit chips. In 2012, Sony announced the first stacked chip CIS camera systems for consumer

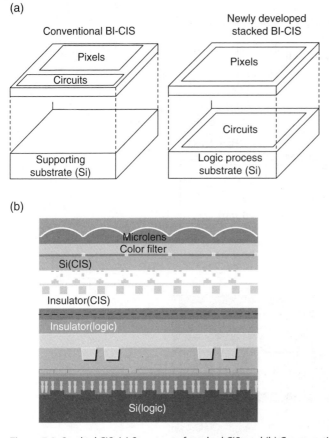

Figure 7.8 Stacked CIS: (a) Structure of stacked CIS; and (b) Cross-sectional view of stacked CIS.

electronics [13]. This technology has both perfected performance and accomplished high levels of sensitivity and a wide dynamic range by increasing the scale of circuits on peripheral circuit chips. Figure 7.8(a) shows shrinkage in the chip area, as the shrunken chips are suitable for wearable devices. It is anticipated that the functions of stacked chip CISs will increase by improving integration technology and embedding more circuits. A cross-sectional view of the stacked BSI CIS is shown in Figure 7.8(b), where the top half of the chip is formed with conventional 1P4M BI-CIS process technology laid upside down, and the bottom half of the chip is formed with 65 nm 1P7M logic process technology. The on-chip color filter and micro-lens are formed on the top surface of the chip. The connection between the interconnect layers of the top and bottom parts is realized by TSV, which are a type of vertical vias-type contact.

7.2.2 Noise and Model

The CIS sensor suffers from non-idealities, defects, and random fluctuations at different levels, thus corrupting the integrity of the signal. These random events occur at the level of the PD, during the charge transfer, and also at the level of the readout circuit electronics. Based on whether the noise is stationary or not, the noise is divided into two categories: temporal noise (or random noise) and fixed pattern noise (FPN) [14]. Temporal noise refers to the time-dependent fluctuations in the signal level. Temporal noise in the pixel includes photon shot noise, dark current shot noise, reset noise (kTC noise), thermal noise, and flicker noise (1/f noise). Each noise component originates from a specific mechanism. Noise appearing in a reproduced image, which is "fixed" at certain spatial positions, is referred to as FPN, usually caused by the CIS readout circuitry.

7.2.2.1 Photon Shot Noise

Shot noise is a statistical phenomenon appearing in nature, for physical processes resulting from a series of independent events occurring with the same probability. In optics and electronics, the quantized nature of light and charge makes a photon or electron flux obey the Poisson process, therefore both the photocurrent and the dark current shot noise have the same mechanism. Particularly for CIS application, the photon incidence obeys the Poisson distribution, thus it can be used to characterize photo sensors [15,16]. This PCT method was first developed at JPL in the 1960s for Vidicon imagers, then applied to CCDs in the 1970s by Janesick *et al.* [15]. The power spectral density (PSD) of the shot noise is constant over all frequencies and given by:

$$S_{shot-photon} = CG^2 \times N_{photo} = CG^2 \times \frac{I_{photo} \cdot t_{int}}{q} \tag{7.1}$$

where I_{photo} represents the average photocurrent and CG is the conversion gain showing how the photon converts electrons. The term t_{int} is the integration time, normally several ms. As shown in Equation 7.1, the photon shot noise has a square root relation with the photocurrent, thus producing the illumination.

Figure 7.9 shows the photon transfer curve (PTC) curve, which contains a typical noise profile seen at the output of a digital camera. There are three distinct noise regions of the camera imaging system: read noise, shot noise, and FPN. Under dark conditions, the noise read coming from readout circuitry is dominant. Consequently, as the incident light intensity increases, the photon shot noise becomes the major noise source of the pixel. Under normal light conditions when photon noise is the dominant noise source, plotting photon shot noise against signal level generates the PTC, which can be used for sensor Conversion Gain.

Figure 7.9 Photon transfer curve (PTC) showing different noise sources at the CIS imaging system.

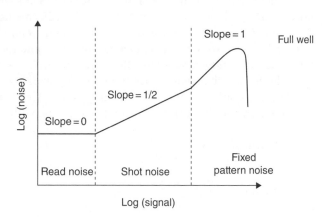

7.2.2.2 Reset Noise

As mentioned in the previous section, the CIS pixel is read out through the CDS, and the signal integrated on a pixel is measured relative to its reset level. The thermal noise uncertainty associated with this reset level is referred to as the reset or kTC noise. This noise comes from the thermal noise of the MOS switch. The noise voltage is given by [17]:

$$\overline{v_{n,kTC}^2} = \int_0^\infty 4kT \frac{R_{on}}{1+\left(2\pi R_{on}Cf\right)^2}df = \frac{kT}{C} \tag{7.2}$$

The noise charge is given by:

$$\overline{n_{n,kTC}^2} = C^2 . \overline{v_{n,kTC}^2} = kTC \tag{7.3}$$

where k is the Boltzmann's constant, T is the temperature, R_{on} is the channel resistance of the RST, and C is the charge sensing node capacitance (FD node capacitance for the pinned photodiode APS). It can be concluded that the noise is a function only of the temperature and the capacitance value, also called "kTC noise". The low frequency thermal noise can be removed by the CDS technique, while the high frequency component is removed by the filtering effects of the large column line capacitance (normally several pF).

7.2.2.3 Thermal Noise

Thermal noise is a fundamental physical phenomenon observed in all conducting devices at a positive absolute temperature. It was first measured by J.B. Johnson in 1928 at the Bell Labs. Thermal Noise (Johnson noise) is primarily the result of random motion of electrons due to thermal effects [18]. The noise signal can be represented by a series voltage source with a PSD:

$$S_{thermal} = 4kTR \tag{7.4}$$

The thermal noise has a white spectral density and a Gaussian amplitude distribution. However, its mean-square value does not depend on the current itself but on the absolute temperature and the resistance of the conductor.

In order to derive the thermal noise of the CMOS imager pixel, an equivalent thermal noise model is drawn, as shown in Figure 7.10. In this figure, i_{SF}, v_{RS}, and i_{bias} are the thermal noise sources associated with SF, RS, and column bias transistor, respectively. $g_{m,SF}$ and $g_{m,bias}$ are the transconductance of the SF and the column bias transistor, $g_{d,RS}$ is the channel conductance of the RS transistor, and C_{col} is the total column capacitance. Both the SF and the column bias transistor are working in the saturation region, and the RS transistor is working in the linear region, so the thermal noise PSD of the SF, the RS transistor, and the current bias transistor can be written as:

$$S_{thermal-SF} = 4kT \frac{2}{3} \frac{1}{g_{m,SF}} \tag{7.5}$$

$$S_{thermal-RS} = 4kT \frac{1}{g_{d,RS}} \tag{7.6}$$

Figure 7.10 Small signal model for the noise analysis in CIS.

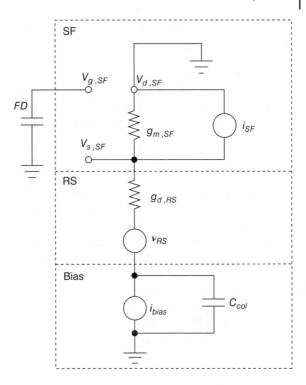

$$S_{thermal-bias} = 4kT \frac{1}{g_{m,bias}}$$ (7.7)

Assuming steady state and neglecting the transistor body effect, the input referenced PSD of the thermal noise can be given by:

$$S_{thermal-SF} = \frac{2}{3} \frac{kT}{C_{col}} \frac{1}{1 + \frac{g_{m,SF}}{g_{d,RS}}} \frac{1}{A_v}$$ (7.8)

$$S_{thermal-RS} = \frac{kT}{C_{col}} \frac{1}{g_{d,RS} \left(\frac{1}{g_{d,RS}} + \frac{1}{g_{m,SF}} \right)} \frac{1}{A_v}$$ (7.9)

$$S_{thermal-bias} = \frac{kT}{C_{col}} g_{m,bias} \left(\frac{1}{g_{d,RS}} + \frac{1}{g_{m,SF}} \right) \frac{1}{A_v}$$ (7.10)

where A_v is the voltage gain of the SF. These equations show that the different noise sources are associated with the different noise bandwidths, and thus have different effects on the noise. The total thermal noise voltage is the mean square sum of the above three integrated from the available frequency bandwidth. However, comparing the three noises, it was found that the thermal noise from the RS transistor is very small and so can be neglected.

7.2.2.4 Flicker Noise

Flicker noise or 1/f noise is due to traps or imperfections in the semiconductor, which capture and release carriers randomly. This noise source only occurs when the DC current is flowing. The PSD of flicker noise is given by [8]:

$$S_{Flicker} = \frac{K_f}{C'_{ox}WL} \cdot \frac{1}{f} = \frac{K'_f}{f} \tag{7.11}$$

where K_f is a process-dependent constant, and C'_{ox}, W, and L denote the gate capacitance per unit area, gate width, and gate length, respectively. Unlike the thermal noise or shot noise, the frequency distribution of the flicker noise is not white, and the amplitude variation is generally a non-Gaussian distribution. At low frequency, the 1/f noise can be the dominant component, but at high frequency the 1/f noise drops below thermal noise.

To estimate the contribution from the SF flicker noise, a transfer function of the CDS operation should be introduced, since the flicker noise has a time-domain correlation. Assuming each sampling operation is expressed by the δ-function, the transfer function of the CDS can be expressed by:

$$H(j2\pi f) = 1 - e^{-2\pi f \Delta t} \tag{7.12}$$

where Δt is the interval between the two samples of CDS.

The resulting output referred flicker noise component is estimated by:

$$\overline{v^2_{Flicker}} = \int_0^\infty \left|H_{CDS}\left(j2\pi f\right)\right|^2 \cdot \left|H_{SF}\left(j2\pi f\right)\right|^2 \cdot \frac{K'_f}{f} \cdot df \tag{7.13}$$

where $H_{SF}(j2\pi f)$ is the transfer function of the SF. Assuming $H_{SF}(j2\pi f)$ is represented by a single-pole, low-pass filter characteristic with the low-frequency cut-off frequency of f_c the above equation can be rewritten as:

$$\overline{v^2_{Flicker}} = 2K'_f \cdot \int_0^\infty \frac{A_v^2}{1+\left(f/fc\right)^2} \cdot \frac{\left(1-\cos\left(2\pi f \cdot \Delta t\right)\right)}{f} \cdot df \tag{7.14}$$

Therefore, the flicker noise coefficient K'_f and the interval between two samples Δt should be examined carefully when designing the readout circuit.

Recent research proved that the 1/f noise induced by traps located at the Si/SiO$_2$ interface in the SF gate region becomes dominant on the pixel read noise floor in CMOS imagers [19,20]. As pixels and transistor sizes shrink, the random telegraph signal (RTS) noise becomes an important factor limiting the performance of the sensor [21,22]. It has been recognized that the 1/f noise is a result of RTS noise.

7.2.2.5 Fixed Pattern Noise

Fixed pattern noise (FPN) refers to a non-temporal spatial variation over the pixel array. The spatial variation is random from chip to chip, but correlated in time for each chip.

FPN can be either coherent or non-coherent, and is mainly due to pixel-to-pixel photon response non-uniform due to device and color filter mismatch, column level gain and offset variations, and analog-to-digital converters (ADCs) variations.

The most problematic FPN in image sensors is associated with easily detectable (or coherent) row-wise and column-wise artifacts due to mismatches in multiple signal paths, and uncorrelated, row-wise operations in the image sensor. Coherent FPN offset components can generally be eliminated by reference frame subtraction. Gain mismatches are more difficult to remove, since this approach requires time or hardware intensive gain correction.

Dark current FPN due to the mismatches in the pixel photodiode leakage currents tends to dominate the non-coherent component of FPN, especially with long exposure times. The low leakage photodiodes are preferable to reduce this FPN component. Dark frame subtraction is an option, but this approach tends to increase the readout time.

7.3 Readout Circuit

The analog-to-digital conversion is an important function block that affects the image quality, frame rate, and cost (chip area) [23]. The CIS architecture can be divided into different readout methodologies by how to implement ADC, as shown in Figure 7.11:

1) *Global serial readout*: When pixel array size is comparatively small (VGA ~8 Meg pixels), the data throughput (industry standard 30 frames/s) is not a design burden. The whole pixel array can share one single ADC and all pixel outputs are time multiplexed to the input node of global ADC to provide digital output in serial, the so-called Global Serial Readout.
2) *Column-parallel readout*: With continuing increase of pixel array size (10 Meg ~ 28 Meg pixels), the speed of chip-shared ADC needs to increase dramatically to reduce

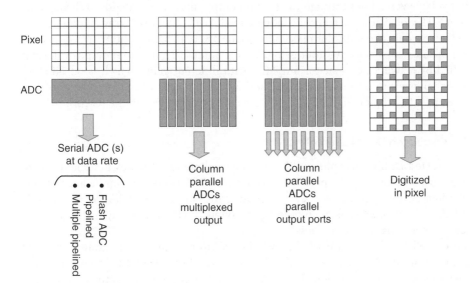

Figure 7.11 CIS readout circuit structure.

the time dedicated to read out the pixel outputs. The global ADC design becomes very challenging, and also the high frame rate leads to large power consumption. Increasing the number of ADCs working in parallel, or even implementing an ADC within each column, will lower the ADC speed limit, so the frame read-out time will be reduced. However, the main challenges are the area constraint, where only simple ADC structures such as single slope ADC can be implemented within small column pitch. Meanwhile the power consumption should also be lower. Nowadays, column-parallel ADC architecture is the dominant readout architecture in the CIS industry; however, the column-to-column FPN is of major concern. The other issue with multiple ADC per sensor is the output data flow and extra memory needed be implemented to digest the data output stream.

3) *Digitized Pixel readout*: Professor A. El Gamal at Stanford University first proposed implementing ADC within the pixel to further increase the frame rate, the so-called Digital Pixel Sensor [24]. Pixel readout operations (sensing, amplification, and digitization) are performed simultaneously within every pixel. Finally, each digitized pixel is read out serially through a shared output bus. DPS offers several advantages over the commonly-used APS structure, including elimination of the column temporal noise and FPN, and high-speed readout. However, while the pixel pitch area is increasing dramatically, it is not practical for the commercial market driven by low-cost and more pixels. Nevertheless, DPS sensors can be implemented for certain applications, such as the line 1-D linear scanner [25], since the pixel layout can be stretched along one dimension. Recently, the development of 3-D TSV stacked technology also makes it possible to dedicate one analog die for ADC integration, connecting the PD die through TSV for each pixel, and having one extra digital die for data storage and processing.

7.3.1 Global Serial Readout

A Global serial readout [26] CIS chip schematic is shown in Figure 7.12, where each pixel output voltage is read out through the column output line further digitized through the column S/H, global amplifier, and 12-bit pipelined ADC. The pixel array readout is controlled by row decoder and column decoder, so the pixel can be read either in sequence or region-of-interest by selective addressing. With column S/H, the pixel output voltage is amplified by a switched-capacitor amplifier with different gains, which is on different input signal levels to improve sensitivity and dynamic range. The analog signal is then digitized by a 12-bit pipelined ADC, and driven off the chip through the IO pad.

7.3.2 Correlated Double Sampling

The Corrected Double Sampling (CDS) readout technique is the most efficient way to reduce sensor noise. Pixel-to-pixel VT mismatch of RST transistor significantly affects the readout accuracy of large arrays, by subtracting the reset voltage V_{rst} at FD node right before the charge transfer and the signal voltage V_{sig}, largely reducing the VT mismatch, thus eliminating the 1/f noise and FPN.

The overall block diagram of the switch-capacitor amplifier integrated with the column sample-hold for CDS operation [27] is shown in Figure 7.13. The pixel output is driven by the column readout line, and sampled at column capacitor C_{rst} and C_{sig}, then amplified through an SC amplifier. The operation of the amplifier is controlled by

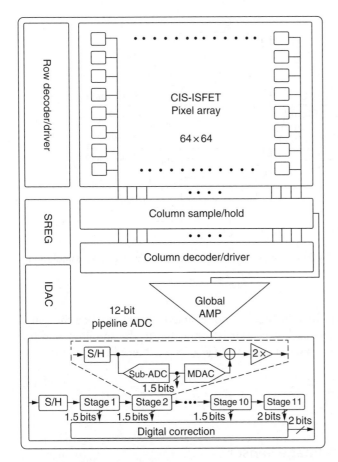

Figure 7.12 CIS Global readout circuit.

the non-overlapping clock signals, phi1 and phi2. During the amplifier reset phase, phi1, both inputs and outputs of the amplifiers are reset to common mode voltage V_{cm} also both sides of the feedback capacitor are connected to the same common-mode voltage. The inputs of the amplifier are controlled by the phi1pp switches, to ensure that both inputs and outputs of the amplifier are reset to the common mode voltage.

During the amplifying phase, phi2, the bottom plate of the sample and hold capacitors C_{rst} and C_{sig} are shorted for the particular column being read out, and the feedback capacitors C_f are connected to the amplifier. The charges on the column sample and hold capacitors are injected into the output buses. Thus, charges are essentially moved from the column sample and hold capacitors to the feedback capacitors. The value of this feedback capacitor sets the stage voltage gain. Here 2 pF capacitors were chosen for the column sample and hold capacitors. A capacitor value of 1 pF was used for the feedback capacitor C_f. When the "gain" switch is not enabled, both feedback capacitors are connected to the amplifier, so the C_f equals 2 pF. The gain of the amplifier can be given by:

$$A_{amp} = \frac{C_{rst}}{C_f + C_f} = \frac{C_{sig}}{C_f + C_f} = \frac{2p}{1p + 1p} = 1 \tag{7.15}$$

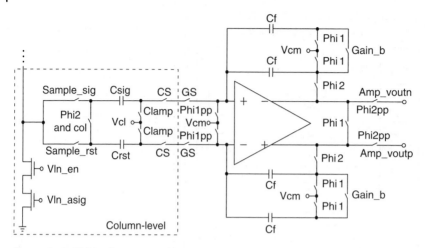

Figure 7.13 CDS implementation by integrating switch-capacitor amplifier with column sample and hold circuitry.

So a unity gain is achieved when the "gain" is not enabled. However, when the "gain" switch is enabled, only one feedback capacitor is connected to the amplifier, and the feedback capacitor is 1pF, such that twice the voltage gain is achieved:

$$A_{amp} = \frac{C_{rst}}{C_f} = \frac{C_{sig}}{C_f} = \frac{2p}{1p} = 2 \tag{7.16}$$

7.4 A 3.2 Mega CMOS Image Sensor

With the benefit of small size, low power, and low cost, CIS technology has been implemented in portable biomedical instruments. One example is the contact imaging system for cell counting; when the blood cells flow through the channel, their shadow images are captured by the image sensor below and further processed for cell detection, classification, and counting [28–30]. However, the main challenge of the contact-imaging-based microfluidic cytometer is the limited resolution of the off-shelf CIS chip. In this section, a 3.2-Mega BI-CIS is developed in the 65-nm process with a 1.1-μm-pitch pixel to capture the small-sized cells. With the improved resolution and contrast of the BSI CIS process, all three types of blood cells can be clearly classified, either from the cell size or internal structure. As a result, the developed microfluidic cytometer becomes a great promising technology for CBC count, with high accuracy and large throughput [31,32].

7.4.1 4-way Shared Pixel Unit

Conventional FSI CIS has poor light sensitivity due to light degradation by stacked metal layers on top of PD, as shown in Figure 7.14. As contact imaging requires a minimum distance between the CIS pixel array and microfluidic channel, we need surface treatments to remove micro-lens and color filters above the pixel array of the FIS CIS.

(a)   (b)

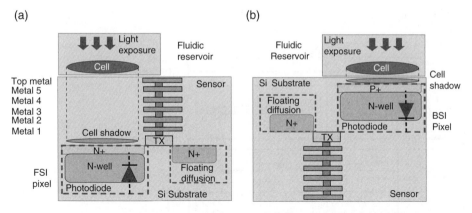

Figure 7.14 Contact imaging using: (a) FSI sensor, where PDs are far from the cell: and (b) BSI sensor, where the PDs are close to the cell.

However, there is the risk of damaging underlying circuits. As an example, in the previous design with the FSI sensor, to minimize the object distance, the protection glass mounted on the sensor chip surface is first removed and then the micro-lens layer above the pixel array is further removed by using oxygen plasma treatment [33,34]. But an extra PDMS thin film is still needed to coat the surface of the sensor chip for die protection, increasing the object distance.

In order to detect the smallest blood cell platelet with a diameter of around $2\,\mu m$, the pixel needs to shrink down to the 1 um range. In the design of this work, the BSI CIS process is implemented to achieve the small pixel size. Different from conventional FSI sensor, where the PD is located at the bottom layers (as in the BSI process shown in Figure 7.14(b)), the light-sensitive PD is fabricated onto the top layers, while the metals are fabricated at the bottom layers [35]. Therefore, the object distance is greatly reduced in this imaging system with the BSI process, improving the image contrast and quality. Besides, the top layer materials in the implemented sensor are silicon and silicon oxide, which are non-corrodible, smooth, and flat, hence suitable for microfluidic channel integration.

Besides the BSI process, the latest 1.1 um 4-way shared No-Row-Select pixel structure is adapted here to further improve spatial resolution. As shown in Figure 7.15, four PDs (PD0–PD3) share a same FD readout through source follower output stage (SF) and reset through the RST. The transfer signals (TX_EVEN) and (TX_ODD) control the charge at four different PDs transferred to FD sequentially, then multiplexed to the shared output data bit line by toggling the VDDPIX signal, which enables or disables SF buffer function. Therefore, the "Row_en" transistor can be removed to further improve the pixel density.

7.4.2 Top Architecture

The top architecture of the developed 3.2-Mega BSI-CIS sensor is shown in Figure 7.16. The chip is composed of six main blocks:

1) a 2056×1600 4-way shared pixel array;
2) 1600 row decoders and drivers;

1.1 by 1.1 um
pixel

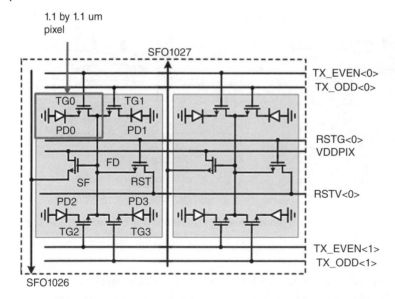

Figure 7.15 Detail 4-way shared no-row-select pixel structure of the BSI image sensor. Four PDs form a unit cell.

3) 2056 column parallel 10 bit ADCs located at both top and bottom;
4) a single-slope ramp generator shared by all columns;
5) digital timing control logic circuit; and
6) high-speed LVDS interface.

In order to realize column ADC within a 4.4 um pitch, area efficient single-slope ADC (SS-ADC) is chosen for the design. Digital double-sampling architecture is proposed to remove device variation and circuit offset that cause vertical FPN. Column readout circuit (shown in Figure 7.17) includes a 10-bit column-level single-slope ADC comprising a three-stage 200-MHz comparator with offset cancellation and a 10-bit ripple counter. The ramp generator drives one input of all column comparators, and the column ripple counters perform the A/D conversion by counting the number of clocks until the comparator output changes, and the counter value presents the digital output value. Digital CDS is obtained by changing up/down counting of the ripple counters during sample reset and sample signal phase. Column-to-column variations of clock skew and counter delay that cause A/D conversion error are corrected by digital CDS. After the data conversion, the digital output is stored in the column-level SRAM, and read out column-by-column sequentially through the sense amplifier. In the design, top-and-bottom readout architecture is implemented to alleviate the physical design constraint of column readout circuit, and also double the frame rate, as data from even and odd columns can be read out separately.

The digital timing of chip operation is illustrated in Figure 7.18. The system operation can be divided into two phases: pixel exposure phase and pixel readout phase. During the pixel exposure phase, the PD is first reset by controlling both the RST and TX switches. The signal RSTG controls the gate of RST to turn on/off the RST switch, and the signal RSTV determines the PD reset voltage. Exposure starts after the reset phase

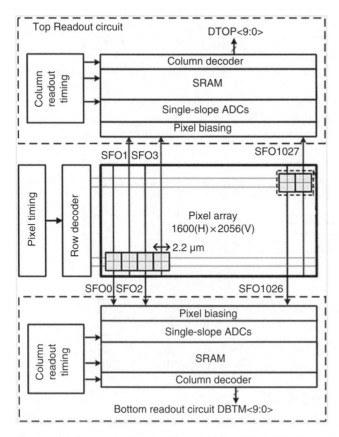

Figure 7.16 System architecture of the 3.2-Mega-Pixels CIS with top-bottom readout scheme and 4.4- column pitch column readout circuit.

Figure 7.17 Block diagram of column readout flow and circuit.

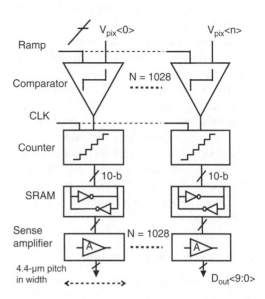

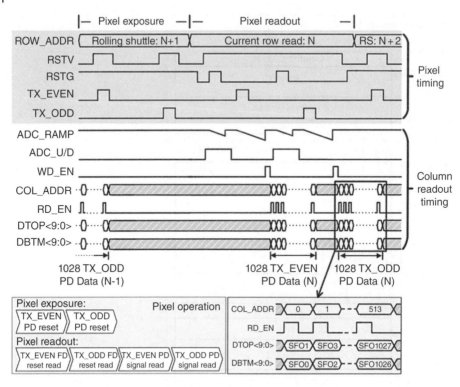

Figure 7.18 Timing diagram of 3.2 Mega BSI-CIS.

when the transmission transistor TX is turned off, and PDs start to collect photons and convert to proportional electrons that lead to the voltage drop of PDs, then TX is turned on, the charge is transferred from PD to FD and ready for read out through the SF buffer. Note here that by toggling the VDDPIX voltage level connected to the source of the SF transistor, the SF can be turned on or off without the "Row_en" transistor, thus the pixel density improves by removing Row_En.

During the pixel readout phase, digital CDS is employed. Reset voltages indicating the starting points of PDs are first sampled by ADCs when the counters are set up for the counting period by the "ADC_U/D" signal. Then the conversion of the reset signal is digitally subtracted from the sensor signal after the charge transfer from the photodiode. By using digital CDS, the analog pixel signal is converted to the corrected digital output signal in the individual columns in parallel. Finally, each row of 1028-even-column PDs managed by TX_EVEN are read out with 514 columns output from DTOP < 9:0 > and DBTM < 9:0 > respectively, following by the readout of odd-column PDs. Then, data read out from DTOP and DBTM are merged to form a complete frame of the raw image.

7.4.3 System Implementation

As shown in Figure 7.19, the prototype microfluidic cytometer includes a PDMS micro-fluidic channel attached to the BSI CIS, a printed circuit board (PCB) with FPGA

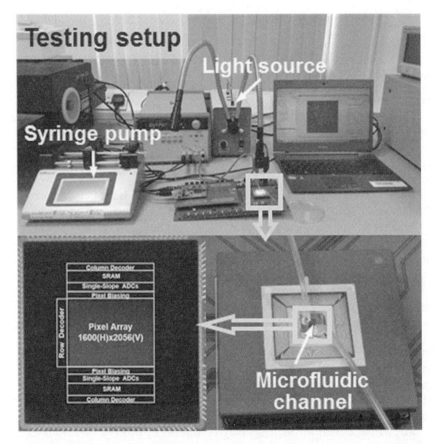

Figure 7.19 Photos of: (a) Setup of the developed microfluidic cytometer system; (b) Die micrograph of BSI CIS; and (c) Microfluidic channel mounted on the ceramic packaged sensor.

control, and a laptop with MATLAB-based GUI. The CIS chip is fabricated in 65 nm BSI CMOS process technology with a die area of 5 mm × 5 mm and a photosensitive area of 1.7 mm × 2.2 mm. It is further bonded to a 144-pin CPGA package with gel covering the surrounding bonding wires for encapsulation. The chip is connected with an Opal Kelly XEM3010 FPGA testing board for timing control, image capturing, and correction.

A PDMS microfluidic channel fabricated by soft-photolithography [27] and the replica molding method [28] is integrated onto the smooth surface of the BSI CIS chip. The channel size and dimension for a transparent mask were designed in AutoCAD. To make full use of the CIS detection area with 3.2-Mega pixels, the microfluidic channel length was designed as 2.6 mm and cut diagonally. A relative wide channel width of 500 μm and a height of 30 μm were chosen, such that a high concentration of blood cells could flow through the channel without clogging [29]. The inlet and outlet of the PDMS microfluidic channel were connected with silastic laboratory tube to a syringe pump and a waste bin, respectively.

Next, the packaged BSI CIS chip with the PDMS channel is soldered onto a PCB that provides the sensor power and digital control signals. The image data of blood cells captured by BSI CIS will be transferred to a laptop through a USB interface on an Opal Kelly XEM3010 FPGA controlled PCB board, which ensures high-speed imaging with a maximum data transfer rate of 56 Mbytes per second. Then a MATLAB-based GUI displays the data as a full-frame image.

7.4.4 Results

7.4.4.1 System Characterization

First, the BSI-CIS chip is characterized. A cold light source L-150A is used to produce illumination with variable light intensity. Under Opal Kelly FPGA control, several groups of output data of the sensor are saved in text files and further processed by a MATLAB program to calculate the characterization parameters.

Chip specifications are summarized in Table 7.1. The CIS has 3.2 mega pixels with a high spatial resolution of 1.1 μm. The on-chip single-slope ADC is first characterized and the output code to input voltage slope can be calculated, as shown in Figure 7.20(a). Therefore, the detected digital code can be translated to the input voltage. Based on this, the FD voltage under different light intensities can be obtained. As shown in Figure 7.20(b), the sensitivity is 1.05 V/lux•s in a 1.1-μm-pitch pixel, leading to a high image contrast for contact imaging. The sensor achieves 10 e/sec dark current at 60 °C junction temperature. The measured power consumption is 182.8 mW at 2.8 V power supply and a frame rate of 45 fps. Conversion gain, full-well capacity, and other performances are also summarized in the table.

7.4.4.2 Digital CDS for FPN Reduction

For a large image sensor array, each pixel has a photon-to-voltage readout circuit and each column of pixels has a digital-to-voltage readout path. When the sensed input voltage is the same, we assume that the array output is uniform. However, in real detection, each pixel reset level may be varied and the ADC in each column may give a different digital code. These circuit mismatches may be caused by process variations that affect the threshold voltage, width/length ratio, parasitic capacitance, etc. These side effects can be regarded as FPN, since they are almost constant during each testing.

Table 7.1 Performances summary of BSI-CIS.

Process	1 P5M 65 nm BSI CMOS
Die size	$5 \times 5 \, mm^2$
Pixel size	$1.1 \times 1.1 \, \mu m^2$
Pixel array	Total: 1600 (H) × 2056 (V)
	Active: 1536 (H) × 2040 (V)
Active area	1.69 mm (H) × 2.24 mm (V)
ADC resolution	10 bit
Maximum frame rate	45 fps
Power consumption	182.8 mW
Power supply	2.8 V
Sensitivity	1.05 V/(lux•s)
Conversion gain	120 μV/e-
Full well capacity	3200 e-

Figure 7.20 Measurement results of: (a) ADC output codes under different input voltages; and (b) BSI-CIS sensor sensitivity.

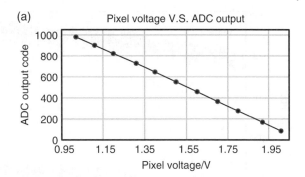

(a)

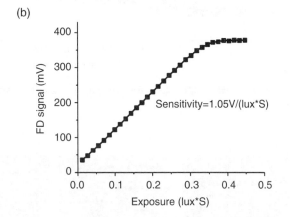

(b)

To obtain a high-quality image, it is important to consider these non-uniformity effects. One main solution is digital CDS where the difference between reset and signal level is measured. As shown in Figure 7.21, one reset voltage and one signal voltage at the FD nodes of one pixel row are measured. A large column mismatch can be observed. However, after performing subtraction of these two voltages, most of FPN is reduced and more uniform outputs are obtained.

7.4.4.3 Blood Cell Imaging Experiments

Experiments are further performed for blood cell imaging. During testing, blood samples are injected and flow through the channel. The flow rate is controlled by a syringe pump. With white light source illumination, cell images are captured by the underlying sensor. The captured raw images of white blood cells (WBC, neutrophils), red blood cells (RBC), and platelets (PLT) are shown in Figures 7.22(a) and (c). It can be observed that even when DDS is employed, pixel mismatches still exist. To alleviate this, a background image is captured and stored in the computer before the experiment. By subtracting the captured raw cell images from the background image, the quality of images is improved, as shown in Figures 7.22(b) and (d).

Figure 7.23 shows a group of captured cell images of RBC, WBC, and PLT with the microscope images as references. For each cell type, different cell morphologies or sizes may be observed. For example, three different shapes of WBC images in Figures 7.23(a–c) and two different sizes of RBC images in Figures 7.23(d–e) are captured. The PLT in Figure 7.23(f) has the smallest size among the three. Nevertheless, each type can still be easily recognized, either from the cell sizes or internal structures.

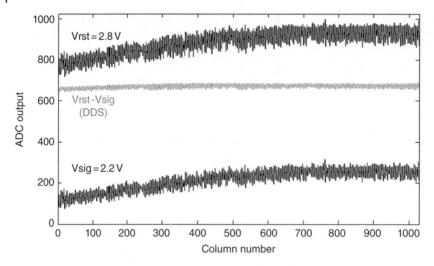

Figure 7.21 ADC outputs of a 2.8V reset voltage, a 2.2V pixel signal and the subtraction of the two voltages.

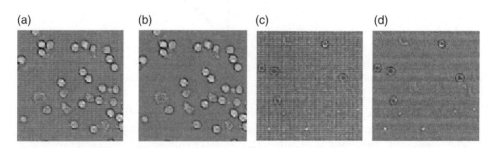

Figure 7.22 Captured raw images of (a) WBC and (c) RBC and PLT. Processed images of (b) WBC and (d) RBC and PLT.

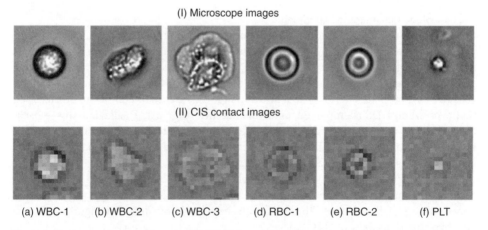

Figure 7.23 Captured contact images of WBC, RBC, and PLT, with microscope images as references.

References

1 G.C. Holst (1996) *CCD Arrays, Cameras, and Displays.* SPIE Optical Engineering Press, Bellingham, WA.
2 M.J. Howes and D.V. Morgan (1979) *Charge-coupled Devices and Systems.* John Wiley & Sons, Ltd, New York.
3 S. Ohba, M. Nakai, H. Ando, S. Hanamura, S. Shimda, *et al.* (1980) MOS area sensor: Part II – Low-noise MOS area Sensor with antiblooming photodiodes. *IEEE Journal of Solid-State Circuits*, 27, 747–752.
4 E.R. Fossum (1995) CMOS image sensors: Electronic camera-on-a-chip. *Electron Devices Meeting IEDM Technical Digest International*, 44, 17–25.
5 N. Teranishi, A. Kohono, Y. Ishihara, E. Oda and K. Arai (1982) No image lag photodiode structure in the interline CCD image sensor. In: *Electron Devices Meeting, 1982 International*, pp. 324–327.
6 B.C. Burkey, W.C. Chang, J. Littlehale, T.H. Lee, T.J. Tredwell, *et al.* (1984) The pinned photodiode for an interline-transfer CCD image sensor. In: *Electron Devices Meeting, 1984 International*, pp. 28–31.
7 R. Fontaine (2015) The state-of-the-art of mainstream CMOS image sensors. In: *International Image Sensor Workshop.*
8 R.H. Walden, R.H. Krambeck, R.J. Strain, J. Mckenna, N.L. Schryer and G.E. Smith (1972) The buried channel charge coupled device. *Bell Labs Technical Journal*, 51, 1635–1640.
9 T. Hirayama (2013) The evolution of CMOS image sensors. *IEEE Asian Solid State Circuit Conference.*
10 K. Itonaga, K. Mizuta, T. Kataoka, M. Yanagita, H. Ikeda, *et al.* (2011) Extremely-low-noise CMOS image sensor with high saturation capacity. *Electron Devices Meeting IEDM Technical Digest International*, 36, 41–44.
11 R. Fontaine (2013) Innovative technology elements for large and small pixel CIS devices. In: *International Image Sensors Workshop.*
12 T. Matsumoto, Y. Kudoh, M. Tahara, N. Miyakawa, H. Itani, *et al.* (1995) Three-dimensional integration technology based on wafer bonding technique using micro-bumps. *Conference on Solid State Devices & Materials*, pp. 1073–1074.
13 S. Sukegawa, *et al.* (2013) A 1/4-inch 8 M pixel back-illuminated stacked CMOS image sensor. *Solid-State Circuits Conference Digest of Technical Papers (ISSCC), 2013 IEEE International*, pp. 484–485.
14 J. Nakamura (2005) *Image Sensors and Signal Processing for Digital Still Cameras.* Taylor & Francis, Inc., Boca Raton, FL.
15 J.R. Janesick (2007) Photon transfer. *SPIE*, August, 49–79.
16 D. Gardner, *Characterizing Digital Cameras with the Photon Transfer Curve.* Summit Imaging. Available at: http://www. couriertronics. com/docs/notes/cameras_ application_notes/Photon_Transfer_Curve_Charactrization_Method. pdf, Accessed 26 June 2012.
17 H. Tian, B. Fowler and A.E. Gamal (2001) Analysis of temporal noise in CMOS photodiode active pixel sensor. *IEEE Journal of Solid-State Circuits*, 36, 92–101.
18 R.J. Baker (2010) *CMOS Circuit Design, Layout, and Simulation*, John Wiley & Sons, Inc., Hoboken, NJ, pp. 1231–1232.

19 J.Y. Kim, S.I. Hwang, J.J. Lee, J.H. Ko, Y. Kim, J.C. *et al.* (2005) Characterization and improvement of random noise in 1/3.2⊠ UXGACMOS image sensor with 2.8 μm pixel using 0.13 μm technology. *IEEE Workshop on CCDs & AIS*, Japan, pp. 149–152.

20 X. Wang, P.R. Rao, A. Mierop and A.J.P. Theuwissen (2006) Random telegraph signal in CMOS image sensor pixels. In: *Electron Devices Meeting, 2006. IEDM '06. International*, pp. 1–4.

21 C. Leyris, F. Martinez, M. Valenza and A. Hoffmann (2006) *Impact of Random Telegraph Signal in CMOS Image Sensors for Low-Light Levels.* In: Proceedings of the 32nd European Solid-State Circuits Conference, ESSCIRC, pp. 376–379.

22 K.M. Findlater, J.M. Vaillant, D.J. Baxter and L.A. Grant (2003), Source follower noise limitations in CMOS active pixel sensors, *Proceedings of SPIE – The International Society for Optical Engineering*, vol. 5251.

23 A. Juan, F.B. Jorge and R.V. Angel (2014) Review of ADCs for imaging, *Proceedings of SPIE*, February.

24 D.X.D. Yang, B. Fowler and A. El Gamal (1998) A Nyquist-rate pixel-level ADC for CMOS image sensors. *Proceedings of the Custom Integrated Circuits Conference*, 34, 237–240.

25 M. Yan, G. Degeronimo, P. O'Connor and B.S. Carlson (2004) A novel CMOS digital pixel sensor for 1D barcode scanning. *Proceedings of SPIE – The International Society for Optical Engineering*, 5301, 213–221.

26 X. Huang, F. Wang, J. Guo and M. Yan (2014) A 64×64 1200 fps CMOS ion-image sensor with suppressed fixed-pattern-noise for accurate high-throughput DNA sequencing. In: Symposium on VLSI Circuits Digest of Technical Papers, pp. 1–2.

27 X. Li (2008) *Mosfet Modulated Dual Conversion Gain CMOS Image Sensors.* PhD Thesis, Boise State University, November 2008.

28 J. Guo, W. Lei, X. Ma, P. Xue, Y. Chen and Y. Kang (2014) Design of a fluidic circuit-based microcytometer for circulating tumor cell detection and enumeration. *IEEE Trans. Biomed. Circuits Systems*, 8(1), 35–41.

29 X. Huang, H. Yu, *et al.* (2015) A single-frame super-resolution algorithm for lab-on-a-chip lensless microfluidic imaging. *IEEE Des. Test. Comput.*, 32(6), 32–40.

30 X. Huang, X. Wang, *et al.* A robust recognition error recovery for micro-flow cytometer by machine-learning enhanced single-frame super-resolution processing, *Integration*, 51, 208–218.

31 X. Huang, J. Guo, *et al.* (2014) A contact-imaging based microfluidic cytometer with machine-learning for single-frame super-resolution processing, *PLoS ONE*, 9(8), e104539.

32 S. Lee and C. Yang (2014) A smartphone-based chip-scale microscope using ambient illumination. *Lab Chip*, 14(16), 3056–3063.

33 G. Zheng, S.A. Lee, S. Yang and C.-H. Yang (2010) Sub-pixel resolving optofluidic microscope for on-chip cell imaging. *Lab Chip*, 10, 3125–3129.

34 S.A. Lee, R. Leitao, G. Zheng, S. Yang, A. Rodriguez and C.-H. Yang (2011) Color capable sub-pixel resolving optofluidic microscope and its application to blood cell imaging for malaria diagnosis. *PLoS ONE*, 6, e26127.

35 R. Nixon, N. Doudoumopoulos and E.R. Fossum (2002) Backside illumination of CMOS image sensor, US Patent 6429036, August 6, 2002.

8

CMOS Dual-mode pH-Image Sensor

8.1 Introduction

In biomedical testing, some properties of a reaction or biological material can be detected optically but not chemically, and vice versa for other properties. In some cases, it is only when these properties are known together that we can draw conclusions about the state of the reaction or biological material. The field of sensor fusion has received much attention recently, as the combining of sensors can improve sensing capability. Thus, multi-modal CMOS image sensors are required.

In this chapter, we develop a dual-mode sensor to provide an image as well as pH information for sample analysis. In addition to the pH sensing, we will introduce optical sensing for the CMOS ISFET. Note that conventional optical microscope imaging systems require intermediate bulky lenses for magnification, which usually constrain the size, weight, and cost with the difficulty of miniaturization. One promising solution is the use of contact imaging, which directly couples the image sensor array with the sample of interest in small proximity (or contact), as shown in Figure 8.1. As such, the sample image can be captured by directly projecting light through it with a detected shadow [1–3].

Contact imaging is kind of near-field sensing without an optic lens [2]. As such, contact imaging systems have different geometrical constraints over spatial resolution compared with lens-based imaging. In conventional optical imaging systems, the image resolution is determined by the number of pixels in the photo detect array as the scene is entirely projected to the sensor array by optics. By increasing the number of pixels, the spatial resolution for the conventional imaging system can be increased. Different to contact imaging, as the image is directly projected from the object to the image sensor array, and the resolution is mainly determined by the pixel dimension as well as proximity distance. Thus, the contact imaging is suitable for miniaturized biomedical applications to detect objects such as microbeads [3] used in DNA sequencing. Thereby, if we can leverage a dual-mode ISFET sensor with both pH sensing to detect H^+ at one microbead and also contact imaging to detect the existence of the microbead, the false pH reporting problem of the existing ISFET sensor can be resolved during DNA sequencing.

We demonstrated a 64×64 CMOS pH-image sensor. First, both pH and image sensing are performed with a dual-mode sensor pixel structure, which integrates the ISFET with a 4T CMOS Image Sensor (CIS) pixel in the standard CIS process. Since the

CMOS Integrated Lab-on-a-Chip System for Personalized Biomedical Diagnosis,
First Edition. Hao Yu, Mei Yan, and Xiwei Huang.
© 2018 John Wiley & Sons Singapore Pte. Ltd. Published 2018 by John Wiley & Sons Singapore Pte. Ltd.

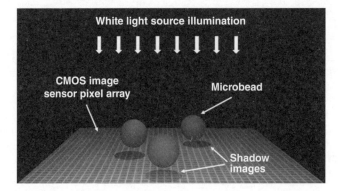

Figure 8.1 Contact imaging principle: with light source illuminated from above; the contact shadow images of microbeads can be captured by the sensor underneath.

microbeads are in direct contact with the sensor surface, the imaging of the microbeads can be detected based on the contact imaging principle without a lens [4]. As such, an accurate pH-image correlation map can be generated to prune the false pH values. Moreover, correlated-double-sampling (CDS) is developed to support both pH and optical modes in the sensor readout circuit to reduce the pixel-to-pixel V_T mismatch (i.e. FPN). The CMOS pH-image sensor is fabricated through standard the 0.18 μm TSMC CIS process with an area of 2.5 mm × 5 mm. Measurements show a sensitivity of 103.8 mV/pH, FPN reduction from 4% to 0.3%, and readout speed of 1200 fps.

8.2   CMOS Dual-mode pH-Image Pixel

Figure 8.2 compares the schematics for (a) 4 T-CIS pixel and (c) ISFET pixel with the proposed (b) dual-mode pixel. The dual-mode pixel contains a 4 T-CIS pixel to sense the shadow image of a microbead by contact imaging [5]. Meanwhile, the source follower (SF) can work as the ISFET to detect the pH value at one microbead.

In the optical mode, the PD first collects photons and converts them to proportional electrons, which are transferred to floating diffusion (FD) by turning on the "TX" switch

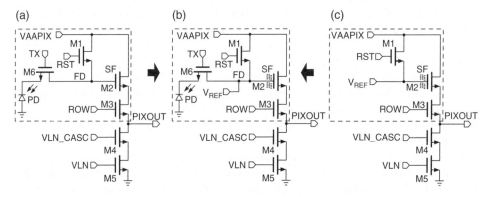

Figure 8.2 Schematic of: (a) 4 T-CIS pixel; (b) Dual-mode pixel; and (c) ISFET pixel.

of M6. The shadow of the microbead is detected through contact imaging. The corresponding voltage signal for the optical image is amplified by SF (M2) and read out through its source under the control of the "ROW" select signal of M3. Since there are multiple rows of pixels that share the same PIXOUT line, the row-select transistor M3 is used to isolate different pixel outputs, and is enabled only when the row is selected for read out. The cascade current source (M4 and M5) provides the biasing current and is shared by the whole column for better current matching.

In the pH mode, the poly-gate of SF (M2) is all-the-way connected to the top metal and Si_3N_4 passivation layer, acting as an ion-sensitive membrane of ISFET. Since the change of ion (H^+) concentration (or pH) can cause a proportional V_T change of the SF, the corresponding voltage signal is correlated to the pH value that is read out through the source of SF. Considering that V_T variation exists in the ISFET transistor, such as with the SF transistor M2 in Figure 8.2, it will show as an offset added at the SF output PIXOUT, that is, $V_{PIXOUT} = \alpha \cdot (V_{FD} - V_T)$, where α is the gain of the SF, and V_{FD} and V_{PIXOUT} are the input and output voltage of the SF. Moreover, note that although the ISFET pixel has a switch to the floating gate, the TX leakage has been reduced through process optimization from the CIS aspect.

As with the cross-sectional and top view of the pixel layout shown in Figure 8.3, a completely depleted pinned photodiode pixel is used, which consists of a pinned diode ($p^+ - n^+ - p$) to reduce the surface-defect noise due to dark current. The depletion layer of a pinned photodiode stretches almost to the $Si–SiO_2$ interface, which is perfectly

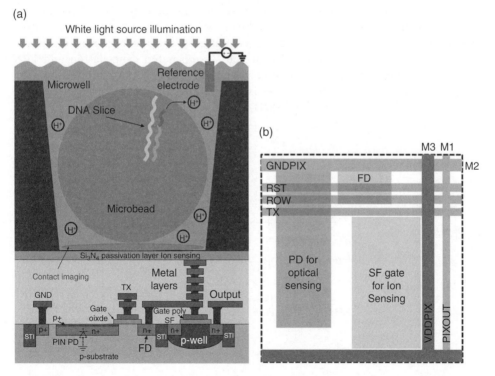

Figure 8.3 (a) Cross-section layout of the dual-mode CMOS ISFET pixel; and (b) The top view of the dual-model pixel.

shielded by the p⁺ layer that keeps the interface fully filled with holes, making the leakage extremely low [6,7]. The existence of a microbead can be detected by contact imaging, and the pH shift caused by nucleotide incorporation can be measured by ion sensing.

When the chip area of a CMOS sensor array is fixed, the only way to improve throughput is to reduce the pixel size and increase the pixel number. But as the sensitivity of the optical imaging is determined by the PD area, and the sensitivity for chemical sensing is determined by the top metal area of SF, the pixel size cannot be too small [8,9]. In this design, we choose a 64×64 array and empirically choose a pixel size of $10\,\mu m \times 10\,\mu m$. Although it is large compared with common commercial CMOS image sensor pixels (ranging from $2\,\mu m$ to $6\,\mu m$), this is to incorporate enough area of the top metal of SF for chemical sensing. There is also a need to optimally partition the pixel area between optical imaging and chemical sensing. As the optical imaging mode is only used to decide the existence of microbeads in the microwells, its sensitivity requirement is not as critical as for chemical sensing. As such, the PD area can be reduced to provide more sensitivity for chemical sensing. To optimally decide the pixel size and partition, detailed modeling needs to be carried out, which will be our future work.

8.3 Readout Circuit

CDS is commonly used in CIS design to reduce the pixel-to-pixel variation and improve the signal-to-noise ratio (SNR) during read out. As a pixel-to-pixel V_T mismatch (or FPN) significantly affects the readout accuracy of a large-arrayed sensor, we are the first to deploy the CDS for the V_T mismatch cancellation and FPN reduction in the ISFET pixel array under dual-mode. The CDS readout schematic supporting both pH and optical modes is shown in Figure 8.4. It consists of a dual-mode pixel, a column sample/hold (S/H) block, a global operation amplifier, and a

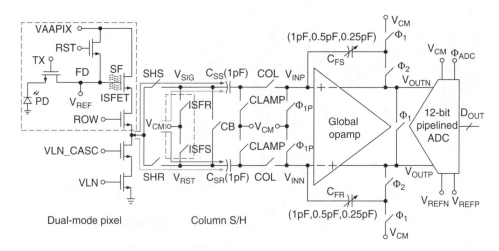

Figure 8.4 CDS readout schematic for dual-mode sensor.

12-bit pipelined analog-to-digital conversion (ADC) block. Pixel reset and signal voltage will be sensed and stored in the two differential terminals of global amplifier. Then the difference between these two voltage levels will be read out and converted to digital data. A series of switches are employed here to operate the readout path in different modes. A properly designed switching behavior can reduce the noise and increase SNR.

The corresponding timing is shown in Figure 8.5. Based on the dual-mode pixel structure, the timing of dual-mode CIS-ISFET pixel sensing control is operated corresponding to the readout timings, shown in Figure 8.5, with following steps:

1) When reaction carrier microbeads are initially distributed into the sensor pixel array, the readout timing is set to optical mode, as shown in Figure 8.5(a), as a normal 4 T-CIS pixel. The shadow images of microbeads can be captured by the contact imaging. Then the existence of a microbead at each pixel can be determined with an address generated.

2) Then the optical mode changes to chemical mode. Before loading the ATCG solution, the reference reset-signal for the whole pixel array is read out using the timing in Figure 8.5(b).

3) After loading the ATCG solution sequentially, the pH readout timing changes to Figure 8.5(c) to obtain the signal of the pixel array with an actual pH value of the individual microbead.

As such, we can obtain the accurate correlation between the measured pH data and the distribution of microbeads. The false pH data at empty microwells can thereby be eliminated by the dual-mode operation.

Note that the timing diagram in Figure 8.5 is for read out only. The exposure phase with PD reset through TX pulse is not illustrated. Moreover, the developed CDS is applied to suppress pixel-to-pixel V_T mismatch by using each pixel itself as a reference, which is intrinsically better than the differential measurement using another REFET device in [10].

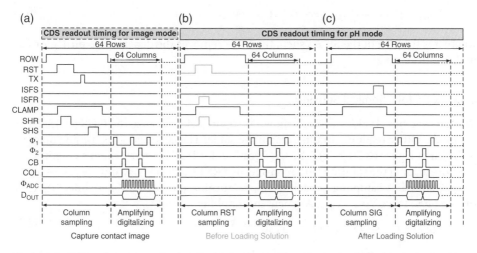

Figure 8.5 CDS readout timing diagram for both: (a) Optical mode; pH mode; and (b) before and (c) after loading solution.

8.3.1 CDS for Optical Sensing

The CDS readout circuit for CIS is realized through the signal chain of CIS pixel, column S/H, and switched-capacitor amplifier. As with the timing shown in Figure 8.5(a), during the pixel to column readout period, the "CLAMP" switch is on so that the top plate of sampling capacitors C_{SS} and C_{SR} are clamped to V_{CM}. The charges on the pixel output line are sampled to C_{SR} when the "SHR" switch is on and to C_{SS} when the "SHS" switch is on. Then during the column to amplifier readout period, the "CLAMP" switch is off. The crow-bar switch "CB" is off during the amplifier reset phase and is on during the charge amplifying phase. The S/H capacitor value is determined by the balance between the KTC noise and speed. A 1 pF poly capacitor is chosen for both C_{SS} and C_{SR}, that is, $C_{SS} = C_{SR} = C_S = 1$ pF. The outputs of the column sample capacitors are successively controlled by the column select signals "COL".

Following the column S/H is the global switched-capacitor amplifier that consists of one non-overlapping clock generator, a fully differential cascode amplifier with switched-capacitor common-mode feedback (CMFB), and several poly capacitors C_{FS} and C_{FR} for programmable gain control. We also have $C_{FR} = C_{FR} = C_F$.

The non-overlapping clock generator produces a pair of non-overlapping clock signals: "Φ_1" and "Φ_2", and also "Φ_{1P}", whose falling edge is slightly earlier than "Φ_1" to reduce the possible charge injection and clock feed-through. "Φ_1" and "Φ_2" work under "CB" to amplify and read out signals of each column. During the reset phase Φ_1, both inputs and outputs of the amplifier as well as the feedback capacitor C_F are reset to V_{CM}, the common mode voltage. During the amplify phase Φ_2, the bottom plates of the S/H capacitors are shorted by turning on CB for the currently selected readout column; and the feedback capitor C_F are connected to the amplifier output. Thus, charges are essentially moved from the column S/H capacitor C_S to the feedback capacitor C_F. As the two input nodes of the differential amplifier connect with the reset level V_{RST} and signal level V_{SIG}, only the difference between them is amplified and output, i.e.:

$$V_{OUT} = V_{OUTP} - V_{OUTN} = \alpha \cdot (C_S / C_F) \cdot (V_{RST} - V_{SIG}) \tag{8.1}$$

where α is the gain of the SF. As such, the V_{OUT} removes the dependence on V_T for CIS in the optical mode.

8.3.2 CDS for Chemical Sensing

We add switches "ISFR"/"ISFS", as shown in Figure 8.4, to realize the CDS for ISFET in pH mode. Other readout circuits remain the same. The corresponding timing diagram is shown in Figures 8.5(b)–(c). The CDS readout for ISFET is performed as follows.

Before loading the solution with microbeads, "RST" is turned on, and the reset voltage V_{RST} is stored at sampling capacitor C_{SR} by turning on "SHR". Meanwhile, "ISFR" is turned on to force $V_{SIG} = V_{CM}$. As such, the amplifier output is:

$$V_{OUT1} = \alpha \cdot (C_S / C_F) \cdot (V_{RST} - V_{CM} + V_T) \tag{8.2}$$

Then the reset voltage level for the whole array is read out and digitized by the 12-bit pipelined ADC at the next stage and saved by external storage.

After loading the solution with microbeads, "ISFS" is turned on to force $V_{RST} = V_{CM}$. The amplifier output now is:

$$V_{OUT2} = \alpha \cdot (C_S/C_F) \cdot (V_{REF} - V_{CM} + V_T - dV) \tag{8.3}$$

where dV is the threshold voltage (V_T) change caused by the chemical reaction between the ion and the passivation layer; and V_{REF} is the voltage of the reference electrode. This output is also converted by the ADC and read out to the external storage for further digital processing.

As a result, we subtract the two outputs and obtain the difference by:

$$V_{OUT1} - V_{OUT2} = \alpha \cdot (C_S/C_F) \cdot (V_{REF} - V_{REF} + dV) \tag{8.4}$$

which removes the dependence on V_T for ISFET in the chemical mode.

8.4 A 64×64 Dual-mode pH-Image Sensor

8.4.1 Top Architecture

The top architecture of the dual-mode sensor is illustrated in Figure 8.6, including a 64×64 dual-mode pixel array, S/H circuit, and global switched-capacitor operational

Figure 8.6 Top architecture of dual-mode sensor.

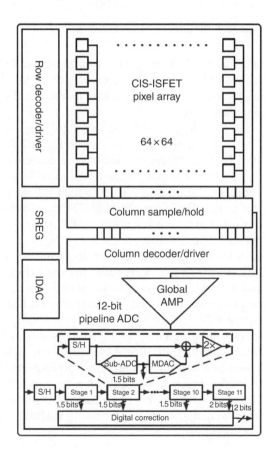

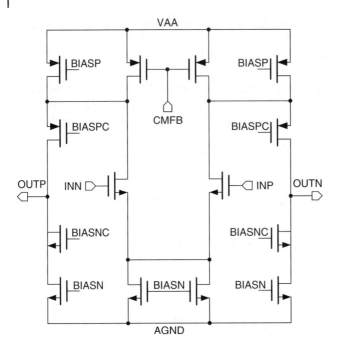

Figure 8.7 The global core amplifier circuit.

amplifier for CDS readout, 12-bit pipelined ADC, and row/column decoders. Other function blocks have also been involved. The SREG block with a series of registers is used to select a different working mode. The IDAC block provides a bias current to the amplifier or ADC.

Basically, there are three testing steps: image sensing, ISFET reset, and ISFET sensing. The pixel timing diagram is given in Figure 8.5. First, the image mode is conducted to identify the microbeads' locations represented by row and column addresses. Then the chemical mode is utilized for pH detection by turning off TX. Before loading any nucleotides, the ISFET gate is reset to high voltage to initiate a uniform sensing condition. During the pH sensing phase, dNTPs are added sequentially, and the local pH change is converted to output voltage by ISFET. As a result, the local pH value is correlated with the microbead address.

As for the global amplifier, the feedback capacitors C_F are adjustable among 1 pF, 0.5 pF, and 0.25 pF, such that the gain C_S/C_F can be selected among 1X, 2X, and 4X under different input signal levels. As such, the sensitivity or dynamic range can be improved. The amplifier utilizes a telescopic structure, as shown in Figure 8.7.

The sensed signal by the ISFET-sensor array is digitized by a 12-bit pipelined ADC before final output. The ADC consists of S/H input stages, ten serially connected 1.5-bit pipeline stages, and one 2-bit flash stage, as shown in Figure 8.8. The digital correction block creates a 12-bit output code by a redundant signed digit (RSD). The 1.5-bit per-stage is chosen because of its immunity to the offsets. A telescopic operational amplifier with gain-boosting is chosen for high dc gain, high GBW, and fast settling times.

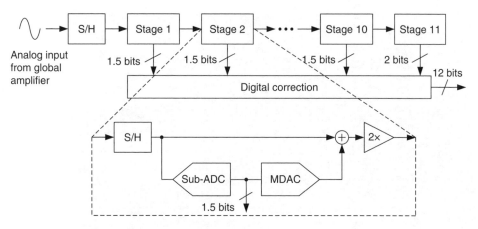

Figure 8.8 12-bit pipelined ADC architecture.

8.4.2 System Implementation

The proposed dual-mode ISFET sensor is fabricated in the standard TSMC 0.18 μm CIS process. After fabrication, the chip is packaged into a 100-pin Pin Grid Array (PGA) package with a size of 33.5 mm × 33.5 mm. As the experimental processes need to be conducted in aqueous environments, proper encapsulation of the sensor chip is necessary to protect the circuits. Thus, we use epoxy to encapsulate the whole chip with the sensing pixel array area open only. Meanwhile, the bonding wires and bonding pads are also covered by epoxy. To retain aqueous samples on the top of the sensor chip, a 3-D-printed plastic reservoir that just fits the PGA package is mounted onto the package with epoxy to fill the gap on all four sides.

The plastic reservoir is also designed to be able to fix the Ag/AgCl reference electrode. The packaged chip is then mounted on a specially designed printed-circuit-board (PCB) through a 100-pin PGA socket. The PCB, which is further connected with a Xilinx Virtex-6 XC6VLX240T FPGA demo board, is designed to provide power supply and digital timing control signals to the sensor chip. We measured the electrochemical characteristics of the chip under the control of a MATLAB-based (Mathworks, Natick, MA) Graphical User Interface (GUI). The chip micrograph with architecture and testing system is shown in Figure 8.9. The design specifications are summarized in Table 8.1.

8.4.3 Results

To evaluate the dual-mode ISFET device fabricated by the standard CMOS image sensor process, we model an N-type ISFET with six metal layers using Synopsys® Sentaurus TCAD (Technology Computer-Aided Design), which is a suite of commercial TCAD tools that simulates the fabrication, operation, and reliability of semiconductor devices. As the electrolyte cannot be directly modeled in the simulation, we change the concentration of the trapped charge in the poly-silicon gate area to try to simulate the charge change in the poly-silicon caused by the ion reaction on the surface of the passivation layer. The change in charge in the poly will result in the change of the V_T of the ISFET.

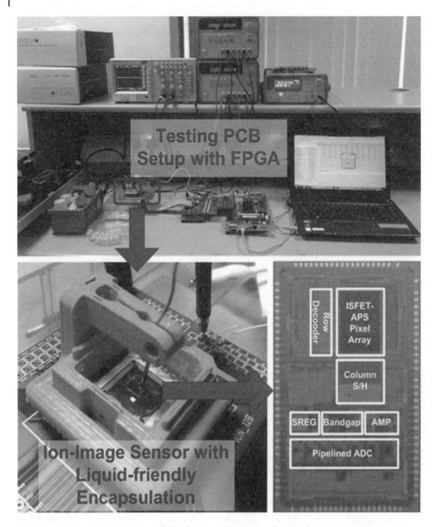

Figure 8.9 Micrograph photo of the dual-mode sensor chip and testing setup.

To evaluate the effect of negative charge, such as the donor, and positive charge, such as the acceptor, we choose $V_{DS} = 1\,V$ with only donor or accepter change in density. The addition of donors and acceptor to semiconductor is similar to the process of adding acids or bases to pure water and altering the balance between H^+ an OH^-.

The cross-sectional structure of the ISFET is modeled in Figure 8.10. The electron concentration is indicated by coloring corresponding to the bar graph on the right. As shown the results shown in Figure 8.11(a), when we increase the concentration of the negative charge donor from $10^{16}\,cm^{-3}$ to $10^{40}\,cm^{-3}$ with acceptors $= 0$, the V_T has a corresponding linear reduction from $1.11\,V$ to $0.06\,V$. As in Figure 8.11(b), when increasing the concentration of the positive charge acceptor from $10^{16}\,cm^{-3}$ to $10^{36}\,cm^{-3}$, with donor $= 0$, the V_T has a corresponding linear increase from $1.13\,V$ to $1.74\,V$. A natural logarithm scale for charge concentrations is used. As such, although the

Table 8.1 Dual-mode sensor chip design specifications.

Parameters	Specifications
Process	Standard TSMC 0.18 μm CIS
Pixel Type	Dual-mode (Optical and Chemical)
Pixel Size	10 μm × 10 μm
Pixel Optical Sensing Area	20.1 μm^2
Pixel Chemical Sensing Area	22.3 μm^2
Array Size	64 × 64
Die Area	2.5 mm × 5 mm
ADC ENOB	11.4 bits
ADC SNDR	70.35 dB
FPN	0.3%
Frame Rate	1200 fps
Total Power Consumption	32 mA @ 3.3 V

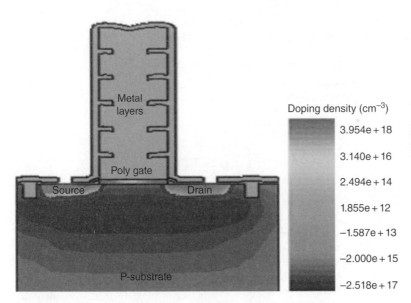

Figure 8.10 Cross-sectional structure of the ISFET, as modeled in Sentaurus TCAD. The electron concentration during ISFET operation is indicated by coloring.

electrolyte is not directly modeled, the effect of changing the surface charge will cause changes in ISFET transfer characteristics, and linearly modulate the ISFET V_T, which is the basic principle of ISFET-based pH sensing.

The AC simulation results in Figure 8.12 show an open-loop gain of 68 dB and bandwidth of 628 MHz. The high GBW enables high-speed readout with 10 MHz column-wise readout speed.

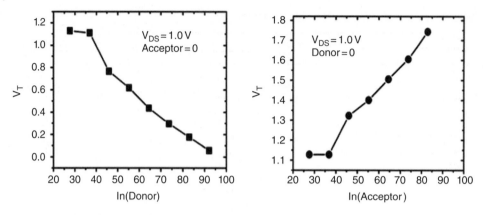

Figure 8.11 ISFET device simulation results showing the V_T change.

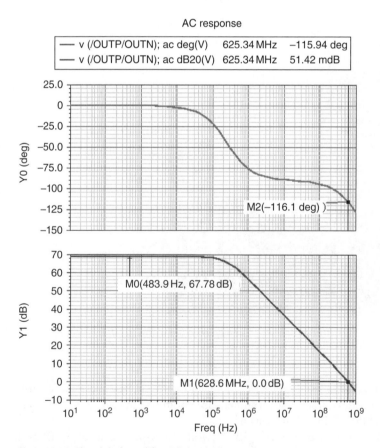

Figure 8.12 The global amplifier AC simulation results.

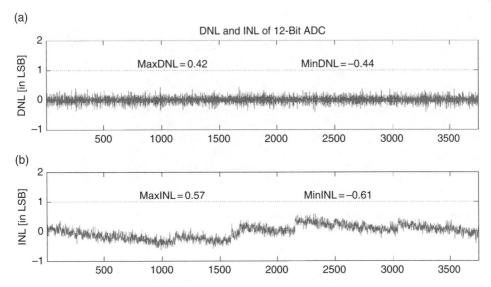

Figure 8.13 12-bit pipelined ADC INL/DNL simulation results.

The simulation results of DNL and INL of the pipelined ADC is shown in Figure 8.13. The maximum DNL is 0.44 LSB and the maximum INL is 0.61 LSB. The ENOB is 11.4 bits, and the SNDR is 70.35 dB. As such, the whole row-readout time is 13 μs, including the pixel sampling, amplification, and digitization. Therefore, for a 64 × 64 array, the whole readout time for 64 rows is 64 × 13 μs = 0.832 ms, with a frame rate of approximately 1/0.832 ms = 1200 fps. Fast readout speed can enable us to capture a chemical image in a shorter time. For DNA sequencing, sampling the signal at high frequency relative to the time of the nucleotide incorporation signal allows signal averaging to improve the SNR.

First, the correlated contact image and pH map of microbeads are shown in Figure 8.14. The microbeads of 45 μm diameter are used (Product# 07314–5, Polysciences, Warrington, PA). Note that we have not fabricated the microwell array on top of the image sensor die to correspond to each microwell with an ISFET pixel. Thus, a relatively larger microbead compared with 10 μm pixel size is selected such that the contrast of shadow imaging can be improved. With the contact shadow imaging, the image size of microbead takes up about a 5 × 5 pixel array area. Due to the diffraction effect, the center pixels show darker intensity and the pixels near the boundary show lighter intensity. For the proof-of-concept verification, the microbeads are first diluted and prepared in acid solution as they are ideally suited for protein binding using passive adsorption techniques, and then dropped onto the sensor surface to test the local pH changes. The contact image determines the existence of microbeads and provides their addressed distribution. The exposure time of the contact imaging is 160 μs. The pH map is thereby locally associated with microbeads by pruning out the uncorrelated pH data. Due to the diffusion effect, the pH map at microbead locations shows a pattern similar to a normal distribution.

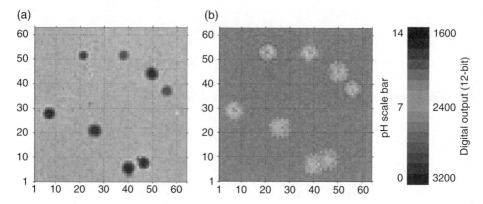

Figure 8.14 The correlated maps of distributed microbeads: (a) Contact images; and (b) pH values.

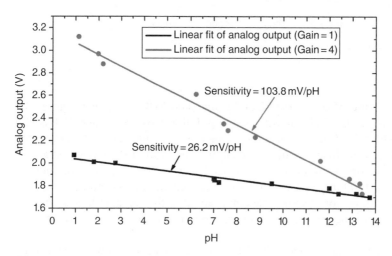

Figure 8.15 Measurement results: pH sensitivity of dual-mode ISFET sensor.

Next, the pH measurement results are shown in Figure 8.15. The pH of solution is changed by adding HCL and NaOH. The readout pH sensitivity of ISFET by CIS process is measured as 26.2 mV/pH with amplifier gain = 1 and as 103.8 mV/pH with amplifier gain = 4. The device sensitivity at gain = 1 is somewhat lower than the commonly observed response of 45–56 mV/pH for Si_3N_4, which can be due to the low-pressure chemical vapor deposition (LPCVD) technique for Si_3N_4 at low temperatures, which generally causes a low-density and porous passivation layer. It can be optimized by the LPCVD at a high temperature or add further depositions, which are still the standard CMOS process [11].

The sensor chip is also calibrated by testing the pH change of a bacteria (*E. coli*) culture solution at different time intervals. The measurement results by the dual-mode sensor can correlate well with the commercial pH meter (Checker, Hanna Instruments, RI, US) in Figure 8.16.

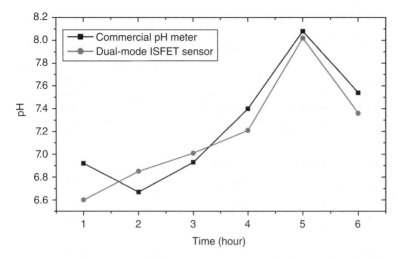

Figure 8.16 The comparison with commercial pH meter for bacteria (*E. Coli*) culture solution with glucose at different time intervals.

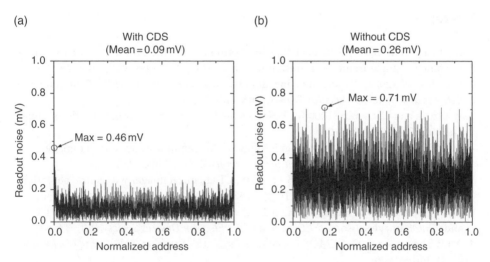

Figure 8.17 Measurement results: spatial FFT of readout voltage variations: (a) with CDS; and (b) without CDS read out.

The comparison of readout voltage variations with and without CDS is shown in Figure 8.17. After performing spatial FFT to the readout voltages with respect to the locations of the sensor array, the mean and peak variations are reduced by 0.17 mV and 0.25 mV, respectively. The FPN is accordingly reduced from 4% down to 0.3%.

Lastly, the comparison with the state-of-the-art ISFET sensors is summarized in Table 8.2. The proposed dual-mode sensor shows the state-of-the-art results: 10 μm pixel pitch, 64 × 64 pixel array, fast frame rate of 1200 fps, and sensitivity of 103.8 mV/pH in the standard CIS process. The pixel pitch can be further reduced and the array size can be scaled to 1 million for higher throughput detection.

Table 8.2 Comparison of state-of-the-art ISFET sensors.

	[12]	[13]	[14]	[15]	This Work
Process	5 μm Non-CMOS	0.35 μm Modified CMOS	0.35 μm Standard CMOS	0.18 μm Standard CMOS	0.18 μm Standard CMOS
Pixel Size (μm × μm)	200×200	12.8×12.8	10.2×10.2	20×2	10×10
Array Size	10×10	16×16	64×64	8×8	64×64
Frame Rate (fps)	30	–	100	–	1200
Sensitivity (mV/ pH)	229	46	20	37	26.2 (gain = 1) 103.8 (gain = 4)
Dual-Mode	No	No	No	No	Yes

References

1 X. Huang, *et al.* (2014) A contact-imaging based microfluidic cytometer with machine-learning for single-frame super-resolution processing. *PLoS One*, 9(8), e104539.

2 H.H. Ji, *et al.* (2007) Contact imaging: Simulation and experiment. *IEEE Transactions on Circuits and Systems I-Regular Papers*, 54(8), 1698–1710.

3 A. Ozcan and U. Demirci (2008) Ultra wide-field lens-free monitoring of cells on-chip. *Lab on a Chip*, 8(1), 98–106.

4 R.R. Singh, *et al.* (2012) A CMOS-microfluidic chemiluminescence contact imaging microsystem. *IEEE Journal of Solid-State Circuits*, 47(11), 2822–2833.

5 C.Z.D. Goh, *et al.* (2011) A CMOS-based ISFET chemical imager with auto-calibration capability. *IEEE Sensors Journal*, 11(12), 3253–3260.

6 E.R. Fossum and D.B. Hondongwa (2014) A review of the pinned photodiode for CCD and CMOS image sensors. *IEEE Journal of the Electron Devices Society*, 2(3), 33–43.

7 A.J.P. Themissen (2008) CMOS image sensors: State-of-the-art. *Solid-State Electronics*, 52(9), 1401–1406.

8 J. Farrell, *et al.* (2006) Resolution and light sensitivity tradeoff with pixel size – art. no. 60690 N. *Digital Photography II*, 6069, N690–N690.

9 L. Shepherd and C. Toumazou (2005) Weak inversion ISFETs for ultra-low power biochemical sensing and real-time analysis. *Sensors and Actuators B-Chemical*, 107(1), 468–473.

10 P.A. Hammond, *et al.* (2004) Design of a single-chip pH sensor using a conventional 0.6-mu m CMOS process. *IEEE Sensors Journal*, 4(6), 706–712.

11 J.M. Rothberg, *et al.* (2011) An integrated semiconductor device enabling non-optical genome sequencing. *Nature*, 475(7356), 348–352.

12 M.J. Milgrew and D.R.S. Cumming (2008) Matching the transconductance characteristics of CMOS ISFET arrays by removing trapped charge. *IEEE Transactions on Electron Devices (TED)*, 55(4), 1074–1079.

13 B. Nemeth, *et al.* (2012) High-resolution real-time ion-camera system using a CMOS-based chemical sensor array for proton imaging. *Sensors and Actuators B: Chemical*, 171–172, 747–752.

14 C. Wai Pan, *et al.* (2010) An integrated ISFETs instrumentation system in standard CMOS technology. *IEEE Journal of Solid-State Circuits (JSSC)*, 45(9), 1923–1934.

15 A. Manickam, *et al.* (2012) A fully-electronic charge-based DNA sequencing CMOS biochip. In: *Symposium on VLSI Circuits (VLSIC)*, pp. 126–127.

9

CMOS Dual-mode Energy-harvesting-image Sensor

9.1 Introduction

Recently, with the benefit of low power, high speed, and feasibility of system-on-chip (SoC) integration, CMOS image sensors (CIS) are replacing power-hungry Charge-coupled Devices (CCD) in many biomedical applications. These advantages become more attractive, especially for personalized diagnosis device and implantable medical system optimization [1,2], which places more emphasis on low power consumption to enable the standalone operation of diagnosis device in isolated environments for extended durations. One application is the endomicroscope, a novel device to obtain non-invasive real-time diagnosis in *in vivo*-imaging environment. Monitoring liver fibrosis progression by liver biopsy is important for disease treatment; however, repeated biopsy is invasive for the patient.

Traditional non-invasive methods [3] use indirect markers to assess liver fibrosis, but are limited by the sensitivity, while the endomicroscope provides better accuracy by transferring second harmonic generation (SHG) imaging into *in-vivo* imaging and real-time monitoring of liver fibrosis directly [4]. The imaging acquisition device is the critical component to the miniature endomicroscope system, and sensitivity is an important parameter, especially in low-light internal environments. Therefore, the CIS technique is a suitable candidate with the advantage of low power consumption, low cost, and small size. The recent development of backside illumination (BSI) technology has dramatically improved the fill factor and quantum efficiency to achieve super low-light performance [5]. Meanwhile, the CIS technique enables on-chip image data analysis to achieve real-time imaging observation based on compatible standard CMOS processes [6].

Besides low-power consumption, the capability to harvesting energy is also desired for implant medical devices. In the retinal implant system [1,7–10], CIS are used as extra ocular units that capture images, and the captured image data is processed by a video processing unit to understand the scene and transmit through either RF or optical links to the intraocular unit. This unit is typically composed of power and data recovery circuits and stimulates the neural system with microelectrode arrays. Thus, the power source, image sensor, and microelectrode arrays are three major components, where complicated structures result in bulky, complex, inefficient, and power hungry intraocular units. By combining all of the aforementioned functional blocks on the same silicon would potentially improve system efficiency, size, power consumption, and the life time

CMOS Integrated Lab-on-a-Chip System for Personalized Biomedical Diagnosis,
First Edition. Hao Yu, Mei Yan, and Xiwei Huang.
© 2018 John Wiley & Sons Singapore Pte. Ltd. Published 2018 by John Wiley & Sons Singapore Pte. Ltd.

of the implant, thereby improving comfort and reducing surgical complexity and complications. Since the retinal implant operates in illuminated environments, photovoltaic (PV) energy harvesting is the natural choice among all the different kinds of energy harvesters. A CIS can achieve energy autonomous operation by harvesting its own energy from the light existing in the environment as required. To achieve this goal, a self-powered, extremely low-power image sensor could be implanted alongside the microelectrode array.

A personalized diagnosis device capable of harvesting ambient energy in the environment can achieve a significantly longer operating lifetime. Among all harvesting energy resources, such as thermal energy, wind energy, and kinetic energy, etc., the solar energy harvester is a viable choice for powering implant medical devices due to the availability of a high-density energy source in environment, relatively good harvesting efficiency, and its compatibility with standard CMOS processes [11–13]. For the image sensor-based medical device, the ambient light required for capturing an image could also be converted into electrical energy to support the sensor operation. In order to achieve this, it is imperative to design the circuitry by using ultra-low power design techniques at all levels, while maximizing the energy harvesting and management efficiencies. Therefore, the solar energy can be sufficient for powering an ultra-low power image sensor if it is harvested efficiently.

There are several approaches to integrate solar power source with an image sensor. A discrete PV (solar) cell could be used for powering the device, where a discrete solar cell and an image sensor could only be placed side-by-side or on the opposite side of the sensor stack as in [14], so that the solar cell does not obstruct the camera view. If size is not critical, then the solar cells could be integrated on the same plane with the node elements and image sensor (i.e. on the same wafer with pixel array or on the same printed circuit board) or detached completely. Placing the solar cell and image sensor on opposite sides is a better choice when size is of primary concern. However, this limits the use of the integrated sensor only to applications where light is incident on both sides of the sensor node. Thus, it is necessary to integrate solar harvesters and the image sensor on the same focal plane while minimizing the area.

In this chapter, an energy harvesting type ultra-low-power CIS design with an integrated power management system (PMS) is introduced towards personal diagnosis application. Section 9.2 explains the design details of the new energy high-energy harvesting image (EHI) pixel structure and pixel operations. Section 9.3 describes the details of the readout circuitry block design, as well as other ultra-low power functional imaging and energy harvesting blocks. Section 9.4 introduces the overall architecture of the EHI imager with PMS. With the 96×96 sensor array under 1-V power supply, the power consumption is only $6\,\mu W$ with 5 fps speed, and simulated and measured performance characteristics of the EHI CIS are also presented.

9.2 CMOS EHI Pixel

Several CIS designs with integrated energy harvesting photodiodes have been reported in the past. The self-powered image sensor (SPS) concept introduced in [15,16] is based on connecting a floating photodiode in series with the battery supply. Thus, it is not self-powered, but rather generates only a boosted supply voltage. Pixels proposed in [17,18] are based on reconfigurable PN-junctions that could perform both image capture and energy harvesting operations. However, drain junctions of the pixel transistors connected to the anode of the energy harvesting photodiode cause significant leakage, decreasing the energy harvesting efficiency. An EHI pixel is first introduced in [1,2] and implemented based on reconfigurable PN-junction photodiodes. Compared to other structures mentioned above, better energy harvesting efficiency was achieved in EHI by decoupling the anode of the energy harvesting photodiode from pixel transistors and other loss paths.

The EHI pixel (shown in Figure 9.1) is based on a three-transistor (3 T) standard active-pixel-sensor (APS) structure, but with an additional photodiode and control-switch to switch between EHM and IM. At EHM (Figure 9.1(b)), the EHB_EN switch is turned on, PD1 is disabled by connecting the FD node to the ground, while the solar cell PD2 generates the current and sends it through the energy harvesting bus (EHB) to an on-chip power management (PM) circuit, thus the solar energy is continuously collected. At IM (Figure 9.1(c)), the switch EHB_EN is turned off and the EHB is connected to the ground. Therefore, both photodiode-1 (PD1) and photodiode-2 (PD2) are reversely biased to work as an image sensor. The signal at the floating diffusion (FD) node generated from imaging PDs is amplified by the source follow transistor and reset by a reset-switch transistor, as in the standard 3 T APS pixel.

The detail description of pixel operation will be described below. Like in standard 3 T CMOS APS, transistors M1-M3 are correspondingly Reset (Rst), Source Follower (SF), and Row Select (RS) transistors associated with PD1. The differences between the EHI and a typical 3 T APS pixel are the reconfigurable PD2 and the mode select transistor M4. Cathodes of PD1 and PD2 are both connected to the FD node. The anode of PD1 is permanently grounded, while the anode of PD2 is connected to the global EHB. During EHM, the mode select transistor M4 is turned, on shorting the FD node to ground. EHB is connected to the PMS, as shown in Figure 9.1(b). In this configuration, PD1 is shorted and the anodes of the PD2 diodes in all pixels are disconnected from the ground. The solar cell array formed by the PD2 diodes delivers the generated energy to the EHB and the on-chip PMS. The PMS controls the load of the solar cell array to harvest the maximum energy from the incident light. In the IM, the EHB is connected to ground, as shown in Figure 9.1(c). Therefore, both diodes (PD1 and PD2) are reverse biased and work like a typical imaging photodiode. The cathodes of PD1 and PD2 connected to the FD node are reset like a regular 3 T APS. The voltage on FD is buffered by the pixel SF transistor to the column sample and hold (CSH) circuits.

As shown in Figure 9.2, a novel layout structure by employing a deep-N-well is proposed in the pixel photodiode to enhance the energy harvesting capacity. The pixel pitch is 23 μm with 27.2% of fill-in factor. Instead of using P diffusion and N-well layers to form the PN junction, here in the EHI pixel the deep-N-well/P-substrate junction forms the PD1 and the N-plus/P-well junction forms the PD2. PD2 is composed of a parallel combination of vertically stacked P-well/N-well and P-well/N-plus photodiodes. Therefore, the effective light-sensitive area is increased for the same silicon area. Vertical stacking of P-well/N-well and P-sub/N-well junctions results in a larger harvesting pixel fill factor. Moreover, the effective junction area for the P-well/deep N-well junction is much larger than the area of a shallow junction with the same lateral silicon area, since the P-well/N-well junction has much deeper sidewalls. Thus, the total junction area is much larger than a P diffusion/N-well junction with the same lateral silicon area.

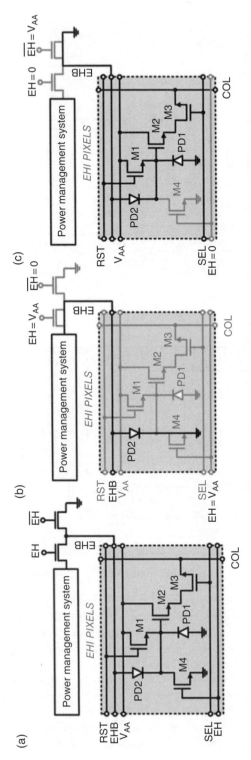

Figure 9.1 Dual-mode CMOS EHI APS pixel: (a) Circuit schematic; (b) Energy harvesting mode (EHM) configuration; and (c) Imaging mode (IM) configuration.

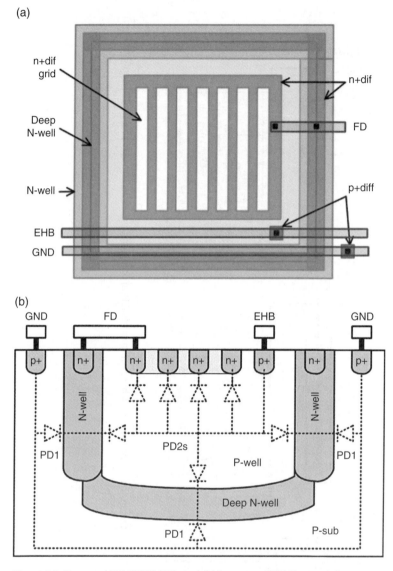

Figure 9.2 Proposed EHI CMOS APS pixel: (a) Layout; and (b) Cross-section.

The total photo-generated current of the proposed EHI structure is considerably higher, since the photo-generated current in a PN-junction is proportional to the total junction area [19]. Since deep N-well and N-plus layers can be placed on top of each other, two photodiodes are built in the same lateral silicon area.

Photons with different wavelengths are absorbed at different depths in silicon. Electron-hole pairs created by the absorbed photon energy recombine, unless they are separated by a built-in electric field in the depleted region. Therefore, only photons absorbed in the vicinity of depleted regions contribute to photoelectric processes. Shallow junctions formed between diffusion layers and substrate or wells absorb photons with wavelengths in the green spectrum with higher efficiency. On the other hand, deeper junctions formed between isolated P-well and N-well, and between P-sub and N-well absorb photons with longer wavelengths, which penetrate deeper. Since short wavelength photons (i.e. blue) cannot penetrate into silicon, depleted regions very close to the silicon surface are needed for capturing them with high efficiency. The added junctions in the proposed EHI pixel structure not only increase the energy harvesting capacity, but also improve the spectral response during IM. Since the sidewalls of every junction reach the surface, the total depletion region at the silicon surface depends on the total length of the junction sidewalls. Therefore, dividing the n + dif into grids improves lateral collection regions [20], and improves blue sensitivity. Moreover, lightly doped junctions (i.e. P-well/N-well and P-sub/N-well) have wider depleted regions that extend to the surface, further improving blue sensitivity.

Besides improving energy harvesting efficiency, the deep-N-well EHI layout structure also reduces pixel fixed-pattern-noise (FPN), thus boosting the sensor performance. As shown in Figure 9.2, the N-type nodes of both PDs are connected by N-well and metal to FD. The P-type node of PD1 is connected to ground by P-substrate, and PD2 is connected to EHB by metal. The deep N-well is covered by N-well surrounding it, such that the PD2 in one pixel is totally isolated from its neighbors. Moreover, the deep-N-well/P-substrate junction provides better isolation between the pixel and its neighbors. As such, the deep-N-well pixel architecture achieves better FPN performance to avoid the crosstalk. It is an important design specification to achieve high-sensitivity personalized diagnosis application, especially under low-light application.

9.3 Readout Circuit

For EHI sensor operation, low-power designing consideration is the main focus. Using column series readout architecture in high-resolution and high-speed imagers is popular to achieve high-speed A/D conversion. However, for low-resolution and low-speed applications, a serial readout architecture is preferred, since it consumes less power, a smaller chip area, and does not introduce additional FPN due to the mismatch between parallel readout channels [21]. Therefore, the readout architecture in the EHI sensor uses a serial readout architecture with a single global charge amplifier (GCA) and an ADC for the whole imager, thus digital conversion is performed sequentially and data is sent out serially. Pixels in the array are read out row by row in column-series architecture. Pixel SFs in the selected row are connected to the column load transistor (M4) through pixel select transistors (M3). Since the SF output can be pulled toward the input level with unlimited current, the SF bias current does not have any effect on the sampling time, as long as the initial voltage on the column capacitor is lower than the input level. Thus, the column bias current in the proposed imager is set as low as possible, reducing the static power consumption of the pixel array.

Pixel outputs are sampled by the CSH and amplified by GCA circuits, as shown in Figure 9.3. The CSH and GCA effectively function as a switched capacitor programmable gain amplifier. The pixel SF outputs in the whole row are sampled on CSH capacitors (C1, C2) at the end of integration (signal level) and right after the pixel reset (reset level) operations. During signal sampling, all CSH (M1), column select (M2), and GCA reset transistors (M3) are turned on simultaneously. The buffered pixel signal voltage is

(a)

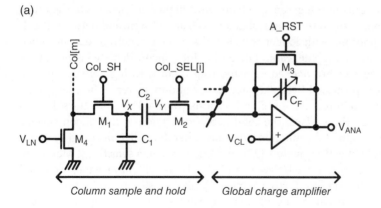

(b)

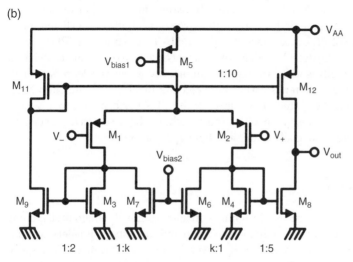

Figure 9.3 (a) Global and column level analog readout circuits; and (b) Current mirror OTA schematic used in GCA.

stored on the CSH capacitor C2 against the clamp voltage (V_{CL}). Consequently, all pixels in the row are reset. Sample and hold switch (M1) in all columns are turned on again, while the column select transistors (M2) are off. The bottom plates of the CSH capacitors (V_x side) are charged to the buffered FD reset level and the floating top plate of C2 is level shifted by the difference between pixel reset and signal levels. Voltage at the top plate of the sample and hold capacitor (C_{SH}) C2 is given by Equation (9.1):

$$V_Y = V_{CL} + V_{rst} - V_{sig} = V_{CL} + V_{eff} \tag{9.1}$$

In an integration-type image sensor, light incidence on the pixel photodiodes is converted to currents proportional to the light intensity. This light-dependent current discharges the pre-charged junction capacitor. The difference between the voltages across the junction capacitor at the beginning and end of the integration period is proportional to the light intensity incident on an individual pixel. If all pixels are reset to exactly the same voltage, the final voltage could be used to extract the light intensity. However, the reset voltage varies pixel-to-pixel due to the threshold voltage, doping concentration, and physical size variations of pixel transistors (M1–M3). Therefore, the final FD node voltage at the end of integration period represents not only the light intensity, but also the FPN caused by the mismatches. Subtracting the signal level from the reset level for each pixel using the differential sampling scheme described above is known as correlated double sampling (CDS). CDS eliminates not only pixel FPN, but also thermal noise and 1/f noise. True CDS is achieved by subtracting the reset level and signal level for the same integration period. True CDS is not possible in 3 T CMOS APS pixels. The CDS described above is a pseudo-CDS, where the signal value is subtracted from the reset level of the next integration period [22–25].

Most of the power in a column readout circuit is consumed during charging and discharging of the CSH capacitors. Reducing the CSH capacitor size reduces the power consumption of the imager. If the capacitor is too small, the voltage drop due to leakage discharge will become significant. Columns that are read out later will appear darker and images will have a brightness gradient. Therefore, capacitor size is picked carefully to achieve a good balance between image quality and power consumption. The leakage increases significantly when semiconductor devices are exposed to light. Thus, special light shields are built above the CSH circuits to protect sensitive column circuits and nodes.

The GCA shown in Figure 9.3 performs several critical functions in the analog signal chain. Since the pixel and column readout circuits attenuate the FD signals, GCA restores signal swing and increases the signal-to-noise ratio (SNR). The GCA also functions as a voltage buffer between the CSH capacitors and the ADC S/H capacitor. Besides, GCA helps CDS operation by forcing the top plates of all CSH capacitors to V_{CL} during signal sampling. Once the differential sampling of the columns is completed, the column select switches are turned on one by one, connecting each CSH circuit to the GCA. When the switch is turned on, the amplifier forces V_y in the column readout circuitry to V_{CL}. The excess charge on the CSH capacitor C_2 is moved to feedback capacitor C_f. The amplifier output voltage considering amplifier non-idealities (V_{offset}) is given by Equation (9.2):

$$V_{out} = V_{CL} - \frac{C_1 C_2}{C_f(C_1 + C_2)} V_{eff} + \left(1 + \frac{C_1 C_2}{C_f(C_1 + C_2)}\right)\frac{V_{offset}}{1 + A_o} \tag{9.2}$$

Designing a very low power charge amplifier is challenging, due to the tradeoffs between power consumption, settling time, and bandwidth. The amplifier has to drive the feedback capacitor, sample, and hold capacitor of the on-chip ADC or the analog output pad if analog output is desired. Therefore, the amplifier has to be capable of providing sufficient output current for driving such a large load capacitance. Since the major part of the voltage gain is achieved at the output node, no compensation capacitor is needed in a single-stage differential amplifier [24]. Removing the compensation capacitor reduces the power consumption significantly. Balanced current mirror-type OTA is a single stage amplifier providing high current driving capability and large output swing. It was shown that the overall power consumption of a balanced current mirror OTA is lower than that of the

Miller compensated two-stage OPAMP with equal gain, slew rate, gain bandwidth product, and phase margin [26].

The circuit diagram of the low-voltage, gain-enhanced current-mirror OTA [27] used in the EHI imager is shown in Figure 9.3. The additional transistors M6 and M7 reduce the current mirrored to the output branches. Therefore, the output impedance of the amplifier is increased, while the transconductance of input transistors remains constant and higher gain is achieved. The gain enhancement ratio is $1/(1-k)$, where k is the ratio of the currents. Gain enhancement reduces the output current. Since only the output stage current determines the bandwidth, slew rate, and settling time, the current mirror ratios are arranged to have an adequate current in the output branch to drive the large capacitive loads, while keeping the current in other branches low, as shown in Figure 9.3.

A 10-bit single ended successive approximation register (SAR)-type ADC is used for converting the GCA output to a digital code in the EHI imager. SAR ADCs consume relatively low power, offering a good balance between chip area and bit resolution. They are suitable for image sensors with medium to high resolutions, where ADCs are required to operate at a relatively medium speed. Even though fully differential SAR ADCs have better rejection of common mode noise and even-order harmonic distortion, they require twice the number of switches, two capacitive DACs, more complicated sample and hold circuits, and consume more power compared to single-ended SAR ADCs. Therefore, single-ended SAR ADCs are preferred for low power applications [28,29].

The schematics of the 10-bit SAR ADC and two-stage dynamic comparator are shown in Figure 9.4. The ADC uses a 10-bit binary-weighted capacitor array to generate quantization levels. Sampled input voltage (V_{in}) is compared with the output of the charge redistributed digital-to-analog converter (DAC). SAR logic implements the binary search algorithm. The direction of the binary search is determined by the comparator output [30]. During sampling, the phase top and bottom plates of all capacitors in the capacitive DAC are connected to ground and GCA output is sampled on to the C_{SH}. After sampling, the bottom plate of the largest capacitor in the DAC is switched to the ADC reference voltage (V_{ref}). In this step, the sampled input is compared to $V_{ref}/2$, determining the MSB bit. During the second step, V_{in} is compared to either $3V_{ref}/4$ or $V_{ref}/4$, depending on the MSB bit determined in the previous step. This process continues until all digital bits are determined and the sampled analog input voltage is converted to the digital domain. Detailed timing diagram and circuit diagrams that implement the binary search algorithm can be found in [31].

The static power consumption of the ADC is ideally zero, if an energy efficient dynamic comparator is used [32]. A true single phase, two-stage comparator is used in the design to reduce the kickback noise. The preamplifier first stage increases the gain for higher sensitivity and faster comparison. The main component of power consumption is the switching power dissipated for charging and discharging the DAC capacitors between GND and V_{ref}. Since V_{ref} is set by the output range of the GCA and the clock frequency is determined by the frame rate, the only way to reduce switching power of the SAR ADC is by minimizing the unit capacitor size. Thus, the minimum allowed capacitor size is used to reduce the ADC power consumption.

(a)

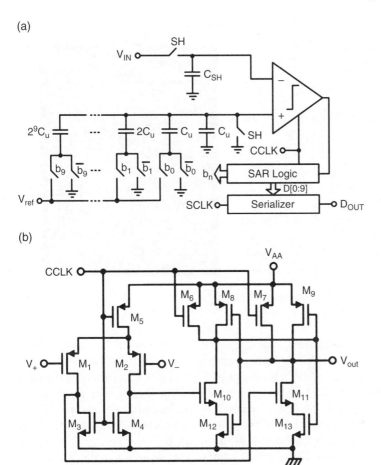

(b)

Figure 9.4 The schematics of the 10-bit SAR ADC and two-stage dynamic comparator.

9.4 A 96×96 EHI Sensing System

In this section, we introduced an ultra-low power CIS design with energy harvesting capability by integrating on-chip PMS. The low power circuit design technique is explored with global readout sensor architecture. What is more, the proposed sensor array has dual operation mode towards extreme low power. The total power consumption is only 6 µW for a 96 × 96 array with 5 fps frame rate.

9.4.1 Top Architecture

A block diagram and die micrograph of the ultra-low power EHI type CIS with an 96 × 96 pixel array is shown in Figure 9.5. The EHI pixel structure achieves improved energy harvesting efficiency and wider spectral response. The design works in two modes sequentially: i) IM; and ii) EHM.

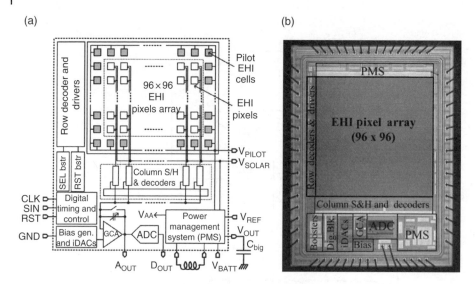

Figure 9.5 (a) Ultra-low power CIS architecture; and (b) Chip photo.

In IM, the pixel photodiodes work as image capturing devices and convert the light incident on them into voltage. A column series readout architecture, with a GCA and an analog-to-digital converter (ADC), is integrated with a pixel array, which is read out sequentially, like a regular CMOS APS imager with rolling shutter. The pixel output from each row is first sampled by CSH circuits. The absolute pixel signal after CDS is amplified by a GCA and converted into digital by a 10-bit SAR type ADC. During EHM, pixel photodiodes are configured as solar cells to harvest the solar energy. It is important to harvest the maximum available power from solar cells in this mode. The maximum power point (MPP) of a solar cell changes with illumination level and ambient temperature. Therefore, a MPP tracking (MPPT) circuit is integrated into the PMS in order to collect energy more efficiently. The PMS monitors the illumination conditions using integrated pilot solar cells, tracks the MPP, and stores the harvested solar energy onto a storage capacitor. Since the solar energy harvester output voltage is less than 0.5 V, an on-chip self-timing boost converter with line regulator is integrated into the PMS to generate the desired supply voltage. The PMS connects the image sensor supply bus to the storage capacitor that holds the harvested energy when sufficient energy is stored. Once the storage capacitor is discharged to a certain level, the PMS connects the imager supply back to battery. During EHM, all blocks related to imaging are turned off to save power.

Power consumption of the imager is scaled down by using additional low-power circuit design techniques. Supply voltage reduction is an effective tool for reducing the power consumption of both digital and analog circuits. Power consumption in digital circuit blocks is proportional to the square of the supply voltage, while in analog blocks it is typically proportional to the supply voltage. Thus, when the supply voltage is reduced from 1.2 V to 1.0 V, the power consumed by digital and analog blocks are reduced by approximately 30% and 17%, respectively. Smart use of low-power design techniques for power-hungry blocks, such as a GCA and on-chip ADC without sacrificing performance, further reduced the power consumption. Power scheduling in active analog and digital blocks were also adopted. Typically, the minimum supply voltage requirement of the pixel electronics is higher than that of other blocks to achieve a good pixel dynamic range. The pixel dynamic range diminishes almost to zero for sub-1 V supply voltages.

In the proposed image sensor, global voltage boosters are used for critical nodes in the pixel array to increase the dynamic range of the pixel instead of increasing the supply voltage. As a result, the whole sensor can work under a 1-V supply without sacrificing the performance metrics. Additionally, an over-rideable digital timing and control block is integrated on-chip to reduce the power dissipated by the digital IO pads. The chip was fabricated in a standard 1.8 V, 1 P6M, 0.18 µm CMOS process. The total power consumption of the proposed EHI CIS is 6.53 µW on a 1 V power supply for a 96 × 96 pixel array while operating at 5 fps frame rates.

9.4.2 System Implementation

In the EHI sensor chip, the pixel array is read out in sequence by controlling the row decoder. The traditional 3 T CMOS APS pixels shown in Figure 9.6 have serious supply voltage limitations and are unsuitable for low-voltage operation. The gate to source voltage drop across the pixel reset and SF transistors limit the dynamic range of the pixel and the readout electronics following it. The dynamic range of a pixel is related to the buffering range of the FD node voltage by the pixel SF. In this design, we adopted the select and reset boosting techniques to extend the dynamic range of the standard 3 T APS pixel electronics. A circuit diagram of the global, row, and pixel level circuits that implement reset and select boosting are shown in Figure 9.6.

The global booster circuit is a single-shot voltage doubler composed of a NAND gate, two inverters, a boosting capacitor, and a PMOS transistor. During pixel readout, all pixels in a row are reset or selected in parallel. Therefore, reset and select boosters drive the gates of all reset and select transistors on the selected row, as well as the parasitic capacitances of the metal interconnects and the row driver circuits shown in the Figure 9.6. Thus, loads for both reset and select booster circuits are mostly capacitive. As long as no active current is drained from the booster output (V_{BST}), the high level of the boosted supply voltage for row drivers is given in Equation (9.3):

$$V_{BST} = V_{AA} + \frac{C_B}{C_B + C_L} V_{AA} \tag{9.3}$$

where C_L is the load capacitance of the booster. If the boosting capacitance (C_B) is large enough, good boosting efficiency is achieved and the boosted voltage level is closer to 2 V_{AA}. When a reset signal with a logic high level equal to V_{AA} drives the reset switch, the maximum voltage at the FD node will be lower than V_{AA} by the threshold voltage (V_{THN}) of the reset transistor. The threshold voltage of the reset transistor will be higher than the nominal threshold voltage due to the body effect. This results in a significant reduction in pixel dynamic range. When the logic high level of the reset signal is larger than $V_{AA} + V_{THN}$, the reset transistor can pull the FD node to V_{AA} with no voltage drop. Boosting the select signal reduces the channel resistance of the select transistor. When the channel resistance is reduced, the voltage drop across the select transistor is reduced.

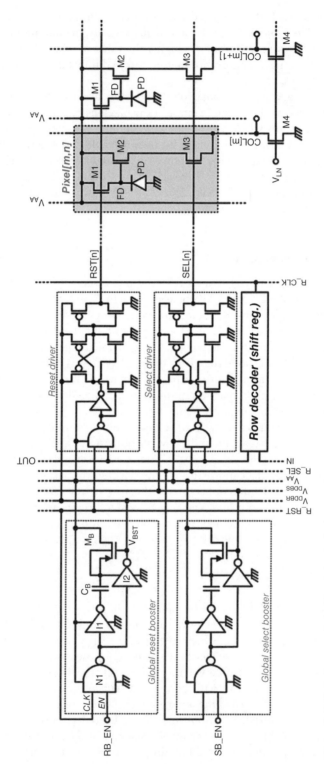

Figure 9.6 Global, row, and pixel level circuits for reset and select boosting in 3 T CMOS APS imagers.

Therefore, boosting the reset and select signals improves the dynamic range, even for lower supply voltages. The use of booster circuits allows reducing the supply voltage from 1.7 V to sub-1 V, which leads to a further reduction of total power consumption.

Since only one row of pixels are accessed at a time, one global reset booster and one global select booster circuit are required in the proposed imager. Each row has a row driver and a select driver circuit to drive the reset and select transistors with boosted RST and SEL signals. A cross-coupled high voltage driver was used for this purpose, as shown in Figure 9.6. A dynamic shift register is used as the row decoder, because of the small pixel array and to reduce the power consumption of the row decoders. The static power consumed by the booster circuits is very low, since no current is drawn from the booster circuit outputs. Their dynamic power consumption is also relatively low, since they are clocked at very low frequencies.

The GCA is one of the most power hungry blocks in the readout chain. Here, a gain-enhanced current-mirror OTA (shown in Figure 9.7) is employed in order to achieve low-power consumption under a 1-V power supply. The OTA only needs two bias voltages, Vb1 and Vb2, to minimize the power dissipation of bias circuits. Note that a big-ratio (10:1) of current-mirror is adopted to increase the output driving capability. It is able to drive at least a 10 pF load at $(15 + 1.5) \times 200$ nA (3.3 µA) bias current, when considering that the amplifier needs to be output directly to a testing board. The gain enhancement is implemented by MN4 and MN5 to distribute the current through MN1 and MN2, which results in the increased resistance load at the input stage. The gain can be increased by $1/(1 - k)$ times and is further adjusted by tuning the value of k [27].

A 1-V supplied 10-bit shift-register-based standard SAR ADC [28,33] is designed to convert the signal to digital output. An energy-efficient dynamic comparator [32] is employed to minimize power consumption of ADC, as shown in Figure 9.8. The comparator does not consume DC-bias current. The amplifier as first stage of comparator can suppress the kick-back noise and also make comparisons faster. Note that the SAR ADC can achieve 100 kS/s speed under a 1-V supply. It meets the requirement of 10 fps full-speed of the image sensor system toward endomicroscope applications. The entire ADC only consumes 900 nW when running at 50 kS/s, which is fast enough for the targeted 5 fps sensor speed.

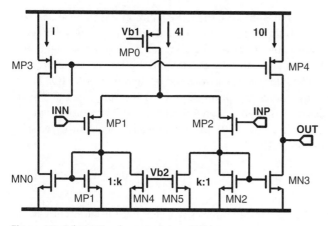

Figure 9.7 Schematic of current-mirror OTA.

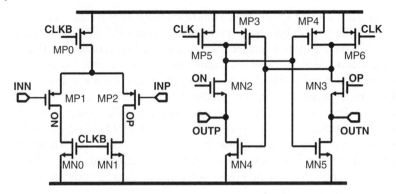

Figure 9.8 Low-power dynamic comparator in SAR ADC.

The digital timing control is also implemented on the same chip to ensure the chip operation. It generates control signals for each individual block, including row decoder, column decoder, amplifier, and ADC. The total layout size is 0.14 mm × 0.14 mm. Compared to use of off-chip IO digital inputs [1], this on-chip implementation of digital control can reduce power consumption by 70% (5.6 μW to 1.6 μW).

The unique integrated PMS consists of a MPPT circuit, a boost converter, a voltage regulator, and a PM decision block. The PMS circuit and its operation principles are shown in Figure 9.9.

Solar cells in the array are operated at the MPP by the MPPT circuit. The output voltage of the solar cell array is boosted by an inductive boost converter. The output of the boost converter is stored in a large off-chip storage capacitor. The storage capacitor voltage is regulated to a level slightly higher than the battery voltage by using an anti-blooming gate. The PM decision block compares the voltage at the storage capacitor V_{OUT} to the battery voltage V_{BATT}. Once V_{OUT} reaches a sufficient level, the chip internal supply voltage (V_{AA}) is switched from battery supply to harvested voltage. In other words, the chip uses the battery voltage for V_{AA} until V_{OUT} is charged to a sufficient level. Once V_{OUT} is charged to this level, the chip is supplied by the harvested energy.

Since the power generated on-chip is limited, the MPPT circuit has to be at as low a power as possible. The on-chip MPPT circuit is implemented using a pilot solar cell, a comparator, and a 4-bit programmable resistive voltage divider, as shown in Figure 9.9. The open circuit output voltage is generated by a distributed pilot cell structure surrounding the EHI pixel array. The pilot cell is constructed using the same CMOS layers as used for building the energy harvesting photodiodes, so that pilot cell and pixel energy harvesting photodiodes have the same open circuit voltage. The resistive voltage divider output is the reference voltage (VMPP) and k_v is ideally equal to the resistive division ratio k_R given in Equation (9.4):

$$k_R = \frac{R_2}{R_1 + R_2} \tag{9.4}$$

Measurements have shown that integrated micro solar cells built in different CMOS processes have a voltage fraction k_v in the range between 0.80 and 0.85. The k_R ratio is

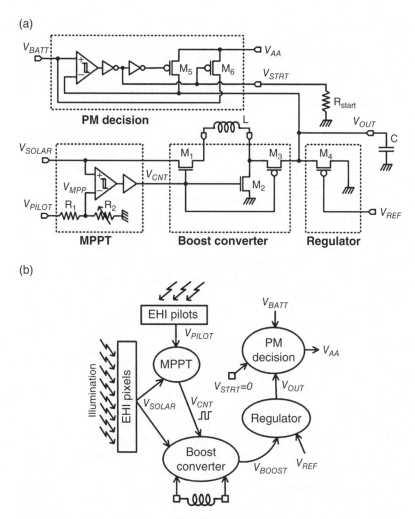

Figure 9.9 (a) Circuit diagram of the PMS; and (b) Operation principle of the PMS.

controlled by the programmable bottom resistor R_2 to set k_v to the correct value. Ideally, pilot cells should not be loaded so that pilot cell output voltage (V_{PILOT}) is equal to the open circuit voltage. The resistive voltage divider is implemented with a very large on-chip resistor string, so that the current drawn from the pilot cell is much smaller than the short circuit current of the pilot cells. Deviation of V_{PILOT} from V_{oc} is insignificant for small output currents, due to the logarithmic dependence of photodiode voltage on the output current. Since the resistive chain is programmable, k_R can be adjusted to include the deviation of V_{PILOT} from V_{oc}. The required value for resistive division ratio is given in Equation (9.5):

$$k_R = k_v \times \frac{V_{OC}}{V_{PILOT}} \tag{9.5}$$

The MPPT block comparator continuously monitors whether V_{SOLAR} is larger than VMPP and generates a control/clock output (V_{CNT}) used by the boost converter. The comparator functions as an asynchronous control signal generator for the boost converter. Since the boost converter is the load for the solar cell array, the comparator controls the amount of current sourced from the solar cell array by switching the boost converter. Therefore, it keeps solar cells operating at MPP, thus optimizing harvesting efficiency.

When M1 and M2 in the boost converter block are turned on, the solar cell current flows through the off-chip inductor to ground. The output voltage of solar cell (V_{SOLAR}) drops as the current drawn from the solar cell increases. If V_{SOLAR} becomes 0 V, the current reaches the maximum available current (short circuit current). The MPPT circuit tries to keep the current at the optimum level by sensing the V_{SOLAR} voltage. When V_{SOLAR} drops one hysteresis voltage below the V_{MPP}, the MPPT comparator turns the NMOS switches (M1, M2) off and turns the PMOS switch (M3) on. At this moment, the inductor is floating with one terminal connected to the storage capacitor. Since the inductor current cannot change instantly, the floating inductor will go on supplying a decaying current. Thus, the solar energy stored in the EMF of the inductor is transferred to a large external storage capacitor. Meanwhile, the V_{SOLAR} voltage rises. When it raises one hysteresis voltage above V_{MPP}, the output of the MPPT comparator is toggled, starting a new cycle. This operation continues indefinitely, charging the V_{OUT} node voltage higher at each cycle with maximum efficiency. The switches in the boost converter are driven by the MPPT circuit. This integrated topology requires no clocks to drive the switches, so the circuit ends up being very simple compared to other switched capacitor charge pump designs. The MPPT algorithm is implemented with no extra power consumption.

In order to regulate the harvested voltage output at the V_{OUT} node with low-power consumption, a charge skimming regulation technique was utilized. As the floating inductor (acting like a current source) pumps charge to the storage capacitor, the voltage across the capacitor increases proportionally and decreases as the load removes charge from it. If the current consumed from the capacitor is larger than the current supplied, the capacitor will eventually discharge. However, when the supplied current is larger, voltage will go on increasing indefinitely. The charge skimming gate is a simple switch that turns on when the storage capacitor voltage reaches $V_{REF} + |V_{THP}|$. When the charge skimming gate turns ON, it will dump the excess charge to ground. As the excess charge is dumped and the voltage level falls, the charge skimming gate will turn OFF. The output voltage might have a small ripple due to transistor switching, but satisfactory performance is achieved using such a simple regulator.

The job of the power management (PM) decision block is to switch the chip power supply (V_{AA}) between the energy storage node (V_{OUT}) and battery (V_{BATT}) voltages. It compares the V_{OUT} and V_{BATT} with a hysteresis. If V_{OUT} is one hysteresis voltage (V_{HYST}) above the V_{BATT} voltage, then M5 turns on, and M6 turns off allowing self-powered operation. Meanwhile, MPPT and the boost converter continue to transfer charge from the solar cells to the external capacitor, keeping V_{OUT} high. If the harvested and transferred energy is more than the energy consumed by the imager, then regulator transistor M4 turns on and skims the excess charge from the V_{OUT} node. Here, the regulator turn-on voltage could be adjusted above the $V_{OUT} + V_{HYST}$, so that more charge is stored on the external capacitor beyond the optimum operating voltage.

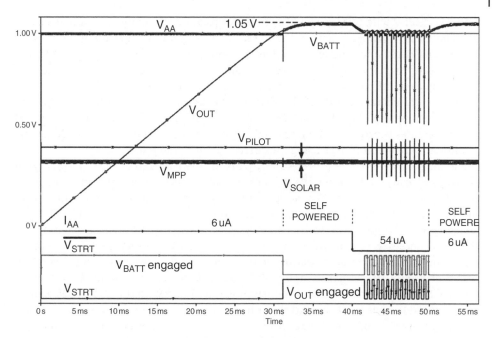

Figure 9.10 Simulation result of the full operating cycles of the PMS.

A simulation representing full operation cycles of the PMS is shown in Figure 9.10. In this simulation, the battery voltage was set to 1 V, while k_R is 0.8, V_{SOLAR} is 400 mV, and the comparators have 50 mV hysteresis. The storage capacitor charges and the system is self powered when the load current is set to 6 μA. Then it is switched to 54 μA to show the adaptive operation of the PMS under larger loading conditions. The PMS repeatedly switches the supply rail between battery and the harvested energy.

Note that the whole chip including the PMS is powered through the internal V_{AA} supply line. Thus, the V_{AA} line has to be connected to an auxiliary power source or a battery when the chip is first powered. This is achieved by grounding the gate of M6 through a large off-chip resistor ($R_{START} > 5$ MΩ). The inverter driving the gate of M6 is made stronger, accommodating this component. In energy autonomous mode of operation, the V_{START} signal is used as the EH signal and the imager is switched to EHM when V_{OUT} drops below V_{BATT} and once V_{OUT} increases above V_{BATT}, the imager switches back to IM. Full energy autonomy is possible in this mode. When the incoming light increases, more power is harvested and the imager will stay in EHM for a shorter time. As harvested power decreases, the imager will need to harvest energy for a longer time to power the imager for the same amount of time.

9.4.3 Results

The proposed self-powered CIS was fabricated in a standard 1.8 V, 1 P6M, 0.18 μm CMOS process. The chip occupies a 3 mm × 4 mm silicon area. The image sensor is composed of a 96 × 96 pixel array with a pixel pitch of 23 μm. Compared to other pixel structures, the new pixel has two vertically stacked high fill factor photodiodes (PD1 with 83.4%, PD2 with 50.6%), resulting in better photoresponsivity in confined spaces. The energy harvesting capacity of the micro solar cell array, composed of the in-pixel energy harvesting photodiodes as well as the power output from the boost converter, are measured to characterize the power consumption and energy harvesting capacity of the EHI imager. IM performance characteristics are also provided in this section.

The general characteristics of the EHI imager are presented in Table 9.1. Overall power consumption of the EHI imager in IM for 1 FPS, 2.5 FPS, 5 FPS, 10 FPS, and 20 FPS frame rates is provided. Tektronix DMM 4040, 6.5 digit multimeters with 100 pA resolution were used for measuring the current input to the power pads.

The imager has separate power supply pads for the pad frame, ADC, PMS, digital block, pixel array, and readout electronics. Detailed power consumption of the main circuit blocks running on a 1 V supply voltage and different frame rates in IM are shown in Table 9.2. The PM decision block is on during IM, so that it can switch the imager power supply back to the battery supply when the storage capacitor discharges. Therefore, it is included in the IM power consumption. The GCA and SAR ADC consume most of the power in the new EHI imager. Power consumption of the amplifier is 2.09 μW with 1 V supply at 5 fps. ADC operates at 50 kS/s conversion speed with 10-bit resolution, while consuming only 1.53 μW in this case. ADC can be reconfigured to have 9-bit resolution for lower power consumption instead of 10-bit resolution. At a 5 fps frame rate, SAR ADC consumes 1.09 μW power with 9-bit resolution.

Even though the imager is designed for a nominal operating supply voltage of 1.0 V, it can operate with satisfactory performance down to 0.8 V. Power consumption of the EHI imager in IM for 0.8 V, 1.0 V, and 1.2 V supply voltages running at different frame rates, are shown in Figure 9.11.

Power consumption of the digital circuit blocks increases linearly as the operating frequency increases. Power consumption in analog blocks is independent of operating frequency. Since the amplifier output settling time decreases at higher operating frequencies, the amplifier bias current is increased to settle to the final voltage faster. Therefore, even though the charge amplifier is an analog block, its power consumption increases with frame rate. Moreover, the power consumed by the amplifier while

Table 9.1 Performance summary of the EHI imager

Process	0.18 μm 1P6M CMOS				
Pixel Type	3 T CMOS EHI APS				
Pixel Fill Factor (PD1)	83.4%				
Pixel Fill Factor (PD2)	50.6%				
Pixel Array Size	96 × 96				
Supply Voltage (V)	1.0				
ADC Type	SAR				
ADC Resolution	10-bit				
Frame Rate (FPS)	1.0	2.5	5.0	10.0	20.0
Power Consumption (μW)	2.09	3.96	6.53	11.16	19.96

Table 9.2 Performance summary of the EHI imager circuit blocks in IM on 1 V supply

Frame Rate (FPS)	1.0	2.5	5.0	10.0	20.0
Pixel Array (μW)	0.11	0.12	0.14	0.17	0.23
Row Decoder (μW)	0.06	0.14	0.25	0.50	1.01
Ref. Gen. and Bias Circuits (μW)	0.16	0.16	0.16	0.16	0.16
Column Circuits (μW)	0.010	0.017	0.028	0.050	0.095
GCA (μW)	0.68	1.40	2.09	2.82	4.22
ADC (μW)	0.31	0.77	1.53	3.07	6.15
Pad Frame (μW)	0.12	0.29	0.53	1.08	2.07
Timing Generator (μW)	0.33	0.77	1.49	3.00	5.72
PM Decision (μW)	0.31	0.31	0.31	0.31	0.31
Total (μW)	2.09	3.96	6.53	11.16	19.96

charging load capacitances also increases with operating frequency. In practice, the only blocks that consume strictly static power are the reference bias generator, bias circuits, and the continuous time comparator in the PM decision block. These blocks consume a small portion of the total chip power. Therefore, power consumption of the EHI imager has an almost linear dependence on the frame rate, due to the frame rate adaptive amplifier bias current.

The energy figure of merit (FoM) is an important performance metric for comparing the power consumption of imagers with different resolutions operating at different frame rates [1]. It is defined as the energy consumed for generating the digital output for a single pixel. FoM is given in Equation (9.6), where P_{Total} is the total power consumption, FR is the frame rate, m is the number of pixel array rows, and n is the number of pixel array columns:

$$\mathrm{FoM} = \frac{P_{Total}}{FR \cdot m \cdot n} \tag{9.6}$$

Figure 9.11 also shows the variation of power consumption with supply voltage. The power consumption of digital blocks has a quadratic dependence on supply voltage, while the power consumption of analog blocks has an almost linear dependence. Since the power supply rejection of the reference current generator is finite, the bias current increases slightly with increasing supply voltage. Switching power consumption dominates the power consumption at higher operating frequencies, so the power consumption dependence on supply voltage is closer to quadratic for higher operating frequencies. At nominal 1 V supply and 5 fps frame rate, the imager achieves 142 pJ/Frame × pixel efficiency. As expected at 20 fps, this drops to 108 pJ/Frame × pixel. Figure 9.12 shows the variation of FoM with frame rate for different supply voltages.

The power generated by the on-chip solar cell array is measured by turning the boost converter off and directly loading the EHB with a variable resistor. The current voltage (IV) and power voltage (PV) curves for various illuminations are shown in Figure 9.13.

Output power from the voltage regulator and the output power from the solar cell array are measured to determine the efficiency of the PMS block under 60 Klux

(a)

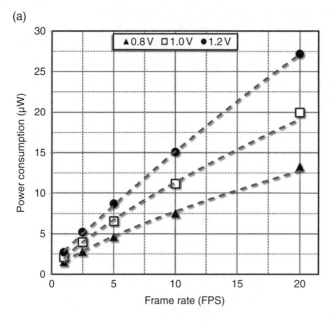

(b)

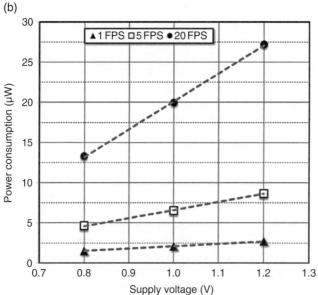

Figure 9.11 Power consumption of the EHI imager for varying frame rates (a) and varying supply voltages (b).

illumination conditions. The measurements are performed by varying the reference input to the MPPT comparator to control the solar cell array output voltage. Boost converter efficiency is the ratio of output power from the boost converter to the input power. However, the input power is not constant and varies for different solar cell voltages. The ratio of output power to the maximum input power is defined as normalized

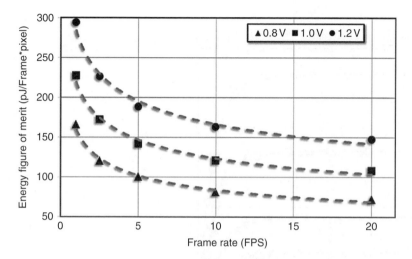

Figure 9.12 FoM performance of the imager under different frame rates and supply voltages.

boost converter efficiency, which is a better metric for characterizing the boost converter. PMS consumes 2.21 µW total power and this power consumption further reduces the overall efficiency of the PM block.

Figure 9.14 shows how the boost converter efficiency, normalized boost converter efficiency, and overall PMS efficiency change for different solar cell voltages. The MPP for the solar cell array and the maximum efficiency point for the boost converter do not overlap. The boost converter operates with maximum efficiency of 60.4% when V_{SOLAR} is 303 mV. The solar cell array delivers the maximum power to the boost converter when V_{SOLAR} is 422.6 mV. The boost converter delivers maximum output power of 17.32 µW for an input power of 28.8 µW when V_{SOLAR} is 362 mV. This input power is less than the maximum output power of 31.2 µW available from the solar cell array. The maximum overall efficiency of PMS is measured as 48.4%. These measurements suggest that by operating the MPPT comparator at this voltage, instead of the MPP of the solar cell array, increases the power delivered by the PMS. These results are summarized in Table 9.3.

The power consumption and energy harvesting capacity of the proposed imager with the other EHI sensors are presented in Table 9.4. The power harvesting capacity of the proposed imager is significantly higher than other imagers and energy FoM is second after [19].

The V_{START} signal becomes high when the output capacitor is charged and the regulated voltage is more than the battery supply, as shown in Figure 9.15, indicating the system is self-powered. The power output from the PMS block is almost three times the power consumed at 5 fps frame rate. This allows the imager to operate with a 72.5% duty cycle. Therefore, the imager can run for 72.5 s autonomously, while disconnected from the battery using the power harvested for 27.5 s.

An ultra-low power EHI-type CMOS APS image sensor capable of energy harvesting with an on-chip PMS is presented. The new energy harvesting photodiodes built with a P-well layer increases the power harvesting capacity significantly compared to the energy harvesting photodiodes built with p-diffusion layer, as reported in other

(a)

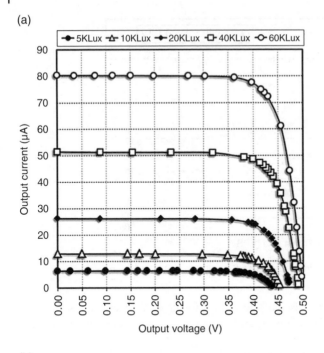

(b)

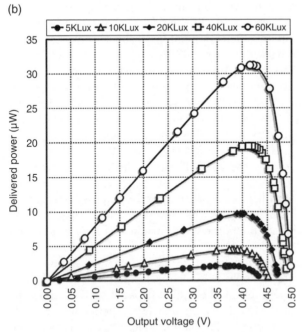

Figure 9.13 Measured output voltage vs. output current (a) and output power of the solar cell array (b).

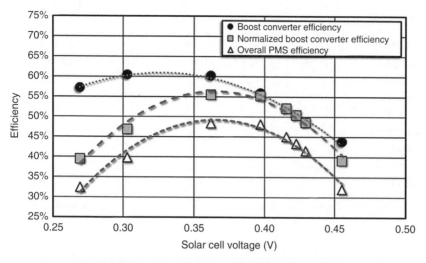

Figure 9.14 Measured efficiency of boost converter and overall PMS block.

Table 9.3 Performance summary in EHM

PM Decision Power (μW)	0.31
MPPT + Boost Converter Power (μW)	1.90
Total PMS Power Consumption (μW)	2.21
Boost Converter Efficiency	60.4%
Normalized Boost Converter Efficiency	55.5%
Overall PMS Efficiency	48.4%

Table 9.4 Comparison of proposed imager to other EHIs

PARAMETER	[1] Ay	[17] Law	[18] Tang	This Work
Technology	0.5μm/5 V(2P3M)	0.35μm (2P3M)	0.35μm (2P3M)	0.18μm/1.8 V(1P6M)
Pixel Pitch	21μm	15μm	10μm	23μm
Array Size	54×50	32×32	128×96	96×96
Fill Factor	PD1-62%/ PD2-32%	21.0%	39%	PD1-83.4%/ PD2-50.6%
ADC Resolution	10 bit SAR	8 bit-Ramp	10 bit-Ramp	10 bit SAR
Supply Voltage	1.2 V	1.5 V	1.35 V	1.0 V
Energy Harvesting (μW)	2.10 @ 20 klx/ 3.35 @ 60 klx	0.0356 @ 29klx	3.7 @ 35 klx *	31.2 @ 60 klx/ 19.5 @ 40 klx
Energy Harvesting (μW/mm²)	1.76 @ 20 klx/ 2.81 @ 60 klx	0.154 @ 29 klx	0.68 @ 35 klx	6.4 @ 60 klx/ 4.0 @ 40 klx

Table 9.4 (Continued)

Frame Rate (FPS)	7.4	21	9.6	1	20
Power Consumption (Whole Chip) (μW)	14.25	15.8	10	2.09	19.96
Power Consumption (Pixel Array) (μW)	0.0264	NA	0.37	0.11	0.23
eFOM (Whole Chip) (pJ/frame * pixel)	713.2	765	84	226.8	108.3
eFOM (Pixel Array) (pJ/frame * pixel)	1.32	NA	3.2	11.9	1.25

Note: Calculated using reported open circuit voltage and short circuit current and assuming 0.76% power fill factor.

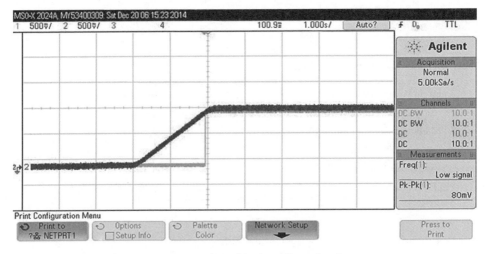

Figure 9.15 Measured storage capacitor voltage (V_{OUT}) and V_{START} signals.

works. The proposed EHI system is capable of harvesting more power than it consumes under normal indoor lighting conditions. Integrated PMS turns the imager on whenever sufficient energy is stored on the storage capacitor and puts it in standby mode when the storage capacitor discharges. The PMS is capable of automatically switching the imager power supply bus between battery and harvested power with a 72.5% duty cycle.

This self-powered structure has great potential for applications requiring extended operation lifetimes with a limited battery supply without the need for any human interference and sufficient light is available. A promising application is a retinal implant. Once the sensor is implanted in the eye, battery replacement is not an option. However, plenty of light is available. Therefore, an image sensor that can use the available ambient light as an energy source is a promising solution for this application.

References

1 S.U. Ay (2011) A CMOS energy harvesting and imaging (EHI) Active pixel sensor (APS) imager for retinal prosthesis. *Transactions on Biomedical Circuits & Systems IEEE*, 5, 535–545.

2 T. Wang, X. Huang, M. Yan, H. Yu, K.S. Yeo, *et al.* (2012) A 96 × 96 1 V ultra-low power CMOS image sensor for biomedical application. In: *2012 IEEE Asia Pacific Conference on Circuits and Systems (APCCAS)*, pp. 13–16.

3 C.T. Wai, J.K. Greenson, R.J. Fontana, J.D. Kalbfleisch, J.A. Marrero, *et al.* (2003) A simple noninvasive index can predict both significant fibrosis and cirrhosis in patients with chronic hepatitis C. *Hepatology*, 38, 518–526.

4 Y. He, C.H. Kang, S. Xu, X. Tuo, S. Trasti, *et al.* (2010) Toward surface quantification of liver fibrosis progression. *Journal of Biomedical Optics*, 15, 056007–11.

5 H. Rhodes, D. Tai, Y. Qian, D. Mao, V. Venezia, *et al.* (2000) The mass production of BSI CMOS image sensors. In: *2000 IEEE Workshop on Signal Processing Systems, 2000 (SiPS 2000)*, pp. 801–810.

6 M. Yan and X. Huang (2012) High-speed CMOS image sensor for high-throughput lensless microfluidic imaging system. *Proceedings of the SPIE – The International Society for Optical Engineering*, 8298, pp. 8298044–12.

7 J. Loudin, J. Harris and D. Palanker (2011) Photovoltaic retinal prosthesis. In: *SPIE BiOS*, pp. 788513–13.

8 W. Mokwa (2010) MEMS technologies for artificial retinas. *Proceedings of the SPIE – The International Society for Optical Engineering*, 7594, 759402–759414.

9 T. Schanze, L. Hesse, C. Lau, N. Greve, W. Haberer, *et al.* (2007) An optically powered single-channel stimulation implant as test system for chronic biocompatibility and biostability of miniaturized retinal vision prostheses. *IEEE Transactions on Biomedical Engineering*, 54, 983–992.

10 G. Roessler, T. Laube, C. Brockmann, T. Kirschkamp, B. Mazinani, *et al.* (2009) Implantation and explantation of a wireless epiretinal retina implant device: observations during the EPIRET3 prospective clinical trial. *Investigative Ophthalmology & Visual Science*, 50, 3003–3008.

11 M. Ferri, D. Pinna, E. Dallago and P. Malcovati (2009) Integrated micro-solar cell structures for harvesting supplied microsystems in 0.35-μm CMOS technology. In: *Sensors, 2009 IEEE*, pp. 542–545.

12 B. Plesz, L. Juhasz and J. Mizsei (2010) Feasibility study of a CMOS-compatible integrated solar photovoltaic cell array. In: *2010 Symposium on Design Test Integration and Packaging of MEMS/MOEMS (DTIP)*, pp. 403–406.

13 E.G. Fong, N.J. Guilar, T.J. Kleeburg, P. Hai, D.R. Yankelevich and R. Amirtharajah (2013) Integrated energy-harvesting photodiodes with diffractive storage capacitance. *IEEE Transactions on Very Large Scale Integration Systems*, 21, 486–497.

14 G. Kim, Y. Lee, Z. Foo and P. Pannuto (2014) A millimeter-scale wireless imaging system with continuous motion detection and energy harvesting, pp. 1–2.

15 A. Fish, S. Hamami and O. Yadid-Pecht (2006) CMOS Image sensors with self-powered generation capability. *IEEE Transactions on Circuits & Systems II Express Briefs*, 53, 1210–1214.

16 C. Shi, M.K. Law and A. Bermak (2011) A novel asynchronous pixel for an energy harvesting CMOS image sensor. *IEEE Transactions on Very Large Scale Integration Systems*, 19, 118–129.

17 M.K. Law, A. Bermak and C. Shi (2011) A low-power energy-harvesting logarithmic CMOS Image sensor with reconfigurable resolution using two-level quantization scheme. *IEEE Transactions on Circuits & Systems II Express Briefs*, 58, 80–84.

18 F. Tang and A. Bermak (2012) An 84 pW/frame per pixel current-mode CMOS Image sensor with energy harvesting capability. *IEEE Sensors Journal*, 12, 720–726.

19 M.A. Green (1981) *Solar Cells: Operating Principles, Technology and System Applications*. Prentice Hall: Englewood Cliffs, NJ.

20 S.U. Ay (2008) Photodiode peripheral utilization effect on CMOS APS pixel performance. *IEEE Transactions on Circuits & Systems I Regular Papers*, 55, 1405–1411.

21 A.I. Krymski, N.E. Bock, N. Tu, D. Van Blerkom and E.R. Fossum (2004) A high-speed, 240-frames/s, 4.1-Mpixel CMOS sensor. *IEEE Transactions on Electron Devices*, 50, 130–135.

22 E.R. Fossum (1995) CMOS image sensors: Electronic camera on a chip. In: *Proceedings of the IEEE International Electron Devices Meeting (IEDM)*, Washington, DC, 10–13 December, pp. 17–25.

23 E.R. Fossum (1997) CMOS image sensors: Electronic camera-on-a-chip. *IEEE Transactions on Electron Devices*, 44, 1689–1698.

24 K.B. Cho, A.I. Krymski and E.R. Fossum (2003) A 1.5-V 550-μW 176 × 144 autonomous CMOS active pixel image sensor. *IEEE Transactions on Electron Devices*, 50, 96–105.

25 K.B. Cho, A. Krymski and E.R. Fossum (2000) A 1.2 V micropower CMOS active pixel image sensor for portable applications. In: *IEEE International Conference on Solid-state Circuits*, pp. 114–115.

26 W. Gao and R.I. Hornsey (2005) Low-power realization in main blocks of CMOS APS image sensor. In: *Photonics North*, pp. 596926–596929.

27 L. Yao, M. Steyaert and W. Sansen (2003) A 0.8-V, 8-μW, CMOS OTA with 50-dB gain and 1.2-MHz GBW in 18-pF load. In: *Proceedings of the European Conference on Solid-State Circuits, Esscirc' 03*, pp. 297–300.

28 M.D. Scott, B.E. Boser and K.S.J. Pister (2003) An ultralow-energy ADC for smart dust. *IEEE Journal of Solid-State Circuits*, 38, 1123–1129.

29 L.S.Y. Wong, S. Hossain, A. Ta, J. Edvinsson, *et al.* (2005) A very low-power CMOS mixed-signal IC for implantable pacemaker applications. *IEEE Journal of Solid-State Circuits*, 39, 2446–2456.

30 Z. Zhou, B. Pain and E.R. Fossum (1997) CMOS active pixel sensor with on-chip successive approximation analog-to-digital converter. *IEEE Transactions on Electron Devices*, 44, 1759–1763.

31 A. Mesgarani and S.U. Ay (2013) A 1.2-V 100 KS/S energy efficient supply boosted SAR ADC. *Midwest Symposium on Circuits & Systems*, pp. 1152–1155.

32 M. Van Elzakker, E. Van Tuijl, P. Geraedts and D. Schinkel (2008) A 1.9 μW 4.4fJ/ conversion-step 10b 1MS/s charge-redistribution ADC. *ISSCC Digest of Technical Papers, February 2008*, pp. 244–245.

33 S.U. Ay (2011) A sub-1 Volt 10-bit supply boosted SAR ADC design in standard CMOS. *Analog Integrated Circuits and Signal Processing*, 66, 213–221.

10

DNA Sequencing

10.1 Introduction

DNA detection, categorized as sequencing and genotyping, plays a significant role for modern human health. Sequencing, the detection of the order of nucleotides in DNA strands, enables studies of metagenomics, genetic disorders, diseases, and genomic medicine. Genotyping, targeted sequencing, or mutation of specific DNA, is deployed for single nucleotide polymorphism (SNP) detections, most of which are associated with diseases and deficiencies [1]. Sanger sequencing has successfully employed DNA detection since the 1970s, which was expensive and time-consuming for large-scale sequencing [2]. Next-generation sequencing technologies were later developed for high-throughput sequencing with low cost, including pyrosequencing, sequencing by oligo ligation detection (SOLiD), and Illumina sequencing [3]. However, these methods require fluorescent labels and bulky optical instruments and hence are not feasible for personalized diagnosis.

A large-array CMOS-compatible sensor foresees a strong potential in future personalized DNA sequencing. The same as computer and communication devices, it follows Moore's law in that it is scalable for millions of DNA strands to be detected simultaneously on a single CMOS chip. As shown in Figure 10.1, since 2008, the development of new sequencing technologies under the continuous semiconductor process scaling leads to dramatic scale-down on the cost of CMOS processing. State-of-the-art CMOS-compatible methods include ion-sensitive field-effect transistor (ISFET)-based [4–8] chemical sensing and nanopore-based [9] electrical sensing.

This chapter introduces the latest development of CMOS-based multi-modal sensor platform for personalized DNA detection, which includes:

- Large-array ISFET-based sequencing;
- THz-based genotyping for SNP detection; and
- Beyond-CMOS single-molecule nanopore sequencing.

10.2 CMOS ISFET-based Sequencing

10.2.1 Overview

In humans, the DNA length is about 3.2 billion nucleotides pairs. For bacteria such as *Escherichia coli*, it is about 4.6 million. For viruses such as HIV, it is about 9700.

CMOS Integrated Lab-on-a-Chip System for Personalized Biomedical Diagnosis,
First Edition. Hao Yu, Mei Yan, and Xiwei Huang.
© 2018 John Wiley & Sons Singapore Pte. Ltd. Published 2018 by John Wiley & Sons Singapore Pte. Ltd.

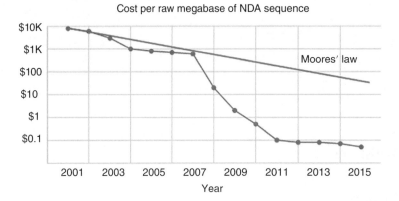

Figure 10.1 The relationship between DNA sequence cost and Moore's law: Data from the NHGRI Genome Sequencing Program (GSP): Available at: www.genome.gov/sequencingcosts.

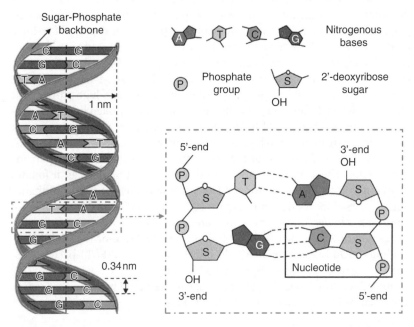

Figure 10.2 A typical DNA molecule structure.

High-throughput DNA sequencing needs to reduce the cost and time of detection, even though human DNA is only 2% in being informative.

Figure 10.2 is the chemical structure of a double-stranded DNA (dsDNA) chain. The fundamental unit is called a nucleotide, which is composed of a nitrogenous base, a 2'-deoxyribose sugar, and a phosphate group. The nitrogenous base is attached to the 1'-end of sugar in place of the –OH group. Four types of bases are involved, including Adenine (A), Thymine (T), Cytosine (C), and Guanine (G). Adenine and Thymine is a pair of bases that can be associated by two hydrogen bonds. Similarly, the Cytosine-Guanine pair is associated by three hydrogen bonds. On the other hand, the phosphate

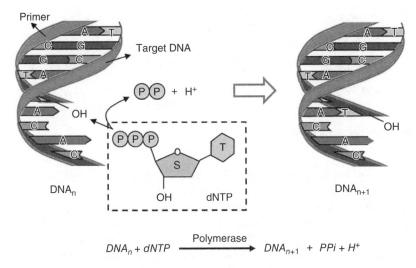

Figure 10.3 ISFET-based sequencing principle.

group is attached to the 5'-end of sugar in the place of the −OH group, after which it can be added to the 3'-end of a sugar, so that the two adjacent nucleotides are connected through phosphodiester bonds. Overall, the DNA structure can be regarded as two helical sugar-phosphate "backbones" bonded together by the attached base pairs.

Polymerization shown in Figure 10.3 is an important reaction in DNA sequencing, where single-stranded DNA (ssDNA) acts as the target sample. Since a new nucleotide can only bind to the carbon-3' of a pre-existing nucleotide, a primer is attached to act as a starting point. A primer is a short ssDNA that can be manufactured to match any sequence on the target DNA. Then nucleotide segments will incorporate and extend from the free 3'-end of primer. To ensure the polymerization process, deoxyribonucleotide triphosphate (dNTP) should be added. It contains a sugar, a nitrogenous base, and three phosphate groups. Incorporation will happen when the dNTP base is complementary to the target nucleotide with the help of a polymerase enzyme. A hydrogen ion and pyrophosphate (the detached two phosphate groups, PPi) are produced, which are equivalent to nucleotides polymerized. By detecting the pH change of solution, DNA incorporation can be recognized. Consequently, the whole strand sequences can be obtained through the detection of each individual nucleotide.

10.2.2 ISFET-based Sequencing Procedure

Template-based DNA polymerase synthesis has been widely used in DNA sequencing. A long ssDNA chain is first fragmented into short templates, then clonally amplified on microbeads by a polymerase chain reaction (PCR).

A high-quality genomic library is important for sequencing. The preparation procedure is shown in Figure 10.4. The first step is to prepare short DNA slices (<600 base pairs). Physical and enzymatic methods, as well as chemical methods can be employed to fragment long double-strand DNA. Non-ideal ends at detached parts may be introduced after fragmentation. The second step performed is end repair, so as to remove

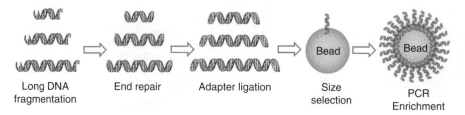

Figure 10.4 DNA sample preparation process.

overhangs and create phosphorylated blunt ends. The third step is where adapters are ligated to both ends of fragmented dsDNA. An adapter is a short dsDNA molecule with known sequence that is complementary to primers used in genomic replication. The adapter and primer combined together make it possible to synthesise any fragmented DNA with uncertain sequence. Since the DNA strand is randomly fragmented, the segment size is also randomly distributed (e.g. Poisson distribution) within a certain range. Therefore, the fourth step is the desired size selection (e.g. 200 base pairs). The agarose gel electrophoresis technique is an effective method to differentiate between different DNA sizes. Since the DNA molecule is negatively charged, when applying a voltage to the gel, the DNA move towards the positive electrode. Since a short strand moves fast and a long strand moves more slowly, different DNA sizes are recognized and selected.

An alternative method used in ISFET sequencing is bead-based selection, in which certain-sized dsDNA will be bonded to a magnetic bead, under the existence of polyethylene glycol (PEG) and salt (NaCl). In order to produce a relatively high signal level for the sensor to detect, sufficient copies of DNA sample are required. Therefore, the last step should be replication of selected DNA on a bead before testing. PCR is a common-used technique for DNA amplification.

PCR is actually a serial temperature change, which affects DNA behavior. As shown in Figure 10.5(a), in order to conduct a PCR experiment, the DNA sample on a bead, heat-stable Taq polymerase, nucleotides, and buffer, as well as primers are needed, which will be first mixed in a tube and then placed in a thermal cycler for reaction. Basically, three main steps are involved in PCR: DNA denaturation, primers annealing, and polymerase extension, as shown in Figure 10.5(b). When the mixture is heated up to 98 °C, dsDNA will be separated into two single DNA strands. The temperature is decreased to 48 °C ~ 72 °C, so that primers will bind to their complementary sequences of ssDNA. Finally, when the temperature is within 68 °C ~ 72 °C, appropriate nucleotides will add to the 3'-end of primes and extend under the effect of polymerase enzyme, until the detached ssDNA is turned into a dsDNA again. In this way, two single DNA strands are actually amplified to four ssDNAs. DNA strands will be sufficiently amplified, when these three steps are repeated multiple times (e.g. 10–12 cycles).

As shown in Figure 10.6, the DNA-templated microbeads are scattered into micro-wells mounted on a chip surface through centrifugal spinning. Microwells are located on top of each ISFET sensing node, which can be formed by the post process. One of the most commonly used materials is photoresist (e.g. SU-8). First, the entire ISFET chip surface will be spin-coated with the photoresist. Second, the chip is exposed under UV light through a mask to pattern the well. Lastly, the chip is washed in a

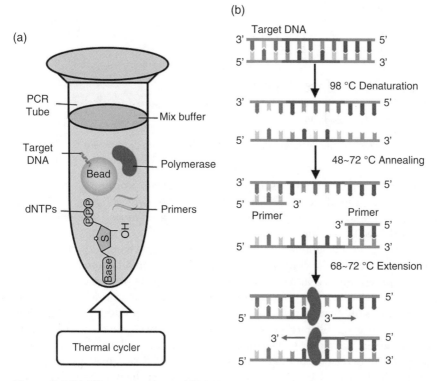

Figure 10.5 (a) PCR components; and (b) PCR process.

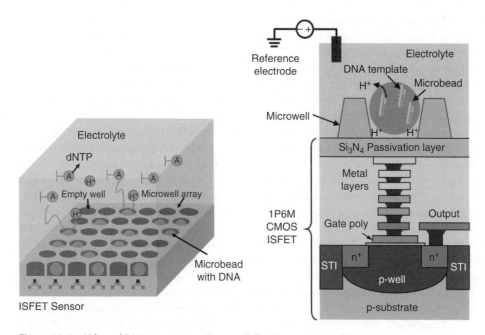

Figure 10.6 pH-based DNA sequencing diagram (left); Cross-section of ISFET during sequencing (right).

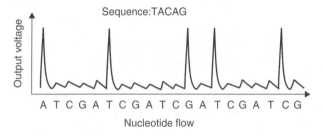

Figure 10.7 Output voltage in one microwell during the DNA sequencing procedure.

certain solution to remove unnecessary parts. After these procedures, microwell arrays are formed on top of the ISFET pixel array. A 1:1 ~ 1.5:1 well height to width ratio is preferred to hold a microbead. Thereafter, H⁺ released during sequencing will be detected by the ISFET sensor.

During detection, four nucleotides (dNTPs) are cyclically delivered. This can be realized by automatic microfluidic control system. A hydrogen ion will be released when one nucleotide is incorporated into its complementary template base. A decreased pH value will be observed, which is proportional to the number of incorporations. ISFET is adopted to detect this pH change, based on the detected output voltage value. The DNA sequence can then be assembled. H⁺ generated in each microwell will produce local pH changes, but these hydrogen ions will eventually diffuse to the bulk solution, therefore the detected pH is not constant but in dynamic change. The period may last for 1 second. Therefore, the ISFET sensor should continuously detect the pH change and find the peak value with the largest signal-to-noise ratio (SNR).

As shown in Figure 10.7, when four nucleotides are added sequentially, the pH-induced voltage in one microwell is observed. When the added nucleotide is incorporated with the target DNA base, an obvious voltage change will be observed. Based on the measurement result, the target DNA sequence "TACAG" is obtained.

Large-array CMOS ISFET sensors have been commercialized by Ion-Torrent™, whose products include 314, 316, 318, Proton I, and Proton III, with array size from 1.5 million to 660 million pixels. In order to integrate more pixels on a single chip, pixel size should be miniaturized. Even though the ISFET array fabricated in the CMOS process with small size and low cost has been realized by industry, sequencing accuracy is a big problem. Especially for a DNA strand with multiple consecutive similar sequences, such as "AA" or "AAAAAAAA", all of the same nucleotides will be complementarily incorporated in one operation. It is obvious to recognize 0-base and 1-base incorporation, but it is a challenge to differentiate 7-base and 8-base incorporation, since the produced pH change is not linearly proportional to the number of nucleotides, as shown in Figure 10.8. Low pH sensitivity is still a major problem remaining to be solved for better sequencing accuracy. Adding more amplification to ISFET sensing would be a possible solution to increase the gap between multi-base incorporations.

For CMOS ISFET-based DNA sequencing, there exists another significant inaccuracy, as illustrated in Figure 10.9(a). As the DNA-templated microbeads are scattered into the microwell array by centrifuge spinning, the distribution of microbeads into the microwell array is unknown [10]. Thus, the measured pH response has no correlation

Figure 10.8 pH changes of different multi-base incorporations.

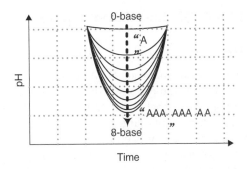

with the physical locations of microwells that contain microbeads. When incorporation happens in one microwell, the locally produced H⁺ ion will diffuse into the bulk solution. It may affect the pH value of other microwells. If there is no microbead in the microwell, due to crosstalk from neighboring microbeads in the solution, it will lead to false pH values being reported. To tackle this problem, a dual-mode image-ion sensor, as described in Chapter 8, is introduced by correlating local pH values with the locations of microwells filled with microbeads. The cross-sectional view of the proposed dual-mode pixel is shown in Figure 10.9(b). Since the microbeads are in direct contact with the sensor surface, the imaging of the microbead distribution can be detected based on the contact imaging principle without a lens [11]. As such, we can determine the existence of the microbead in optical mode and detect the pH value in chemical mode. Thus, an accurate pH-image correlation map can be generated to prune the false pH values due to crosstalk for empty microwells.

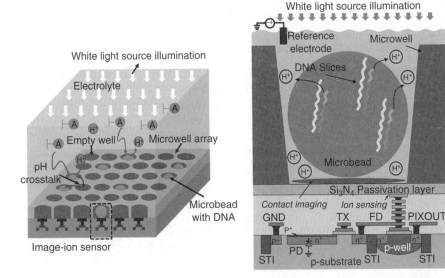

Figure 10.9 Dual-mode sensor to deal with pH crosstalk (left); Cross-section of dual-mode pixel with microbead contact imaging and ion sensing (right).

10.3 CMOS THz-based Genotyping

10.3.1 Overview

Genotyping is also an important DNA detection that focuses on recognizing base mutations of specific DNA, most of which are associated with diseases and deficiencies [1]. In most situations, a single base difference would be observed, which is called SNP found in more than 1% of a large population. Unlike sequencing, genotyping is fast and highly focused, saving a lot of effort.

The DNA microarray is widely used in genotyping, where thousands of artificially produced DNA probes are attached to a glass or plastic plate. When the array is exposed to a solution with DNA samples, the matching probes hybridize with target DNA strands, so that target DNA sequences can be inferred by their given complementary probes. Unlike the detection of the nucleotides' order in whole-genome sequencing, the identification of hybridization that relies on labeling and optical detection is the main issue to be solved in genotyping. Recently, the CMOS THz-based electrical detection sensor has aroused great interest in DNA detection, especially genotyping.

The development of the THz-based DNA sequencing method has become one possible new solution to tackle the aforementioned challenges [13,14]. THz-sensing has attracted a lot of research activities in the past decades, as numerous materials can exhibit unique spectrum signatures in THz range. In [15], Brucherseifer *et al.* first demonstrated that the binding state of DNA can be directly probed through its complex refractive index in the THz range. A free-space detection and an integrated detection based on planar waveguides are initially realized [15,16]. To increase the sensitivity and reduce the amount of sample needed to characterize the sequence, metamaterial THz sensors based on electrical/magnetic resonance are proposed with sub-wavelength scattering [17]. More recently, one silicon nano-sandwich pump device was proposed that can provide both the excitation of the DNA strands' self-resonant modes and feedback for current-voltage measurements to identify the strands' sequences [18].

10.3.2 THz-based Genotyping Procedure

Figure 10.10 illustrates the diagram of THz-based genotyping. The hybridized DNA strand can be identified by resonant frequency shift to ssDNA probes. Several ssDNA probes and a hybridized dsDNA are shown on the surface of detector. The probes are

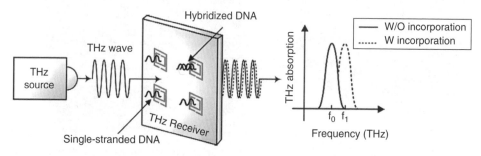

Figure 10.10 Diagram of THz-based genotyping.

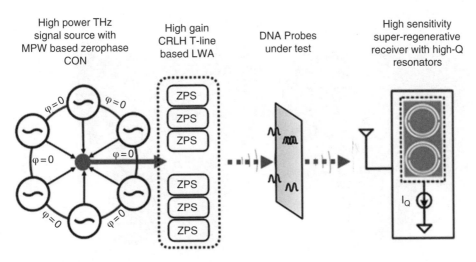

High power THz signal source with MPW based zerophase CON

High gain CRLH T-line based LWA

DNA Probes under test

High sensitivity super-regenerative receiver with high-Q resonators

Figure 10.11 Realization diagram of metamaterial based THz-sensing system.

illuminated with a THz wave generated by an on-chip source and the resonant frequencies are recognized by the THz detector. It is reported that a probe at which hybridization takes place exhibits a reduced resonant frequency in the THz range [19]. Thereby binding states of DNA strands can be recognized by the THz-based sensor.

High-performance THz-sensing systems can be constructed by on-chip metamaterial-based signal sources, receivers, and antennas, as described in Chapter 4. The block diagram is shown in Figure 10.11. A high power THz signal source is first generated by magnetic plasmon waveguide (MPW)-based zero-phase coupled oscillator network (CON) and then radiated by the composite right/left-handed (CRLH) T-line based on-chip leaky wave antenna (LWA). After penetrating through the DNA probes mounted on a high-Q resonator array, the resulting THz signal is received by a high sensitivity super-regenerative differential transmission-line (T-line) loaded with a split-ring- resonator (DTL-SRR). In this article, a high power CON-based signal source and a DLT-SRR based super-regenerative receiver (SRX) are proposed, which combined together consist of a highly sensitive and wide band THz-sensing system at 140 GHz. Different from the optics-based THz-sensing systems that are bulky and expensive, with lack of portability with low detection resolution by electro-optic sampling techniques, the proposed CMOS THz-sensing system demonstrates both high sensitivity and wideband THz sensors at 140 GHz.

10.4 Beyond CMOS Nanopore Sequencing

10.4.1 Overview

Conventional DNA sequencing techniques have limitations of short read length (70–400 bp) and slow read speed (1 min/cycle–1 hour/cycle). As a result, single-molecule nanopore sequencing has aroused great interest by industries, due to its long read length (100 Kbp) and fast run time (1 ms/cycle). Since late 2013,

(a)   (b)

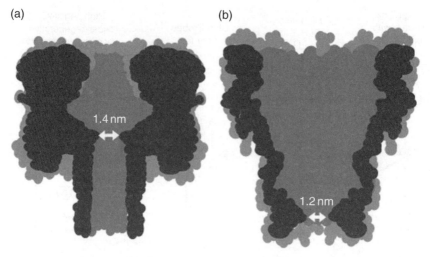

Figure 10.12 Structure of (a) α-HL protein; and (b) MspA protein;

representative companies, including Oxford Nanopore Technologies (ONT) and Genia Technologies. ONT^{TM}, have launched a product named MinION that can be plugged into a computer's USB 3.0 port with an array of 512 MspA biological nanopores, 100 K bp (base pairs) read length, and $1/Mbp (cost per 1 M base) real timing sequencing [12].

As the name indicates, a nanopore is a tiny pore in the nanometer scale sitting on a thin membrane. Based on the material, the nanopore can be categorized as a protein nanopore or a solid-state nanopore. Protein nanopores can be found in nature, such as α-haemolysin (α-HL) and *Mycobacterium smegmatis* porin A (MspA). The protein pore has well-defined and highly-reproducible size and structure. For ssDNA, the helical width is about 1 nm, and the space between two nucleotides is 0.34 nm. The narrowest pore diameters of α-HL (2.6 nm) or MspA (1.2 nm) protein are similar to ssDNA, as shown in Figure 10.12.

Since the environment has a great impact on the protein pore's stability, the solid-state pore is an alternative choice. Its excellent tolerance to chemical, thermal, or mechanical impact makes it a promising substitution. Materials such as single-layer membrane BN or MoS_2 and graphene, as well as silicon materials SiO_2, Si_3N_4, and Al_2O_3, can be used to fabricate a solid-state nanopore. It can be easily integrated with a semiconductor readout chip, so as to reduce sequencing costs and miniaturize sensing systems. An Si_3N_4 nanopore is shown in Figure 10.13. Reported diameter is typically within 2 nm ~ 20 nm. Due to the processing limitation, a solid-state pore diameter cannot be made as small and repeatable as a protein pore.

Nanopore sequencing makes use of an ion current. A typical testing system is shown in Figure 10.14. A membrane with a nanopore sitting on it is placed in a conducted salt solution. It can be regarded as two separated chambers connected by the pore. A pair of Ag/AgCl electrodes are emerged in solution located on both sides of the nanopore. When the voltage drop is applied to the electrode pair, an ion current will flow through the pore that forms an electrophoretic force. Since the DNA strand is negatively charged, it will be pulled through the tiny nano-channel. Regarding that the four nucleotides are

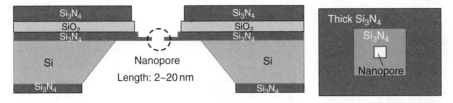

Figure 10.13 Structure and cross-section view of a Si₃N₄ nanopore.

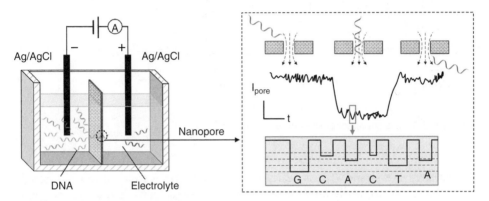

Figure 10.14 A typical nanopore sequencing principle.

different in physical size, the ion current will be modulated caused by their different blocking capacity. By detecting the current values, nucleic acid sequences of the target ssDNA can be identified.

10.4.2 Nanopore-based Sequencing Procedure

To realize high-throughput sequencing, a large nanopore array can be integrated with a CMOS readout chip to reduce the cost and size of the system. Therefore, it is quite demanding to develop a CMOS-compatible nanopore platform, which is also scalable for millions of DNA strands to be detected on a single chip simultaneously. The large-array CMOS-compatible nanopore sensor foresees a promising cost-efficiency, timing-saving, and portable solution in future personalized DNA sequencing.

For a single nanopore, a shared electrode in the bulky electrolyte and an individually-specific read electrode are used. The equivalent protein/solid-state nanopore model is shown in Figure 10.15. It involves electrolyte resistances R_{dl} between each electrode and nanopore membrane, a nanopore resistance R_{pore}, a nanopore capacitance C_{pore} (mainly membrane capacitance), and a parasitic capacitance C_{para} coming from the input of readout circuit. R_{pore} is the key parameter to differentiate nucleotides. After applying a voltage drop across it, an ion current I_{pore} is generated. Other parameters, such as R_{dl}, C_{pore}, and C_{para}, contribute to current readout performance, such as SNR and bandwidth.

In a certain electrolyte such as 1 M KCl, a typical R_{dl} value is 1 KΩ. The R_{pore} value depends on nanopore size and nucleotide type. For example, when a protein is empty

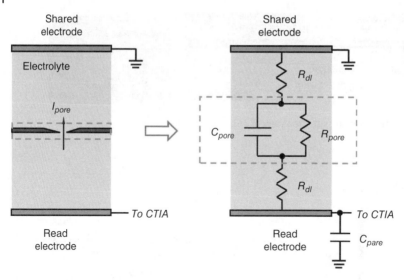

Figure 10.15 Equivalent nanopore model with a pair of electrodes.

without any DNA strand, R_{pore} is nearly 1 GΩ. When a DNA strand is forced through, R_{pore} is increased to nearly 6 GΩ as a result of the sugar-phosphate-base nucleotide structure. Due to base size difference, each nucleotide has respective contribution to R_{pore}. R_{pore} is a combined value of several nucleotides, since the nanopore thickness is larger than a single nucleotide (0.34 nm). C_{pore} value ranges from $1 \sim 100$ pF, which depends on the area of membrane holding the nanopore in the electrolyte. Similarly, the C_{para} value depends on the read electrode area and input device of the readout circuit.

Capacitor transimpedance amplifier (CTIA) is a commonly-used circuit to provide a bias voltage to read the electrode and senses the generated ion current I_{pore} with enough gain. A typical nanopore ion current sensing diagram is shown in Figure 10.16. The CTIA block provides a bias voltage V_{ref} to read the electrode, and integrates an ion current on the feedback capacitor C_{fb}. When C_{fb} is sufficiently small, a large amplification, determined by $I_{pore}*t_0/C_{fb}$, can be achieved in a certain sampling time t_0. Correlated double sampling (CDS), together with the sample/hold (S/H) blocks, are employed to reduce noise by subtracting reset and sampled signal values. The resulting voltage is converted to digital data by on-chip ADC that is immune to noise and interruption.

For a nanopore array, pairs of electrodes are needed. Apart from the shared electrode in the electrolyte, an electrode array on a readout chip surface can be fabricated in the semiconductor process. They are directly placed on top of CTIA blocks. In a standard CMOS process, multiple-layer metals are used for circuit routing. A passivation layer (Si_3N_4) will cover the chip surface to protect it from environmental contamination and oxidation. For the area where the top metal will be exposed to air for pad bonding, a passivation open window will be employed. As shown in Figure 10.17, an electrode array can be fabricated by this process with an array of top metal pads. Since top metal material is always aluminum (Al), it is not a desired electrode. Instead, an Ag/AgCl reference electrode is widely used due to its high stability in solution. Therefore, post process is applied to remove the top Al metal and deposit Ag/AgCl through

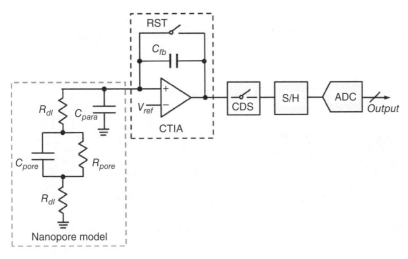

Figure 10.16 A typical nanopore ion current sensing diagram.

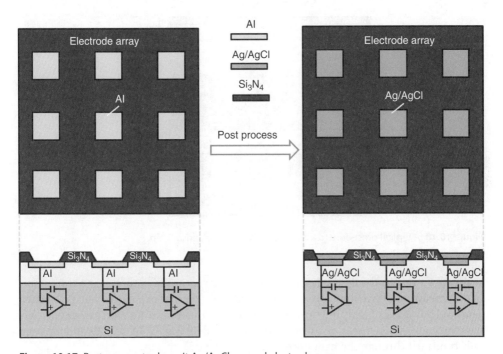

Figure 10.17 Post process to deposit Ag/AgCl on read electrode array.

electroplating and chemical reactions. Then the chip can be used to integrate the protein or solid-state nanopore array for sequencing.

The procedure to assemble protein pores and readout chip involves the formation of a lipid bilayer and insertion of proteins, as shown in Figure 10.18. The lipid bilayer-protein idea comes from the membrane structure of a biological cell. A lipid molecule, also referred to as "fat", is composed of a hydrophilic head region and a hydrophobic tail

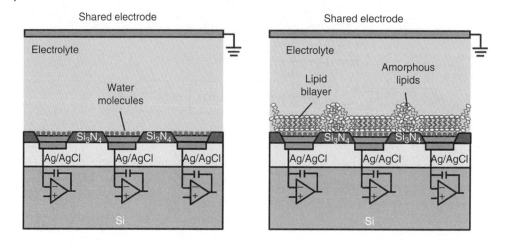

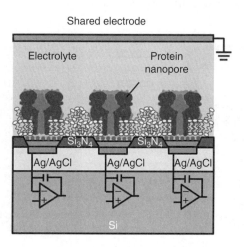

Figure 10.18 A typical procedure to assemble proteins and a sensor chip.

region. As a result, the lipid bilayer is a common structure in nature. It is a thin membrane consisting of two lipid layers, so as to hide the tails and expose the heads to water. The lipid bilayer is a highly impermeable membrane that only water and gases can easily pass through. When inserting a protein into the lipid bilayer, DNA strands and ions can only transport through the nanopores.

The protein nanopore integration procedure is as follows. First, a water molecule membrane will be absorbed onto the Ag/AgCl electrode surface when immersing the readout chip in liquid (Figure 10.18(a)). Second, lipid-coated bubbles are distributed onto the chip surface. With the help of the water film, a lipid bilayer membrane can be deposited on the electrode in good order, whereas for the hydrophobic Si_3N_4 passivation layer, the lipids are amorphous (Figure 10.18(b)). Due to their poor conductivity, the disordered lipids on the Si_3N_4 surface are used to isolate each nanopore sensing node. Lastly, proteins are added and inserted into the lipid bilayers (Figure 10.18(c)).

The lipid bilayer is temporarily disrupted to facilitate nanopore insertion by applying a stimulus voltage to electrode pairs.

A solid-state nanopore array should be first fabricated before integration with a readout chip. As an example, the fabrication process for an Si_3N_4 nanopore array is shown in Figure 10.19. The starting material is a 500-μm-thick silicon wafer. The process is as follows:

a) High-quality 50-nm Si_3N_4 is deposited on both sides of a silicon wafer for nanopore formation using low-pressure chemical vapor deposition (LPCVD);
b) A square cavity is etched as a common-shared chamber;
c) A 200-nm SiO_2 layer and then a 500-nm Si_3N_4 layer are deposited on the original 50-nm Si_3N_4 membrane using plasma-enhanced chemical vapor deposition (PECVD);
d) A 2-μm diameter well array in Si_3N_4 can be defined using focused ion beam (FIB), and then SiO_2 is etched;
e) The 50-nm Si_3N_4 is thinned using plasma etcher; and
f) A 2~20-nm diameter nanopore array is drilled into the Si_3N_4 layer.

Waterproof Teflon or polydimethylsiloxane (PDMS) can be used to integrate a solid-state nanopore array and a readout chip, as shown in Figure 10.20. In this way, each nanopore sensing node is separated to form an array of individual chambers. After nanopore and readout chip integration, the DNA strand can be added to the common chamber. The sensor can continuously read the current values when the DNA is traversing the pore. A software algorithm is employed to recognize and map each current value to its related nucleotide.

Challenges still remain in nanopore sequencing, including the small ionic current differences between each nucleotide (e.g. 1 pA/base type for the protein nanopore), and the rapid DNA translocation velocity (e.g. 1–3 us/base for the protein nanopore and 50 ns/base for solid-state nanopore). With the help of biological adapters or enzymes, the DNA traversing speed through a protein pore can typically reach 100 us/base ~ 1 ms/base. For solid-state nanopores, smaller-diameter and thin-thickness nanopore size would be a better way to slow down the speed. Other solutions include solution temperature, viscosity, and pH value optimization, as well as voltage drop modification.

Typical parameters of protein and solid-state nanopore are summarized in Table 10.1. It can be concluded that a high-sensitivity and high-speed current sensing circuitry is required to improve the quality of sequencing.

10.5 Summary

DNA sequencing shows great promise to life sciences, biotechnology, and medicine, changing the lives of humans. The first sequencing method was introduced by Sanger in the 1970s. Since then, new technologies have been developed from first- to third-generation Illumina and Ion Torrent sequencing, and more recently single-molecule nanopore sequencing that is regarded as the coming fourth-generation has aroused industry's interest. The existing DNA detection methods are summarized in Table 10.2, including the contribution from this chapter: the CMOS pH-TVC ISFET sensor; the CMOS dual-mode sensor; and the CMOS THz-sensor. Such a lab-on-CMOS integration-based approach has shown great potential for label-free personalized DNA sequencing at low cost in the future.

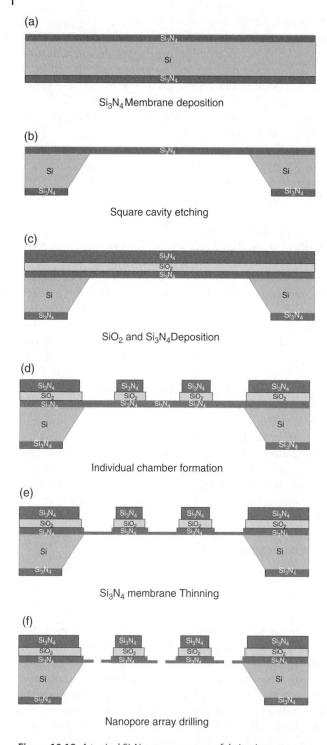

Figure 10.19 A typical Si_3N_4 nanopore array fabrication process.

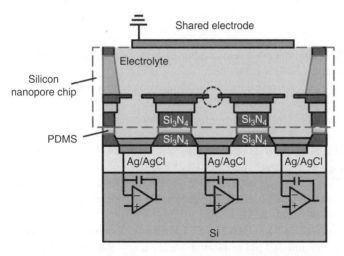

Figure 10.20 Si_3N_4 nanopore array and IC readout chip integration.

Table 10.1 Summary of protein and solid-state nanopore parameters.

Parameters	Protein Nanopore	Solid-state Nanopore
Diameter	$1.2 \sim 1.4\,nm$	$2 \sim 20\,nm$
Base nanopore current (without DNA)	$\sim 60\,pA$	$1 \sim 5\,nA$
Nanopore current with DNA	$\sim 30\,pA$	$1 \sim 2\,nA$
Electrode pair voltage drop	$100 \sim 800\,mV$	$100 \sim 800\,mV$
DNA velocity	$100 \sim 1000$ us/base	50 ns/base

Table 10.2 Summary of DNA detection methods.

Category	Method	Sample Labeling (Complex)	Optical System (Bulky, Costly)	CMOS Compatible (Scalable)	Throughput
Sequencing	Sanger	Yes	Yes	No	Low
	454	No	Yes	No	Moderate
	SMRT	Yes	Yes	No	Moderate
	SOLiD	Yes	Yes	No	Moderate
	Illumina	Yes	Yes	No	High
	Nanopore	No	No	Yes	Potentially High
	pH-based (ISFET/ Dual-mode)	No	No	Yes	Potentially High
Genotyping	Microarrays	Yes	Yes	No	N/A
	THz sensing	No	No	Yes	N/A

References

1 J.M. Rothberg, *et al.* (2011) An integrated semiconductor device enabling non-optical genome sequencing. *Nature*, 475(7356), 348–352.

2 F. Sanger, *et al.* (1977) DNA sequencing with chain-terminating inhibitors. *Proceedings of the National Academy of Science USA*, 749(12), 5463–5467.

3 M.L. Metzker (2010) Sequencing technologies – the next generation. *National Rev. Genetics*, 11(1), 31–46.

4 C. Toumazou, *et al.* (2013) Simultaneous DNA amplification and detection using a pH-sensing semiconductor system. *Nat. Methods*, 10(7), 641–646.

5 X.W. Huang, *et al.* (2015) A dual-mode large-arrayed CMOS ISFET sensor for accurate and high-throughput pH sensing in biomedical diagnosis. *IEEE Transactions on Biomedical Engineering*, 62(9), 2224–2233.

6 Y. Jiang, *et al.* (2016) A 512×576 65-nm CMOS ISFET sensor for food safety screening with 123.8 mV/pH sensitivity and 0.01 pH resolution. In: *IEEE Symposium on VLSI Technology, Honolulu, HI*, pp. 1–2.

7 X. Huang, *et al.* (2014) A 64×64 1200 fps CMOS ion-image sensor with suppressed fixed-pattern-noise for accurate high-throughput DNA sequencing. In: *Symposium on VLSI Circuits Digest of Technical Papers, Honolulu, HI*, pp. 109–110.

8 Y. Jiang, *et al.* (2015) A 201 mV/pH, 375 fps and 512×576 CMOS ISFET sensor in 65 nm CMOS technology. In: *IEEE Custom Integrated Circuits Conference (CICC)*, San Jose, CA, pp. 1–4.

9 S. Kumar, *et al.* (2012) PEG-labeled nucleotides and nanopore detection for single molecule DNA sequencing by synthesis. *Science Reports*, 2, 684.

10 J.M. Rothberg, *et al.* (2012) *Methods and Apparatus for Measuring Analytes*. Life Technologies Corporation (Carlsbad, CA).

11 X. Huang, *et al.* (2014) A contact-imaging based microfluidic cytometer with machine-learning for single-frame super-resolution processing. *PLoS One*, 9(8), e104539.

12 V. Marx (2015) Nanopores: A sequencer in your backpack. *Nat. Methods*, 12(11), 1015–1018.

13 P. Haring Bolivar, *et al.* (2004) Label-free THz sensing of genetic sequences: Towards THz biochips. *Philos. Trans. A Math. Phys. Eng. Sci.*, 362(1815), 323–333; discussion 333–335.

14 X. Huang, *et al.* (2015) A CMOS THz-sensing system towards label-free DNA sequencing. In: *IEEE 11th International Conference on ASIC (ASICON)*, pp. 1–4.

15 M. Brucherseifer, *et al.* (2000) Label-free probing of the binding state of DNA by time-domain terahertz sensing. *Applied Physics Letters*, 77(24), 4049–4051.

16 M. Nagel, *et al.* (2002) Integrated THz technology for label-free genetic diagnostics. *Applied Physics Letters*, 80(1), 154–156.

17 N. Zheng, *et al.* Metamaterial sensor platforms for terahertz DNA sensing. pp. 315–320.

18 A.L. Chernev, *et al.* (2015) DNA detection by THz pumping. *Semiconductors*, 49(7), 944–948.

19 C. Cao, *et al.* (2013) Metamaterials-based label-free nanosensor for conformation and affinity biosensing. *ACS Nano*, 7(9), 7583–7591.

11

Cell Counting

11.1 Introduction

In the elderly population, complete blood cell counting is one of the most informative blood tests reflecting metabolic syndrome and hence indicating the overall health status [1,2]. For example, the counts of red blood cells (RBC, erythrocytes), white blood cell (WBC, leukocytes), and platelets help to diagnose anemia; the CD4$^+$ lymphocyte count is used to monitor the progression of HIV/AIDS [3]. Existing techniques for blood cell counting mainly include manual counting using high magnification optical microscopy with high-numerical-aperture objective lenses, or automated counting using commercial flow cytometers. However, manual counting is time-consuming, has low throughput, and the accuracy is easily affected by operators' experiences, whereas commercial flow cytometers with bulky and sophisticated optics are prohibitively expensive. Hence, both are not suitable for the future personalized diagnosis applications.

With the recent development of microfluidic-based lab-on-a-chip (LOC) technology and mass production of inexpensive CMOS image sensors (CIS), miniaturized optofluidic contact imaging systems without lenses become competitive solutions [4,5]. In this chapter, we present one miniaturized optofluidic imaging system for cell counting based on CIS and the super-resolution (SR) image processing. The demonstrated technique is promising for personalized diagnosis.

11.2 Optofluidic Imaging System

11.2.1 Contact Imaging

A contact imaging system has a basic hardware setup, which directly integrates a microfluidic channel onto a small CIS, and a white light source illuminating from above at a distance of D_{ls} to a sensor array [4]. When blood cell samples flow through the microfluidic channel at an objective distance D_{obj} to the sensor array, their diffracted shadow images are recorded by the CIS underneath without any magnification by lens elements, as shown in Figure 11.1. Since both the cell size and D_{PIX} are similar in scale ($\sim$μm), the captured cell shadow images are typically pixilated and suffer from low resolution (LR), limiting the detection and recognition accuracy [6]. The detailed contact imaging principle can be analyzed using the system resolution model presented in the following section.

CMOS Integrated Lab-on-a-Chip System for Personalized Biomedical Diagnosis,
First Edition. Hao Yu, Mei Yan, and Xiwei Huang.
© 2018 John Wiley & Sons Singapore Pte. Ltd. Published 2018 by John Wiley & Sons Singapore Pte. Ltd.

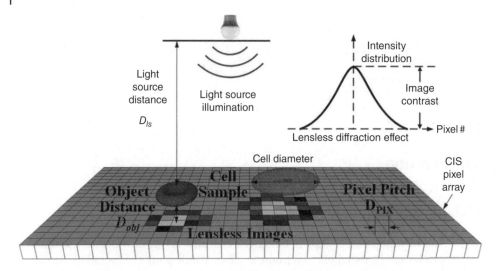

Figure 11.1 General lensless cell counting system setup based on CMOS image sensor (CIS): (a) Lensless cell imaging principle; (b) Cross-sectional view of the lensless system; and (c) Concept of the machine-learning based single-frame super-resolution (SR) processing.

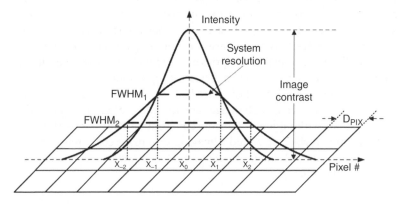

Figure 11.2 Resolution model for lensless microfluidic imaging system.

11.2.2 Optofluidic Imaging System Model

11.2.2.1 Resolution Model

For the lensless optofluidic imaging system in Figure 11.1(a), the image is projected directly from the object onto the CIS. Due to the diffraction effect, the center part of the image shows a higher intensity and so the intensity of the peripheral part is lower. As shown in Figure 11.2, the intensity profile $I(x)$ of the projected image in one dimension can be assumed as a Gaussian distribution [7]:

$$I(x) = \frac{j}{\sqrt{2\pi}\sigma} e^{-\frac{x^2}{2\sigma^2}} \tag{11.1}$$

where σ is the resolution factor, j is the light intensity factor, and x is the pixel coordinate, all to be characterized from the specific setup of the microfluidic imaging system. The

Full-Width-at-Half-Maximum (FWHM) under one image intensity profile can be utilized to represent the imaging system resolution R by:

$$R = FWHM = 2\sqrt{2ln2}\sigma \tag{11.2}$$

Since the resolution and contrast are relevant, if we define the image contrast C as the maximum intensity in the projected image intensity profile, that is $C = I(0) = j/\sqrt{2\pi}\sigma$, the relationship between system resolution R and contrast C thus becomes:

$$R = 2\sqrt{\frac{ln2}{\pi}} \cdot \frac{j}{C} \tag{11.3}$$

Note that the image contrast C has a relationship with D_{obj}, the distance between the object and the sensor [4]. We have:

$$C = \frac{j}{\sqrt{2\pi}\sigma} = \frac{a}{1 + \left(\dfrac{D_{obj}}{d}\right)^b} \tag{11.4}$$

where a, b, d, and j are all constants to be characterized from the setup of the lensless microfluidic imaging system. Once the microfluidic channel is placed close to the sensor within the characteristic distance d, the best achievable system resolution R stays small; but when D_{obj} becomes larger than d, R is exponentially degraded.

As shown in Figure 11.2, the best achievable system resolution R is defined when successfully covering the FWHM with the minimum number of pixels. Hence, we can determine the distance between the two pixels each with effective pixel size D_{PIX} from $x - 1$ to $x1$, which can be thought of as using pixels to sample and digitize the image intensity profile. The minimum number of three pixels is usually enough to capture the peak intensity, but also the two points at the FWHM can be used. Therefore, the optimal spatial resolution R is obtained as the length of $2D_{PIX}$. Thus, the best system spatial resolution R under a specific D_{obj} is given by:

$$2D_{PIX} \leq FWHM = R, \quad \text{or} \quad D_{PIX} \leq \frac{R}{2}. \tag{11.5}$$

Therefore, a smaller pixel size D_{PIX} can result in a much easier case to satisfy Equation (11.5) for design consideration of resolution.

11.2.2.2 Dynamic Range Model

In optofluidic contact imaging system, the dynamic range (DR) quantifies the ability of a CIS to response under both bright highlight and dark shadow conditions. It can be defined as the ratio of the largest current signals i_{max} to the smallest detectable current signal (or noise) i_{min} [7,8]:

$$DR = \frac{i_{max}}{i_{min}} = \frac{q_{max} - i_{dc}t_{int}}{\sqrt{\sigma_r^2 + qi_{dc}t_{int}}} \tag{11.6}$$

where $q_{max} = C_{PD}V_s$ is the well-capacity, C_{PD} is the photodiode capacitance, and V_s is the voltage swing; q is the electron charge; i_{dc} is the dark current; t_{int} is the integration time; and σ_r^2 is the variance of the temporal noise (or KTC) [8]. Note that here only the pixel-sized dependent noises are considered.

Since photodiode capacitance C_{PD}, dark current i_{dc}, and KTC noise all increase approximately linearly with pixel size D_{PIX}, that is $C_{PD} = C_j D_{PIX}$, $i_{dc} = I_d D_{PIX}$ and $\sigma_r^2 = KTC_{PD}/q^2$, DR increases roughly as the square root of pixel size $\sqrt{D_{PIX}}$ by:

$$DR = \frac{C_j D_{PIX} V_s - I_d D_{PIX} t_{int}}{\sqrt{KTC_j D_{PIX}/q^2 + qI_d D_{PIX} t_{int}}} = \varepsilon \sqrt{D_{PIX}} \tag{11.7}$$

where C_j and I_d are the unit junction capacitance and dark current for the photodiode, and ε is the DR factor. Note that the parameters such as C_j, I_d, and ε are all process dependent that can be characterized.

The system model work in [9] assumes that the pixel DR performance is good enough to cover the image intensity range, and the pixel size D_{PIX} is smaller than FWHM of the intensity profiles. However, the pixel DR needs to cover the maximum image intensity range. Otherwise, even when the object distance D_{obj} is very small, high contrast images cannot be captured due to the poor DR. Therefore, a larger pixel size D_{PIX} can result in a much easier case to satisfy the design consideration of DR.

11.2.2.3 Implication to SR Processing

Considering both resolution and DR system models, we show that with the utilization of SR processing, we can optimize the overall system performance as follows.

First, we can design a large pixel size 3 for a high DR. Though it results in a pixel with poor resolution, with a magnification factor of n introduced by the SR processing, we can still reach an equivalent SR image with an effective pixel size:

$$D_{SR} = \frac{D_{PIX}}{n} \tag{11.8}$$

As such, Equation (11.5) becomes:

$$D_{PIX} \leq \frac{nR}{2} \tag{11.9}$$

which means that there is an n-time magnification of resolution. Therefore, the deployment of SR processing can help reach smaller effective subpixels with better resolution without sacrificing DR performance.

11.3 Super-resolution Image Processing

Super-resolution (SR) is one effective image processing technique to reconstruct high-resolution (HR) images [10–13] from observed LR images. Assume that the desired HR image is of size $nL_1 \times nL_2$, where L_1 and L_2 are the row and column numbers of the sensor; and n is the down sampling factor or magnification factor, in both horizontal and vertical directions. Thus, the HR image vector, when denoted in lexicographic notation, is $x = [x_1, x_2, \ldots, x_{nL_1 \times nL_2}]^T$. Similarly for LR images, they can be denoted as $y_k = [y_{k,1}, y_{k,2}, \ldots, y_{k,L_1 \times L_2}]^T$, where $k = 1, 2, \ldots, M$, and M is the total number of LR frames. The observed LR images usually result from wrapping, blurring, and down-sampling by [11]:

$$y_k = DB_k W_k x + V_k, 1 \leq k \leq M \tag{11.10}$$

where W_k is a warp-matrix of size $nL_1nL_2 \times nL_1nL_2$, which is obtained through motion estimation between reference images y_k $(2 \leq k \leq M)$ and the chosen current frame y_1 (assuming the first LR frame is chosen as the current frame). B_k is the $nL_1nL_2 \times nL_1nL_2$ blur-matrix, which represents the point spread function of the image sensor. D is the $(L_1L_2)^2 \times nL_1nL_2$ down-sampling matrix, standing for the decimation operation to reduce the number of observed pixels in the measured images. V_k represents the noise vector.

The aim of SR is to estimate x based on the known images y_k. In the optofluidic contact imaging system, a series of images are captured when samples are flowing in a relatively controlled manner due to the laminar flow effect, making it similar to the case of video sequences where the photographed scene is static and the images are obtained with slight translations [14,15]. Thus, the SR processing for lensless microfluidic imaging becomes a special case, that is, the warping between the measured images is purely translational so that W_k is the block-circulant; the blurring is the space invariant for all the measured LR images, that is $\forall\ k,\ B_k = B$; and the additive noise is white noise, that is autocorrelation of the Gaussian random vector $E\{V_k V_k^T\} = \sigma_v^2 I$ [5]. Thus, the Maximum-Likelihood estimation of x to generate the best HR image can be done as follows [10]:

$$\hat{x} = argmin_x \left\{ \sum_{k=1}^{M} [y_k - DBW_k x]^T [y_k - DBW_k x] \right\} \qquad (11.11)$$

11.3.1 Multi-frame SR Processing

Existing SR processing techniques applied in lensless imaging systems are mainly based on multi-frame reconstruction, in which multiple LR cell images with sub-pixel motions of the same object are synthesized into one single HR cell image. The working steps of the multi-frame SR implemented for optofluidic contact imaging is illustrated in Figure 11.3. Assume that there are M captured images, which are LR-based on the large pixel size D_{PIX}. Each LR image is composed of $L_1 \times L_2$ pixels, where L_1 and L_2 are the row and column numbers. The reconstruction processing includes interpolation, motion estimation, data mapping, and deblurring. In M frames of images, one image is to be chosen as the current frame, and the other $(M - 1)$ images are to be the reference frames. In order to map all the $(M - 1)$ reference LR frames into the current frame and create the final HR frame, the SR processing first needs to interpolate the current LR frame to obtain enough HR pixel grids. Thus the interpolation time defines the final magnification factor n, which is chosen by the user [11]. Since there are $(M - 1)$ reference frames, the interpolation time, that is the magnification factor n, can also be chosen as $(M - 1)$. As such, the HR image array size becomes $(M - 1)L_1 \times (M - 1)L_2$.

In the example shown in Figure 11.3, $L_1 = L_2 = 2$, and n = 4, M = 5. After mapping the reference frames, the data for the remaining HR grids where no LR frames are mapped will be obtained through bilinear interpolation. Note that more reference frames could be used for the SR reconstruction, but that may also introduce a larger implementation cost. The sub-pixel motions can be generated by either flowing the cell samples through the microfluidic channel, shifting the light source, or sequentially activating multiple light sources at different locations [14,16,17]. However, the main problem for

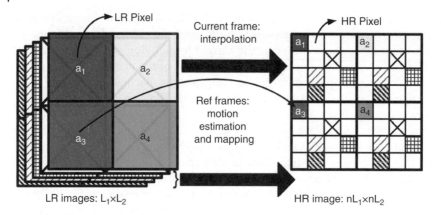

Figure 11.3 Working principle of multi-frame SR processing.

multi-frame SR is that the system needs to continuously capture, store, and process multiple LR images in order to recover one HR image, which not only limits the practical detection throughput but also requires large storage. Hence, it is not applicable for on-chip hardware implementation [14].

11.3.2 Single-frame SR Processing

Due to the disadvantages of multi-frame SR processing, an alternative single-frame SR processing is thereby imperative.

In [18], we proposed a single-frame SR approach that only utilizes one single LR-frame to reconstruct the HR image with bilinear interpolation processing. The advantage of more efficient memory usage makes this approach possible for on-chip implementation with significantly reduced hardware implementation resources as well as reduced latency. Figure 11.4 shows an overview of the proposed system working principle for the single-frame SR. The digital output data from the whole sensor array in terms of the L_1-row and L_2-column is transferred in serial into a data buffer within the SR block. They are then processed as follows:

Step 1: *Data pumping*: The output data from the first row (N_1, N_2 ... N_{L2}) and the first two pixels of the second row (($N+1)_1$, $(N+1)_2$) are pumped into the data buffer array.

Step 2: *Data processing*: In this step, the first original pixel (N_1) will generate HR pixel data of 4×4 pixels (N_1, P_1, P_2 ... P_{15}) by bilinear interpolation with the other three reference pixels (N_2, $(N+1)_1$, $(N+1)_2$); then the 4×4 processed pixel data are driven to the SR pixel frame buffer as outputs.

Step 3: *Data pumping*: The data is continuously pumped in and the second original N_2 moves to the processing position. With another three reference pixels (N_3, $(N+1)_2$, $(N+1)_3$), it will generate another group of 4×4 pixels in a similar way, which are driven to the SR frame buffer after processing.

When one full LR frame is processed, the corresponding SR image is obtained. Compared to the multi-frame SR, the single-frame SR requires much less storage with

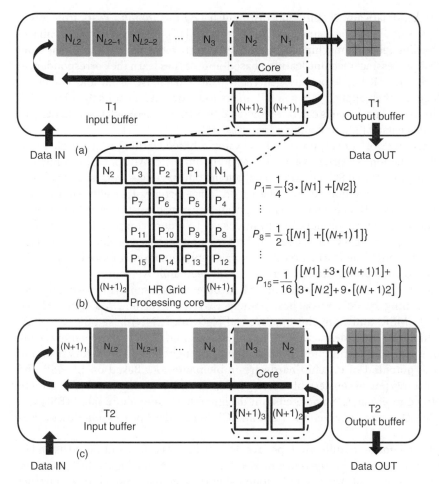

Figure 11.4 Working principle of the proposed single-frame SR algorithm.

less computation. The whole processing block only needs one processing core and one row data buffer to store the data for processing with significantly reduced latency.

However, in such interpolation-based single-frame SR processing, the recovered images are usually overly smooth, the sharpness of the edges cannot be maintained, and the high frequency (HF) details cannot be recovered.

11.4 Machine-learning-based Single-frame Super-resolution

Recently, another category of machine learning-based SR approaches is developing quickly [19–26]. Machine learning has very good performance and applications on a variety of problems such as visual/speech recognition, natural language processing, and biomedical imaging, etc. For example, in a point-of-care testing (POCT) cell imaging system for waterborne pathogen detection, a machine learning algorithm has been adopted to automatically classify and distinguish *Giardia lamblia* cysts from other micro-objects based on the trained statistical features [19]. Also in cell biology, image-based screening relies on machine learning to efficiently recognize various phenotypes [20]. For SR processing, machine learning based-approaches learn the correspondences between LR and HR image patches generated from a database of LR and HR image pairs, which are then applied to a new LR image to recover its most likely original HR image. The exemplary patches can be extracted either from external datasets [21,22], or the input image itself [23], or combined sources [24].

The pioneering work of [21] proposed an example-based learning strategy where the LR to HR prediction is learned via a Markov Random Field (MRF). [25] extends this work by using the Primal Sketch prior to enhancing blurred edges, ridges, and corners. However, the above methods directly based on image patches typically require large databases of LR and HR patch pairs to incorporate any possible patterns encountered in testing, and are therefore computationally intensive. To reduce computational cost, [26] proposed a single image SR via sparse signal representation based on compressed sensing theory. Although the learned dictionary pair representation is more compact, its learning speed and optimization performance still need improvement.

Here, we tackle the aforementioned SR problems by employing two efficient machine-learning based approaches, namely Extreme Learning Machine (ELM)-based SR (ELMSR) and Convolutional Neural Network (CNN)-based SR (CNNSA) [28,29]. Similar to the widely used CNN in deep learning, ELM is also a general suite of machine-learning techniques. Both of them are lightweight, feed-forward, and possess the potential of on-chip hardware implementation. Based on ELMSR and CNNSR, prototypes of lensless blood cell imaging and counting are demonstrated using both commercial CIS and a custom designed back-side illuminated (BSI) CIS with smaller D_{PIX} and D_{obj}. Generic ELM and CNN-based SR processing flows are as follows.

Static HR cell images of different types are first off-line classified and stored as an HR image library to train an SR reference model. Next, with on-line input LR flowing cell images, single-frame SR processing is done using the reference model to reconstruct their corresponding HR images. Then, those cells can be accurately recognized and counted by only checking for the strongest structure similarity (SSIM) [30] referring to the off-line HR image library. Therefore, the developed microfluidic lensless cell counting system can achieve high single-cell image quality without throughput limitation, offering a cost-effective and portable solution for personalized diagnosis.

11.4.1 ELMSR

The ELM, which was developed for single-hidden-layer feed-forward neural networks (SLFNs), has only one input layer, one hidden layer, and one output layer, as shown in Figure 11.5. It has a major merit of randomly generated weights between the input layer and hidden layer, making it tuning-free without expensive iterative training process [28]. This advantage over other machine learning approaches, such as the support vector machine [31] and back propagation [32], makes it suitable for SR processing and recognition error recovery in microfluidic lensless imaging, since the number of training cell images can be large if we need to cover all different cell types under different conditions.

Figure 11.5 Structure of the ELM model.

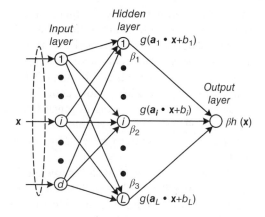

As shown in Figure 11.6, the ELMSR includes off-line training and on-line testing. In the training step, a reference model is trained that can map the interpolated LR images with the HF components extracted from the HR images from the training library. The off-line HR training image library is first generated by taking the grayscale HR images of cells with an inverted microscope camera (Olympus IX71, Tokyo, Japan). For one type of cell to generate an HR library, the cell solution is prepared and dropped into

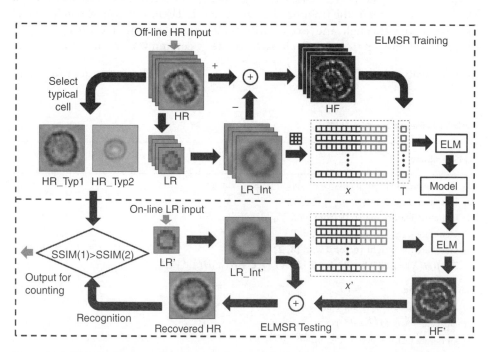

Figure 11.6 ELM-SR processing flowchart. The training is performed off-line to generate a reference model that can map the interpolated LR images with the HF components from the HR images; and the testing is performed on-line to recover an SR image from the input LR image with the reference model.

the inlet of one microfluidic channel that is bonded onto a cover glass. This helps mimic the environment of the microfluidic channel bonded onto the CMOS image sensor.

Cells suspended in the channel can have different rotations or details in appearance. Thus, to ensure a more complete library, a large number of typical images are taken to generate an HR image library for one cell type under different conditions. Thereby, the trained reference model is more generic (as a cell neuron) when used for on-line SR recovery. Note that this work is toward automatic cell counting such that we assume that the cell types in the sample solution are known or to be pre-characterized in advance. If a new pattern appears, we need to train a new ELM-SR model, which is off-line.

The pseudo code for ELMSR is shown in Table 11.1. First, p HR cell images are stored as the training library. For one HR image $HR_{M \times N}$, where M and N are the row and column pixel numbers, it is first bicubically down-sampled to one LR image, $LR_{m \times n}$. Note that the down-sampled LR image is similar to the captured lensless LR image. The down-sampling factor t determines the SR improvement factor, that is, $M = m \times t$, $N = n \times t$. To obtain HF components, the LR image $LR_{m \times n}$ is bicubically interpolated to $LR\_Int_{M \times N}$, which is of the same size as $HR_{M \times N}$ but blurred with lost HF details. Then the HF component $HF_{M \times N}$ can be generated by subtracting the HR image $HR_{M \times N}$ with the interpolated LR image $LR\_Int_{M \times N}$:

$$HF_{M \times N} = HR_{M \times N} - LR\_Int_{M \times N} \tag{11.12}$$

After obtaining all p HF images $HF_{M \times N}$, their pixel intensity values will form a $p \cdot MN \times 1$ row vector as the training targeting value T. Then, a 3×3 pixel patch $P(i,j)$ is used to search through and extract the feature vector from $LR\_Int_{M \times N}$, where $1 \le i \le M - 1$ and $1 \le j \le N - 1$. Each patch creates a column vector consisting of nine pixel intensity values and $\left(\dfrac{\partial P}{\partial x}, \dfrac{\partial P}{\partial y}, \dfrac{\partial^2 P}{\partial x}, \dfrac{\partial^2 P}{\partial y}, \dfrac{\partial^2 P}{\partial x \partial y} \right)$, which indicates the four first- and

Table 11.1 Pseudo code for ELMSR.

ELMSR Training

---

1) Downscale the input p $HR_{M \times N}$ to obtain p $LR_{m \times n}$ images
2) Upscale p $LR_{m \times n}$ images to p $LR_{Int\,M \times N}$
3) Generate feature matrix X from p $LR_{Int\,M \times N}$
4) Generate p $HF_{M \times N}$ and row vector T
5) Generate the weight vector $\boldsymbol{\beta}$ with $[X, T]$
   $$T = \beta H(X) = \beta G(AX + B), \, \beta = T \cdot H(X)^T [I/C + H(X)H(X)^T]^{-1}$$

ELMSR Testing:

6) Input LR image $LR'_{m \times n}$ for testing
7) Upscale $LR'_{m \times n}$ to $LR\_Int'_{M \times N}$
8) Generate feature matrix X' from $LR\_Int'_{M \times N}$
9) Calculate $HF'_{M \times N}$ image,
10) $T' = \beta H(X') = T \cdot H(X)^T [I/C + H(X)H(X)^T]^{-1} H(X')$
11) Generate final SR output with HF components $HR'_{M \times N} = LR\_Int'_{M \times N} + HF'_{M \times N}$

---

second-order derivatives in the horizontal and vertical directions, as well as one second-order mixed derivatives. The column vectors extracted from all patches in p interpolated images $LR\_Int_{M \times N}$ form the feature matrix X. Now, X and T form the ELM training dataset (X, T).

Next, after input of the training dataset (X, T) to the ELM model, a row vector β containing the weights between all the hidden nodes and the output node are to be calculated. The ELM model has d input nodes, L hidden nodes, and one output node. The output of the i-th hidden node is:

$$h_i(x) = g(a_i \cdot x + b_i) = \frac{1}{1 + \exp(-a_i \cdot x - b_i)},$$ (11.13)

where a_i is a row vector of weights between all input nodes and the i-th hidden node; b_i is a randomly generated bias term for the i-th hidden layer; and g is a Sigmoid activation function of hidden layer. The output of ELM is:

$$f(x) = \beta \cdot h(x)$$ (11.14)

where $h(x) = [h_1(x), h_2(x), \cdots, h_L(x)]^T$ is the output of the hidden layer. The output matrix of hidden layer is:

$$H(X) = G(AX + B)$$ (11.15)

where A is the weight matrix between input layer and hidden layer, B is the bias matrix, and G is the same sigmoid function. Thus:

$$T = \beta H(X)$$ (11.16)

In ELMSR, both training error and the norm of output weights should be minimized, i.e.:

$$min \begin{cases} \|\beta H(X) - T\| \\ \|\beta\| \end{cases}$$ (11.17)

Thus, the orthogonal projection method can be applied to obtain β:

$$\beta = T \cdot H(X)^T \left[\frac{I}{C} + H(X)H(X)^T \right]^{-1}$$ (11.18)

where C is a tuning parameter for the weight between $\|\beta H(X) - T\|$ and $\|\beta\|$, and I is the identity matrix with the same size as $H(X)H(X)^T$. The training data A, B, and β will be used as the ELMSR reference model.

In on-line testing, when an LR cell image $LR'_{m \times n}$ is captured for processing, the corresponding HR image can be recovered using the same matrix A, B, and the trained weights β as follows. The $LR'_{m \times n}$ is first bicubically interpolated by t times to $LR\_Int'_{M \times N}$. The same patch searching used in ELMSR training is employed to extract the feature matrix X' from $LR\_Int'_{M \times N}$. Hence, the output vector can be obtained:

$$f(X') = \beta H(X') = T \cdot H(X)^T \left[\frac{I}{C} + H(X)H(X)^T \right]^{-1} H(X')$$ (11.19)

Now $f(X')$ contains the recovered HF components $HF'_{M \times N}$. As such, the final HR image $HR'_{M \times N}$ is recovered with sufficient HF details by:

$$HR'_{M \times N} = HF'_{M \times N} + LR\_Int'_{M \times N} \tag{11.20}$$

As the resolution of lensless cell images is relatively low, we implemented a 4× magnification. Thus, a single cell LR shadow image of spatial size 12×12 can be improved to a 48×48 HR cell image. In the implemented ELM model, we set the node number in input, hidden, and output layer as d = 14, L = 20, and 1, respectively. Each 48×48 interpolated single cell image contains $46 \times 46 = 2116$ patches. The p training images will generate a feature matrix X of 2116p columns, and an HF intensity vector T with 2116p row. In testing, we set tuning parameter C = 512 to achieve a satisfied performance.

11.4.2 CNNSR

As an alternate solution for optimized learning, CNNSR was proposed. Recently, CNN has been widely adopted in deep learning when dealing with large datasets of images. In CNNSR, the deep CNN can find a mapping function between LR and HR images. Similar to ELMSR, there is also one off-line training for optimized model parameters that correlate the LR cell images with HR cell images, and one on-line testing to improve the resolution of captured lensless image. The overall architecture of CNNSR is shown in Figure 11.7.

In CNNSR training, assume there are n training images, and the LR cell images in the training library are first scaled up through bicubic interpolation to the same size as HR images. The interpolated images are denoted as Y_i. The corresponding ground truth HR images are X_i. The up-scaling factor is the SR magnification factor. An end-to-end mapping function F will be learned so that $F(Y_i)$ is as similar as possible to the original HR image X_i. The mean squared error (MSE) between Y_i and X_i is applied as the loss function $L(\theta)$ to be minimized:

$$L(\theta) = \frac{1}{n} \sum_{i=1}^{n} \left\| F(Y_i; \theta) - X_i \right\|^2, \tag{11.21}$$

where n represents the number of training samples, and θ is the grouped network parameters of CNN that should be learned in the training step.

The pseudo code for CNNSR is shown in Table 11.2. The CNNSR mainly comprises three training layers, as shown in Figure 11.7. The first layer randomly and densely extracts the overlapping patches from interpolated LR image Y and represents each patch as a high-dimensional vector:

$$F_1(Y) = \max\left(0, W_1 * Y + B_1\right) \tag{11.22}$$

where W_1 represents n_1 filters of spatial size $f_1 \times f_1$ that convolute the input image Y; '*' is the operation of convolution; B_1 is an n_1-dimensional vector indicating the biases, and each element that is associated with a filter. The output vector $F_1(Y)$ consists of n_1 feature maps. The rectified linear unit function ReLU(max(0, x)) is employed for the filter responses.

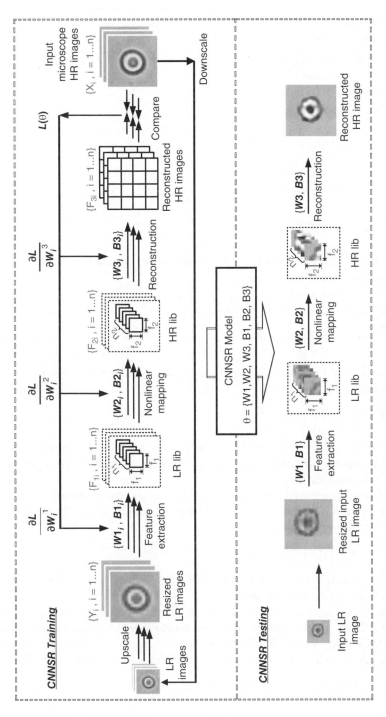

Figure 11.7 CNNSR processing flow including one off-line training and one on-line testing step.

Table 11.2 Pseudo code for CNNSR.

CNNSR Training

Input: LR cell images $\{Y_i\}$ and corresponding HR cell images $\{X_i\}$

Output: Model parameter $\theta = \{W_1, W_2, W_3, B_1, B_2, B_3\}$

  1) **θ** are initialized by drawing randomly from Gaussian Distribution ($\mu = 0, \sigma = 0.001$)

  2) **For** $i = 0$ *to* n//n is the number of training image

  3) **For** $l = 1$ to 3//3 layers to tune

  4) Calculate $F_i(Y)$ based on Equations (11.22)–(11.24)

  5) **End For**

  6) **Calculate** $L(\theta) = \dfrac{1}{n}\sum\limits_{i=1}^{n}\left\|F\left(Y_i;\theta\right) - X_i\right\|^2$

  7) **If** $L(\theta) < \varepsilon$ //ε is closed to zero

  8) **Calculate** $\Delta_{i+1} = 0.9 \times \Delta_i + \eta \times \partial L/\partial W_i^l$, $W_{i+1}^l = W_i^l + \Delta_{i+1}$

  9) **End If**

10) **End For**

CNNSR Testing

Input: LR cell image $\{Y'\}$ and Model parameter $\theta = \{W_1, W_2, W_3, B_1, B_2, B_3\}$

Output: Corresponding HR cell images $F\{Y'\}$

11) **For** $l = 1$ to 3//3-layer network

12) Calculate $F(Y')$ based on Equations (11.22)–(11.24)

13) **End For**

The second layer performs non-linear mapping of the n_1-dimensional vectors to n_2-dimensional ones, where the operation is:

$$F_2(Y) = \max\left(0, W_2 * F_1(Y) + B_2\right) \tag{11.23}$$

where W_2 represents n_2 filters of size $n_1 \times f_2 \times f_2$, and B_2 is an n_2-dimensional bias vector. Hence, each output n_2-dimensional vector is a representation of one HR patch that will reconstruct the final HR image.

The third layer performs the final HR image reconstruction by aggregating the previous HR patches and generates one HR image that is as similar as possible to the original HR image X. Its operation is:

$$F_3(Y) = W_3 * F_2(Y) + B_3 \tag{11.24}$$

where W_3 represents one set of filters of size $n_2 \times f_3 \times f_3$, and B_3 is a 1-D bias vector. The overlapping HR patches are averaged.

All the above three operations compose a CNN. The grouped network parameters $\theta = \{W_1, W_2, W_3, B_1, B_2, B_3\}$ shall be optimized together to obtain the mapping function F that minimizes the loss $L(\theta)$ function. This is achieved by stochastic gradient descent with the standard back propagation. In addition, the weight matrices are updated as:

$$\Delta_{i+1} = 0.9 \times \Delta_i + \eta \times \partial L/\partial W_i^l, \, W_{i+1}^l = W_i^l + \Delta_{i+1} \tag{11.25}$$

In an on-line testing step, when a new LR cell image Y' is captured by the lensless imaging system and input to CNNSR, the corresponding HR cell image $F\{Y'\}$ can be recovered through the trained group network parameters θ. The input LR cell images are first extracted by n_1 linear filters $(f_1 \times f_1)$. The extracted LR patches are then subtracted by its mean and projected into a dictionary with size n_1. Later, a sparse coding solver is applied on the projected n_1 coefficients to obtain n_2 coefficients as representative of the HR patch. The sparse coding solver acts as a non-linear mapping operator that is fully feed-forward. After sparse coding, the n_2 coefficients are projected into another HR dictionary for producing HR patches. Then, these overlapping patches are averaged and reconstructed to obtain the final HR images.

In CNNSR, the magnification factor is also implemented as 4×. Due to the limited array size of single cells, the filter size $f_1 \times f_1$ was set as 5×5, and $n_1 = 64$. The $f_2 \times f_2$ filter size was set as 1×1 with $n_2 = 32$. In addition, the filter of the third layer set is $f_3 = 3$. Therefore, the calculation of an HR pixel adopts $(5 + 3 - 1)^2 = 49$ LR pixel information, which leads to the high-restoration quality of CNNSR.

As a comparison for ELMSR and CNNSR, both ELM and CNN are feed-forward neural networks. Thus, they are computing efficiently with little pre- or post-processing optimization. There is no need to resolve optimization problem on usage. A major merit of ELM is that the weights between the input layer and hidden layer are randomly generated, hence it is tuning-free without iterative training. Since the image number can be large if various cell types under different appearances are to be trained, ELMSR is suitable to speed up the training process. The advantage of using CNNSR is that the patch extraction and aggregation are directly formulated as convolutional layers. Hence, LR dictionary, HR dictionary, and non-linear mapping and averaging are all involved in the filter optimization toward higher restoration quality. Note that the training of the ELMSR and CNNSR model is done off-line. After the model is trained, the computation would not need so much computation costs during testing. Moreover, ELMSR and CNNSR have the potential to be hardware implemented on-chip in the future. In that case, computations would be much faster.

11.5 Microfluidic Cytometer for Cell Counting

11.5.1 Microfluidic Cytometer System

11.5.1.1 System Overview

The proposed contact-imaging based microfluidic cytometer for flowing cell recognition and counting is shown in Figure 11.8. It includes one PDMS microfluidic channel attached on top of a CMOS image sensor, through which cells flow continuously. A syringe pump continuously drives the sample solution of interest into the channel and controls the flow rate. A conventional white LED lamp is applied as the light source above to project flowing microbeads or cells into the solution. The CMOS image sensor can continuously capture shadow images beneath. The captured digital image frames are then rapidly processed with a machine-learning-based single-frame SR algorithm, which can improve resolution of shadow images such that we can recognize and count the flowing cells.

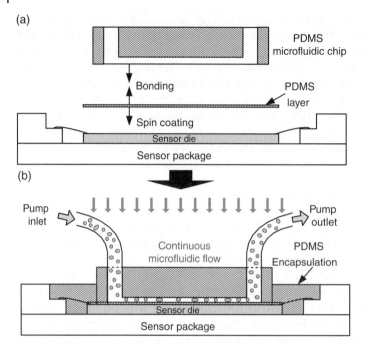

Figure 11.8 Contact-imaging based microfluidic cytometer for flowing cell recognition and counting, (a) Process of bonding with PDMS chip; and (b) Microfluidic cytometer system diagram.

11.5.1.2 Microfluidic Channel Fabrication

The PDMS-based microfluidic channel was fabricated by the conventional soft-lithography [33]. The channel features were designed in AutoCAD (Autodesk, San Rafael, CA) and then written to a transparent mask. Then negative photoresist SU-8 (SU-8 25, Microchem, MA) was spin-coated (SCS G3P-8, Indianapolis, IN) on a 3-inch polished silicon wafer to fabricate the SU-8 mold. Afterwards, a volumetric ratio of 10:1 mixture of PDMS (Sylgard 184, Dow Corning, MI) and curing agent were poured onto the SU-8 mold. After degassing and curing, the PDMS replica was peeled off from the master and punched on top for inlet and outlet holes, which were connected with silastic laboratory tubes to a syringe pump and a waste bin.

11.5.1.3 Microbead and Cell Sample Preparation

In the experiment, HepG2 cells (American Type Culture Collection, MD) were cultured in Minimum Essential Media (MEM) (Gibco, cat# 11095-080) supplemented with 10% fetal bovine serum (FBS) (Gibco, cat# 10270-106), 1 mM sodium pyruvate (Gibco, cat# 11360-070), 0.1 mM MEM non-essential amino acids (Gibco, cat# 11140-050), and grown at 37 °C under a 5% CO_2 atmosphere in a T75 flask. The harvested cells were washed and re-suspended in phosphate-buffered saline (PBS) (Fisher Scientific, Pittsburgh, PA). The blood cell samples were collected from donators, also suspended in PBS. Note that all volunteers signed written informed consent forms before enrollment, and all procedures comply with relevant laws and institutional guidelines, with the approval from the Ethics Committee on our research. The polystyrene microbeads of 6 μm diameter (Product# 07312, Polysciences, Warrington, PA) were selected for calibration experiments, as they were of similar size to RBC. The microbeads were suspended in PBS. All the samples were sonicated in an ultrasonic benchtop cleaner (Branson 2510E-DTH, Danbury, CT) for 10 min before pumping into the microfluidic channel to prevent aggregation.

11.5.1.4 Microfluidic Cytometer Design

To build the contact-imaging based microfluidic cytometer with higher spatial resolution, a grayscale CMOS image sensor (Aptina MT9M032, San Jose, CA) is selected with a pixel size of 2.2 μm × 2.2 μm. The active sensing area is 3.24 mm (H) × 2.41 mm (V) by a 1472 (H) × 1096 (V) pixel array. The hardware design is shown in Figure 11.9.

First, the protection glass of the image sensor chip was removed before bonding with the PDMS microfluidic channel. In addition, the microlens layer above the pixel array was removed by treating the sensor under oxygen plasma (PDC-32G, Harrick Plasma, Ithaca, NY) for 45 min (18 W). However, as the developed system utilized the continuous microfluidic flow, which generates higher pressure to the channel wall than the one using capillary or electroosmotic flow [14,15], a thin PDMS layer was also spin coated on top of the sensor die. A tight PDMS-PDMS bonding [34] is required, as in the process shown in Figure 11.9(a). The spin speed of 9000 rpm is set to generate a thickness

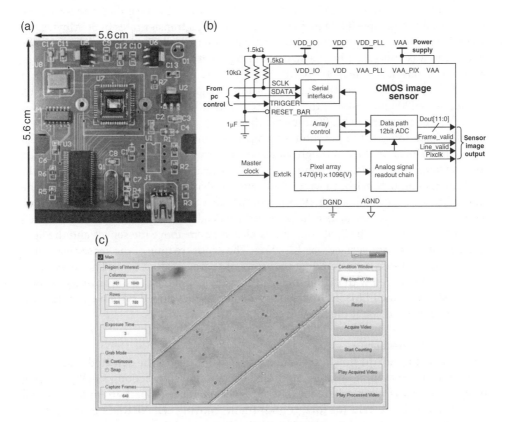

Figure 11.9 Hardware design of the microfluidic cytometer: (a) PCB schematic; (b) PCB hardware with size of 5.6 cm × 5.6 cm; and (c) Control GUI of the microfluidic cytometer.

of 6 µm [35] for PDMS. Therefore, the object distance of our system is 6 µm to enable enough contrast for the microfluidic contact imaging. After spin coating and baking, the surfaces of the microfluidic channel and the image sensor were cleaned with ethanol and oxygen plasma and finally bonded together. Note that after bonding the PDMS coated sensor chip and the microfluidic chip, we also filled the PDMS and curing agent mixture into the gap to encapsulate the bonding wires.

Moreover, to make full use of the active pixel area, the channel length was designed as 4.6 mm and cut diagonally. Thus, when bonded on top of the sensor die, the rectangle microfluidic chip was just within the die area of the bonding wire. A relative wide channel width of 500 µm was chosen such that a high concentration of cells could flow through the channel without clogging [36]. The height of the microfluidic channel was 30 µm, just higher than the normal cell diameters. This ensures that the cells flow close to the sensor surface with better projected image contrast. Besides, in order to improve the wettability of the channel, the channel was coated with bovine serum albumin (BSA) by flowing a 1% solution of BSA in PBS through the channel for an hour [37].

Next, the CMOS image sensor chip was soldered on one low-cost 5.6 cm × 5.6 cm printed circuit board (PCB) that provides the sensor with power supplies and digital control signals, as shown in Figure 11.9(a). The data transferred from the CMOS image sensor to PC was through a USB interface (CY7C68013-56 EZ-USB FX2, San Jose, CA), which ensures high-speed imaging with maximum data transfer rates of 56 Mbytes per second. The sensor working status such as exposure time, ROI, and number of frames to capture was controlled by the status registers that can be accessed through a two-wire serial interface, such as SCLK and SDATA, as in the schematic shown in Figure 11.9(b). They are set through the custom designed GUI shown in Figure 11.9(c). We set 640 × 480 image ROI of the sensor to capture the flowing specimens at a sensor frame rate of approximately 200 frames/s (fps).

In the experiments, the microfluidic chip was connected to a syringe pump (KDS Legato180, Holliston, MA) through silastic laboratory tubes and samples were pumped into the microfluidic chamber continuously at a typical flow rate of approximately 5 µL/min under illumination from a white light source (Olympus LG-PS2, Tokyo, Japan). The thin tube of 0.64 mm i.d. and 1.19 mm o.d. (product no. TW-96115-04, Cole-Parmer, Vernon Hills, IL) was used, as it helps to reduce dead volume and cells loss compared with a thick channel. The light source was placed 12 cm above the sensor and the light intensity at the sensor surface was 1.5 k Lux. The exposure time of the sensor was set at approximately 75 µs, corresponding to 3 rows of sensor readout time. The readout LR frames were buffered with digital image processing conducted to improve the resolution by single-frame ELM-SR processing. As such, the developed system can automatically recognize and count the flowing cells.

11.5.1.5 Cell Detection

For cell counting, all the flowing cells in each LR frame need to be detected first. This is realized by the temporal-differencing-based background subtraction [38–39]. Starting from the first two frames, where the first one is the reference (or background) frame and the second is the current (or foreground) frame, moving cell contours in the current frame is detected by subtracting it with its previous reference frame to obtain a pixel-by-pixel intensity difference. After subtraction, the regions where the intensity differences are zero indicate no moving cells; and those non-zero difference regions are caused by the motion of cells in the channel, or by the addition and removal of a cell from the sensor field-of-view (FOV). A suitable intensity threshold can be set to identify the contours of moving cells from the background in all frames [38]. The time-difference between each two consecutive frames is determined by the sensor frame rate. Note that each detected cell in one frame will be assigned with one unique identification number, which means the cell count of the current frame.

11.5.1.6 Cell Recognition

After recovering the SR image $SR'_{M \times N}$ from the input LR image $LR'_{m \times n}$, cell type recognition in the developed microfluidic cytometer is performed. The recognition process is shown in Figure 11.10 Assuming that the samples of interest include two types of cells, two reference models need to be trained for each type of cell. Then when a detected LR cell $LR'_{m \times n}$ is input, two SR images, $SR1'_{M \times N}$ and $SR2'_{M \times N}$, can be recovered, each corresponding to one reference model. Afterwards, $SR1'_{M \times N}$ and $SR2'_{M \times N}$ are compared with the typical HR images $HR1_{M \times N}$ and $HR2_{M \times N}$ in the training libraries, where the mean structural similarity (MSSIM/SSIM) index [30] is employed to characterize the similarity. The SSIM is a full reference metric between 0 and 1 to indicate the similarity between one SR image with one distortion-free reference HR image by:

$$\text{SSIM}(SR, HR) = \frac{(2\mu_{SR}\mu_{HR})(2\sigma_{SR,HR})}{(\mu_{SR}^2 + \mu_{HR}^2)(\sigma_{SR}^2 + \sigma_{HR}^2)} \quad (11.26)$$

where μ_{SR} and μ_{HR} are the means of the SR and HR images, σ_{SR}^2 and σ_{HR}^2 are the variances of the SR and HR images, and $\sigma_{SR,HR}$ is the covariance of the SR and HR images. It is proven to be consistent with human eye perception compared with traditional metric,

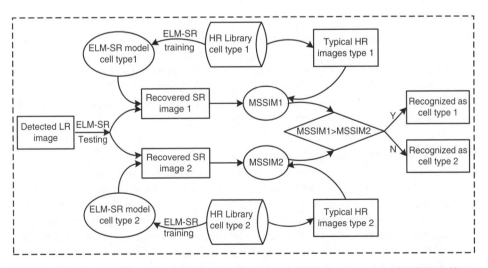

Figure 11.10 Flowing cell recognition flowchart. The detected LR image is processed with ELM-SR to obtain SR images according to different off-line trained models. Then, the SR images are compared with typical HR cell images in the library with cells categorized to one type that has the largest MSSIM.

such as peak signal-to-noise ratio (PSNR) and MSE. The MSSIM is the average of the SSIMs for one SR image with all the typical HR images:

$$\text{MSSIM}\left(SR, HRlib\right) = \frac{1}{K}\sum_{k=1}^{K} SSIM\left(SR, HR_k\right) \tag{11.27}$$

where K is the number of typical HR images in the HR training library. For $SR1'_{M \times N}$ and $SR2'_{M \times N}$, MSSIM1 and MSSIM2 can be calculated. Then we categorize the cell to the type that has the stronger MSSIM. Thus, with the machine-learning-based single-frame SR processing, the developed microfluidic cytometer can have much better imaging capability to distinguish cell details in the continuously flowing microfluidic channel.

11.5.1.7 Cell Counting

After recognizing the type for all the detected cells flowing through the channel, the total number of each cell type in the sample of interest can be enumerated. For one cell type, as the cell number in each frame is already known after the temporal-differencing-based cell detection step, we subtract the cell number of the current frame with its previous reference frame to obtain a difference value. If this difference is larger than zero, this means that new cells have flown into the sensor FOV to increase the cell count over the previous frame. As such, we add this difference to the total cell count. By adding all the positive differences after processing the whole series of frames, the total number for one cell type is obtained. For other cell types, the counting procedure is processed in the same way and hence their concentration ratio can eventually be obtained.

As such, the detection, recognition, and counting for all the flowing cell types in the testing sample can be achieved, realizing the function of the contact-imaging based microfluidic cytometer.

11.5.2 Results

To evaluate the accuracy of the developed contact-imaging microfluidic cytometer with machine-learning for single-frame SR processing, both of the microbead solution and mixed RBC and tumor cell solution were tested with measurement results compared with a commercially available flow cytometer (BD Accuri C6, NJ). The resolution enhancement factor of 4× was selected. The Structural Similarity is employed as a metric to evaluate the quality of reconstructed images.

11.5.2.1 Counting Performance Characterization

First, the 6 μm polystyrene microbead solution was prepared with a concentration of $100\,\mu\text{L}^{-1}$ measured by the commercial flow cytometer. The 6 μm sample was flushed through the microfluidic channel at a flow rate of 5 μL/min by a syringe pump. Then, a series of 640 frames were captured by the CMOS image sensor for a period of 1 min. The total number of microbeads was automatically counted by the developed image processing algorithm. The same process was repeated for 6 min, and the measured concentrations of the microbeads are shown in Figure 11.11. The final microbead concentration is calculated by averaging the counting results of each group, which was $91\,\mu\text{L}^{-1}$ with only 8% error when compared with the result of $99\,\mu\text{L}^{-1}$ by the commercial flow cytometer.

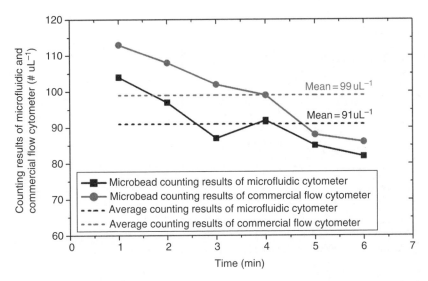

Figure 11.11 Comparison of concentration measurement results for 6 μm microbead solution between the developed microfluidic cytometer and the commercial flow cytometer.

To further evaluate the developed microfluidic cytometer, five microbead samples of different concentrations, ranging from ~50 uL^{-1} to ~800 uL^{-1}, were prepared. The flow rate and imaging time were used under the same settings. As shown in Figure 11.12(a), the measurement results of the developed microfluidic cytometer correlated well with the commercial flow cytometer with a correlation coefficient of 0.99. Moreover, in order to assess the agreement between the two methods, the Bland-Altman analysis was also performed. As with the results shown in Figure 11.12(b), a systematic mean bias of −13 cells uL^{-1} was obtained for the developed microfluidic cytometer compared with the commercial flow cytometer. The under-counting performance was due to the dead volume in the channel inlet/outlet, as well as the cell loss and sedimentation in the tube.

11.5.2.2 Off-Line SR Training

For the microfluidic cytometer prototype with ELMSR and CNNSR, the off-line training image libraries of blood cells and HepG2 tumor cells were first built. The HR training image of HepG2 and blood cells were captured using a microscope camera (Olympus IX71, Tokyo, Japan) and saved into the HR image library, as shown in Figures 11.13 (a1–a3), (e1–e3). Note that we also used the 3-Mega array CIS with the smaller pixel size introduced in Chapter 7 to build one microfluidic cytometer prototype. Since there are two prototypes with different CIS, the original HR images are saved as two different sizes, 48 × 48 and 80 × 80, corresponding to the ELMSR and CNNSR training image libraries. As the enhancement factor is 4, we bicubically down-sampled the 48 × 48 HR cell images to 12 × 12 LR cell images, as shown in Figures 11.13(b1–b3), and down-sampled the 80 × 80 HR cell images to 20 × 20 LR cell images, as shown in Figures 11.13(f1–f3). Then, these LR cell images were interpolated back to 48 × 48 and 80 × 80, as shown in Figures 11.13(c1–c3), (g1–g3).

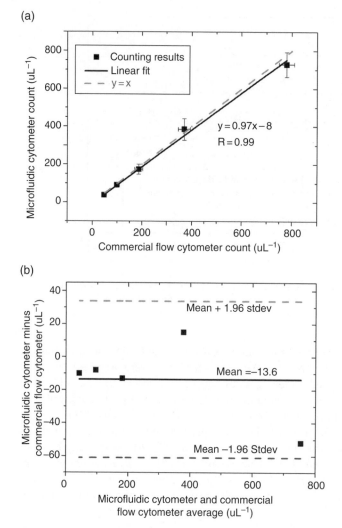

Figure 11.12 Comparison of counting results of different microbead concentration solutions between the developed microfluidic cytometer and the commercial flow cytometer: (a) Measurement results correlate well between the developed system and the commercial one (y = 0.97x – 8, correlation coefficient = 0.996); (b) The Bland-Altman analysis of the measurement results between the developed one and the commercial one show a mean bias of –13.6 uL^{-1}, the lower 95% limit of agreement by –61.0 uL^{-1}, and the upper 95% limit of agreement by 33.8 uL^{-1}.

Now, the detailed structures were already lost in the interpolated images as simple interpolation could not recover the HF components. Next, as shown in Figures 11.13(d1–d3), (g1–g3), the HF components for each training cell image were obtained by subtracting the original HR images with the interpolated cell images. Thus, the training library for ELMSR and CNNSR to train a reference model was generated. Different features in various cell types, such as HepG2 tumor cell, RBC, and WBC, could be clearly seen from the difference in their HF images. For the mixed HepG2 and blood samples, there are 30 HR images selected for each cell type to build the training library.

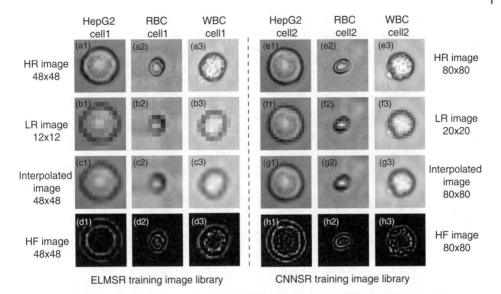

Figure 11.13 Example images of HepG2, RBC, and WBC in ELMSR and CNNSR training image libraries: (a) Original HR images with all HF details in ELMSR library; (b) Down-sampled LR images with HF information lost in ELMSR library; (c) Interpolated LR images whose HF cannot be recovered in ELMSR library; (d) HF components that are lost during down-sampling in the ELMSR library; (e) Original HR images with all HF details in the CNNSR library; (f) Down-sampled LR images with HF information lost in the CNNSR library; (g) Interpolated LR images whose HF cannot be recovered in the ELMSR library; and (h) HF components that are lost during down-sampling.

Note that both interpolated images and HF images were used in ELMSR training to generate ELM reference models, but in CNNSR interpolated images, HR images were directly employed to train the mapping function. We still keep Figures 11.13 (g1–g3) in order to show the different HF features.

11.5.2.3 On-line SR Testing

After building the off-line training image library and obtaining the training model, the on-line SR processing was performed when new lensless LR cell images were captured. As two CIS of different pixel sizes (2.2 μm vs. 1.1 μm) were used to build the lensless imaging systems, the directly captured LR cell images were compared, as shown in Figures 11.14(a,d). Due to the smaller pixel pitch of BSI CIS over the commercial FIS CIS, the captured LR RBC in Figure 11.14(d1) was much clearer than Figure 11.14(a2). The LR RBC images covered about 4 and 8 pixels at the diameter using FSI CIS and BSI CIS, respectively. These results demonstrated the advantage of using CIS of the smaller pixel pitch in generating LR lensless images of higher spatial resolution.

After the raw LR cell images were captured, the interpolated HR images could be generated, as shown in Figures 11.14(b,e). The recovered HR images of one HepG2 cell and one RBC using the ELMSR model are shown in Figures 11.14(c1,c2). The recovered HR images of one RBC and one WBC using the CNNSR model are shown in Figures 11.14(f1,f2). Comparing the interpolated images in Figured 11.14(b,e) with SR recovered images in Figures 11.14(c,f), it can be clearly observed that no matter which SR was used, the recovered images show more cell internal and edge information.

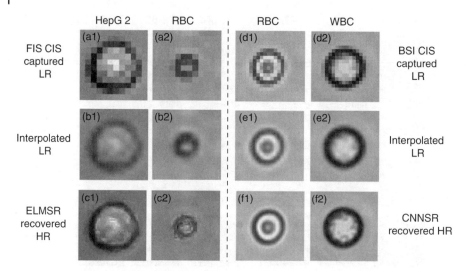

Figure 11.14 Example of HepG2, RBC, and WBC images in ELMSR and CNNSR testing: (a) Raw LR images captured by FSI CIS with pixel pitch 2.2 um; (b) Interpolated LR images; (c) ELMSR recovered HR images; (d) Raw LR images captured by BSI CIS with pixel pitch 1.1 μm; (e) Interpolated LR images; and (f) CNNSR recovered HR images, showing better performance in resolution improvement.

Comparing the performance of resolution improvement for CNNSR and ELMSR, it can be seen that the HR images recovered by CNNSR have less noise compared with ELMSR. In Figure 11.14(c2), the cell edge recovered by ELMSR still had some blurred effect. However, in the CNNSR recovered HR images in Figures 11.14(f1,f2), there was no such effects. Especially in the recovered WBC HR image in Figure 11.14(f2), the cell membrane and nucleolus can be clearly seen.

As shown in Figure 11.15, the MSSIMs for HepG2 in Figure 11.14(c1), RBC in Figures 11.14(c2,f1), and WBC in Figure 11.14(f2) with the corresponding HR image libraries are obtained as 0.5190, 0.7608, 0.8331, and 0.8102, respectively. Thus, CNNSR has 9.5% improvement over the ELMSR on resolution improvement quality. This is possibly due to the fact that the filter optimization in CNNSR includes all the three CNN processing layers, while in ELMSR, there was no such joint optimization in training the network model. Note that although the input LR images for ELMSR and CNNSR are different due to the different CIS used, the improved HR images are compared with their respective original HR images in their off-line training image libraries. Thus, the performance of SR improvement is directly evaluated by comparing the MSSIM metric.

11.5.2.4 On-line Cell Recognition and Counting

The on-line cell recognition and counting performances of the developed prototype were further evaluated using mixed tumor cells and RBC samples. The RBC/HepG2 cell sample was prepared and measured by the commercial flow cytometer (BD Accuri C6, San Jose, NJ). The absolute counts of RBC and HepG2 are 1054 and 978, the ratio of which is about 1.08:1 (51.9%:48.1%). The sample was tested at a flow rate of 5 μL/min using the developed lensless system for six groups, with each group being tested for 1 min. The cell counts were obtained, as shown in Table 11.3. The mean RBC/HepG2 ratio is 52.60%:47.40% = 1.11:1, and the coefficient of variation (CV) is 0.10, which

Figure 11.15 The mean structural similarity (MSSIM) results for on-line recover cell images.

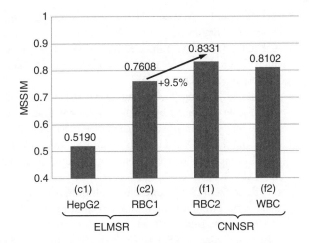

Table 11.3 Measured counting results of mixed RBC and HepG2 sample.

Group	RBC (# μL^{-1})	HepG2 (# μL^{-1})	RBC/HepG2
1	239 (54.32%)	201 (45.68%)	1.19
2	338 (50.22%)	335 (49.78%)	1.01
3	260 (53.72%)	224 (46.28%)	1.06
4	435 (52.98%)	386 (47.02%)	1.12
5	340 (55.74%)	270 (44.26%)	1.26
6	334 (49.85%)	336 (50.15%)	0.99
Mean	324 (52.60%)	292 (47.40%)	1.11
Stdev	70	72	0.11
CV	0.22	0.25	0.10

matches well with the commercial flow cytometer result (1.08:1). Based on the current sample concentration, the average throughput was 3080 min^{-1}. Although the throughput was relatively low compared with commercial flow cytometry, it can be further improved by increasing the sample concentration and flow rate, as the cells captured in each image and the total cells captured in a certain number of images are increased.

References

1 W. Jung, J. Han, J.-W. Choi and C.H. Ahn (2015) Point-of-care testing (POCT) diagnostic systems using microfluidic lab-on-a-chip technologies. *Microelectronic Engineering*, 132, 46–57.
2 C. van Berkel, J.D. Gwyer, S. Deane, N. Green, J. Holloway, *et al.* (2011) Integrated systems for rapid point of care (PoC) blood cell analysis. *Lab on a Chip*, 11(7), 1249–1255.

3 A. Ozcan and E. McLeod (2016) Lensless imaging and sensing, *Annual Review of Biomedical Engineering*, 18(1), 77–102.

4 X. Huang, J. Guo, M. Yan, Y. Kang and H. Yu (2014) A contact-imaging based microfluidic cytometer with machine-learning for single-frame super-resolution processing. *PLOS ONE*, 9(8).

5 X. Huang, X. Wang, M. Yan and H. Yu 2015) A robust recognition error recovery for micro-flow cytometer by machine-learning enhanced single-frame super-resolution processing. *Integration, the VLSI Journal*, 51, 208–218.

6 X. Huang, H. Yu, X.Y. Liu, Y. Jiang and M. Yan (2015) A single-frame superresolution algorithm for lab-on-a-chip lensless microfluidic imaging. *IEEE Design & Test*, 32(6), 32–40.

7 E.H.K. Stelzer (1998) Contrast, resolution, pixelation, dynamic range and signal-to-noise ratio: Fundamental limits to resolution in fluorescence light microscopy. *Journal of Microscopy*, 189(1), 15–24.

8 J. Farrell, F. Xiao and S. Kavusi (2006) Resolution and light sensitivity trade-off with pixel size. In: *Proceedings of the SPIE*, pp. 60690 N.

9 H. Ji, D. Sander, A. Haas and P.A. Abshire (2007) Contact imaging: Simulation and experiment. *IEEE Trans. Circuits Syst. I: Reg. Papers*, 54(8), 1698–1710.

10 O. Bowen and C.S. Bouganis (2008) Real-time image super resolution using an FPGA. *International Conference on Field Programmable Logic and Applications (FPL)*, pp. 89–94.

11 P. Sung Cheol, P. Min Kyu and K. Moon Gi (2003) Super-resolution image reconstruction: A technical overview. *IEEE Signal Processing Magazine*, 20(3), 21–36.

12 E. Choi, J. Choi and M.G. Kang (2004) Super-resolution approach to overcome physical limitations of imaging sensors: An overview. *International Journal of Imaging Systems and Technology*, 14(2), pp. 36–46.

13 M. Elad and Y. Hel-Or (2001) A fast super-resolution reconstruction algorithm for pure translational motion and common space-invariant blur. *IEEE Transactions on Image Processing*, 10(8), 1187–1193.

14 G. Zheng, S.A. Lee, S. Yang and C. Yang (2010) Sub-pixel resolving optofluidic microscope for on-chip cell imaging. *Lab on a Chip*, 10(22), 3125–3129.

15 S.A. Lee, R. Leitao, G. Zheng, S. Yang, A. Rodriguez and C. Yang (2011) Color capable sub-pixel resolving optofluidic microscope and its application to blood cell imaging for Malaria diagnosis. *PloS ONE*, 6(10), e26127.

16 W. Bishara, U. Sikora, O. Mudanyali, T. Su, O. Yaglidere, *et al.* (2011) Holographic pixel super-resolution in portable lensless on-chip microscopy using a fiber-optic array. *Lab on a Chip*, 11(7), 127–1279.

17 A.C. Sobieranski, F. Inci, H.C. Tekin, M. Yuksekkaya, E. Cobra, *et al.* (2015) Portable lensless wide-field microscopy imaging platform based on digital inline holography and multi-frame pixel super-resolution. *Light Science Applications*, 4, e346, 2015.

18 T. Wang, X. Huang, Q. Jia, M. Yan, H. Yu and K.S. Yeo (2012) A super-resolution CMOS image sensor for bio-microfluidic imaging. *IEEE Biomedical Circuits and Systems Conference (BioCAS)*, pp. 388–391.

19 H.C. Koydemir, Z. Gorocs, D. Tseng, B. Cortazar, S. Feng, *et al.* (2015) A rapid imaging, detection and quantification of *Giardia lamblia* cysts using mobile-phone based fluorescent microscopy and machine learning. *Lab on a Chip*, 15(5), 1284–1293.

20 C. Sommer and D.W. Gerlich (2013) Machine learning in cell biology – Teaching computers to recognize phenotypes. *Journal of Cell Science*, 126(24), 5529–5539.

21 W.T. Freeman, E.C. Pasztor and O.T. Carmichael (2000) Learning low-level vision. *International Journal of Computer Vision*, 40(1), 25–47.

22 W.T. Freeman, T.R. Jones and E.C. Pasztor (2002) Example-based super-resolution. *IEEE Computer Graphics and Applications*, 22(2), 56–65.

23 G. Freedman and R. Fattal (2011) Image and video upscaling from local self-examples. *ACM Trans. Graph.*, 30(2), 1–11.

24 J. Yang, Z. Lin and S.D. Cohen (2013) Fast image super-resolution based on in-place example regression. *Proceedings of the 2013 IEEE Conference on Computer Vision and Pattern Recognition*, pp. 23–28.

25 J. Sun, N. Zheng, H. Tao and H. Shum (2013) Image hallucination with primal sketch priors. *Proceedings of the 2003 IEEE Computer Society Conference on Computer Vision and Pattern Recognition*, 16–22.

26 J. Yang, J.C. Wright, T.S. Huang and Y. Ma (2010) Image super-resolution via sparse representation. *IEEE Transactions on Image Processing*, 19(11), 2861–2873.

27 H.C. Koydemir, Z. Gorocs, D. Tseng, B. Cortazar, S. Feng, *et al.* (2015) Rapid imaging, detection and quantification of *Giardia lamblia* cysts using mobile-phone based fluorescent microscopy and machine learning. *Lab on a Chip*, 15, 1284–1293.

28 G. Huang, Q. Zhu and C.K. Siew (2006) Extreme learning machine: Theory and applications. *Neurocomputing*, 70(1), 489–501.

29 C. Dong, C.C. Loy, K. He and X. Tang (2016) Image super-resolution using deep convolutional networks. *IEEE Transactions on Pattern Analysis and Machine Intelligence*, 38(2), 295–30.

30 Z. Wang, A.C. Bovik and H.R. Sheikh (2004) Image quality assessment: From error visibility to structural similarity. *IEEE Transactions on Image Processing*, 13(4), 600–612.

31 C. Cortes and V. Vapnik (1995) Support-vector networks. *Machine Learning*, 20(3), 273–297.

32 B. Yegnanarayana (2004) *Artificial Neural Networks*. PHI Learning Pvt., Ltd., New Delhi.

33 G. Wu, W. Shih, C. Hui, S. Chen and C. Lee (2010) Bonding strength of pressurized microchannels fabricated by polydimethylsiloxane and silicon. *Journal of Micromechical. Microengineering*, 20, 115032.

34 S.C. Lin, P.W. Yen, C.C. Peng and Y.C. Tung (2012) Single channel layer, single sheath-flow inlet microfluidic flow cytometer with three-dimensional hydrodynamic focusing. *Lab on a Chip*, 12, 3135–3141.

35 W.Y. Zhang, G.S. Ferguson and S. Tatic-Lucic (2004) Elastomer-supported cold welding for room temperature wafer-level bonding. *Proceedings of IEEE International Conference on Micro Electro Mechanical Systems*, pp. 741–744.

36 H.M. Wyss, D.L. Blair, J.F. Morris, H.A. Stone and D.A. Weitz (2006) Mechanism for clogging of microchannels. *Physical Review E*, 74, 061402.

37 A.J. Lipton, H. Fujiyoshi and R.S. Patil (1998) Moving target classification and tracking from real-time video. *Proceedings of Fourth IEEE Workshop on Applications of Computer Vision*, pp. 8–14.

38 M Piccardi (2004) Background subtraction techniques: A review. *Proceedings of IEEE International Conference on Systems, Man and Cybernetics*, 4, 3099–3104.

12

Conclusion

12.1 Summaries

The world population is rapidly aging, with the proportion of people aged 60 years old and over growing faster than any other age group. Along with the current aging society, also come special personalized healthcare needs and challenges. It is imperative to prepare healthcare and diagnosis systems to meet the needs of personalized bio-imaging diagnosis of this aging populations. Over the past several decades, biomedical diagnostic techniques such as microscopy, ultrasound, flow cytometry, and even optical genetic sequencing have improved the early diagnosis and accurate monitoring of existing diseases, and an understanding of the underlying causes and mechanisms of disease. However, current biomedical diagnosis instruments are usually bulky, expensive, and hence are not scalable for multiple functionality diagnosis.

This book introduces CMOS-based scalable integration of multiple different types of sensors from different domains, or so-called multi-modal sensors, including impedance, terahertz, ultrasonic, optical, and electrochemical sensors, etc. They are presented from working principle, circuit design, and system implementation, as well as biomedical applications. We have particularly reported the recent progress in the CMOS-integrated multimodal biomedical sensor platform for personalized diagnosis. The CMOS multimodal sensors we developed include:

1) CMOS electronic impedance sensor for rare cell detection and counting;
2) CMOS Terahertz sensor for non-invasive imaging;
3) CMOS (capacitive-micro-machined-ultrasonic-transducer) CMUT sensor for non-invasive 3-D ultrasound imaging;
4) CMOS (ion-sensitive-field-effect-transistor) ISFET sensor for ion imaging towards the DNA sequencing application; and
5) CMOS optical sensor for microfluidic imaging towards cell detection, recognition, and counting applications.

As such, many new design challenges have been raised, such as how to develop multimodal sensors for system integration; how to integrate with MEMS and microfluidic channels from device technology perspective; as well as data fusing and smart processing of multiple domains from the system application perspective. One main research challenge that has been observed is mainly for the CMOS readout circuit design, that is how to deal with the weak signal detection, noise cancelling, and non-uniformity

CMOS Integrated Lab-on-a-Chip System for Personalized Biomedical Diagnosis,
First Edition. Hao Yu, Mei Yan, and Xiwei Huang.
© 2018 John Wiley & Sons Singapore Pte. Ltd. Published 2018 by John Wiley & Sons Singapore Pte. Ltd.

reduction? This book has summarized the common readout circuit design with a number of demonstrated readout circuit designs for each different type of CMOS sensor in different domains.

Moreover, dual-mode sensors are also developed, such as optical-electrochemical sensor. The traditional single-mode ISFET sensor has poor pH detection sensitivity as well as faulty pH values when reporting pH values of micro-reads trapped at the micro-well array during DNA sequencing. The proposed dual-mode (chemical + optical) ISFET sensor can improve the reported pH accuracy significantly by correlated readout of chemical pH values of location-determined micro-beads via optical contact imaging. As such, we can eventually realize a multimodal CMOS sensor platform for personalized diagnosis application, as shown in Figure 12.1. The CMOS sensor chip here involves a large multimodal sensor array, where sensor pixels can detect multiple signals from different domains. Such a CMOS-based multimodal sensor can integrate ISFET pH sensor pixels to detect chemical values, CMOS image sensor pixels to detect images, near-infrared sensor pixels to detect thermal images, ultrasound front-end sensors to detect ultrasound images, THz detectors to detect THz images, and electro-impedance sensors to detect impedance changes. After the CMOS sensor chip is fabricated and packaged, it can then be integrated with the microfluidic channel, allowing a contact-sensing of samples such as molecules, tissues, cells, and bacteria. Therefore such a CMOS-based multimodal sensor provides a promising biomedical diagnosis platform for all biological sample detection needs, from DNA, molecular to cell, and tissue, etc.

Thereby, in the next five years, individual microfluidics, MEMS, electronics, electro-magnetics, and multimodal sensors will continue to develop rapidly. The advancing CMOS-based lab-on-a-chip technology will further integrate them and possibly other new technologies together to form cheaper, smaller, and smarter lab-on-a-chip systems, to better serve the scalability of the future personalized diagnosis.

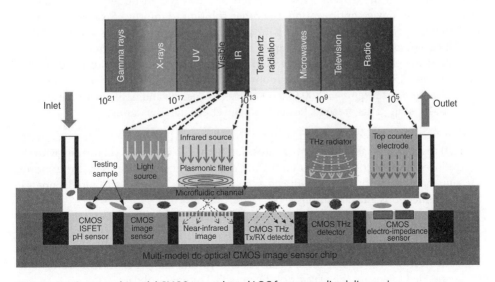

Figure 12.1 Smart multimodal CMOS sensor based LOC for personalized diagnosis.

12.2   Future Works

The CMOS-based multimodal sensor platform has shown a promising future to integrate microfluidics, MEMS, and CMOS sensors, as well as smart data analysis for personal biomedical diagnosis. There are still technological challenges for the CMOS-based approach.

The first challenge is the continued scaling-down of device-dimension to the nanometer. As discussed in previous chapters, a biosensor mainly consists of a probe that interacts with biological materials, such as DNA, cells, etc., and a transducer that converts biological interaction into the measurable signal at optical, electrical, or other domains. The further scale-down of the probe and transducer would benefit the detection resolution but also reduce the sensitivity. This book has shown many new solutions, such as time-integral detection at the sub-threshold region, plasmonic amplification, etc. The nanoscale probe and transducer would present fundamentally different physical and chemical properties and usually exhibit size- and shape-dependent interactions with electrons, photons, and electromagnetic fields. Therefore, we need to utilize the correct new device structure at nanoscale to improve the sensitivity. The other problem relevant to the scalability is CMOS-compatible integration. The 3-D-TSV-based integration method has shown great potential for this need.

For example, the fluorescence detection has attracted great research attention, such as DNA fluorescence detection for early diagnosis of genetic decreases. However, low concentration of bio-markers might be difficult for the detection due to the weak signal-to-noise ratio. By incorporating metallic nanostructures, which can provide highly focused and enhanced signal (optical) fields, we can boost the SNR by several orders of magnitude, thereby resulting in highly enhanced detection of the fluorescence signal. As commonly used for biomolecular fluorescence imaging, nanostructures made of plasmonic device can have resonance interaction with signal fields over a range of spectrums at the nanoscale. However, how to integrate such an artificial nanomaterial or nano-device with the CMOS sensor chip has already brought up new technical challenges. Besides device optimization, the other solution to improve SNR is to optimize the circuitry performance with high gain and noise reduction, such as special readout circuit design for nano-pore, nano-gap, and nano-filter device integration.

The second challenge is the continued scaling-up of data-dimension to the Peta-bit. Among all clinic applications, genomics has the biggest data generation. For the human genome, it requires 3 200 000 000 bases to analyze and easily generates data at the Peta-bit scale. This presents key technology challenges, including:

1) *Data acquisition*: how to design a high-throughput CMOS sensor (high-speed ADC, I/O) that can help genomics data acquisition with high accuracy, yet dealing with the explosive growth of data. Moreover, for many medical applications, the time for sequencing must further be reduced even in real time, especially to rapidly analyze acute infections and conditions.

2) *Data storage*: emerging technologies such as high-bandwidth-memory (HBM) help support large data storage. We also expect algorithmic developments that can extract feature and compress unnecessary data, which can build an efficient window for cloud access. Meanwhile, authentication, encryption, and other security safeguards are needed to ensure the privacy of the personal biomedical data.

3) *Data analysis*: let us still utilize genomics as the example here. The ultimate goal of genomics is to interpret genomic sequences, so as to explain DNA mutations, expression changes related to disease, development, behavior, or evolution. In order to achieve this goal, it requires data analysis using machine learning to search for patterns over very large data collections in very high dimensions. The whole genome alignment (base call) is another important data analysis application. The offline CPUs or GPUs have a large gap to link with the sensor. The biggest bottleneck is the input/output (IO) hardware that shuttles data between storage and processors. Therefore, on-chip machine learning such as data compression, data extraction, and data recognition is needed in a hardware form, within or close to sensor and storage.

As a conclusion, our thorough study to explore CMOS multimodal sensors for lab-on-chip (LOC) integration has demonstrated great potential for the portable personalized biomedical diagnosis system. Taking them further for clinical diagnostics and medical treatment still faces technical challenges, such as how to achieve signal enhancement with CMOS-integration with a nano-device, how to design the efficient signal amplification circuitry at the pA or fA scale, and how to integrate machine-learning-based data analysis within the sensor platform. It requires a knowledge fusion from physical and life sciences, clinical research, engineering development, and the manufacturing industry. But we can foresee that the rapid technology development in this field will result in huge benefits for the improvement in health of the aging world.

Index

Page references to Figures are followed by the letter 'f' in italics, while references to Tables are followed by the letter 't'.

CMOS Integrated Lab-on-a-Chip System for Personalized Biomedical Diagnosis,
First Edition. Hao Yu, Mei Yan, and Xiwei Huang.
© 2018 John Wiley & Sons Singapore Pte. Ltd. Published 2018 by John Wiley & Sons Singapore Pte. Ltd.